Metropolitan College of NY
Library - 7th Floor
60 West Street
New York, NY 10006

The Last Children's Plague

THE LAST CHILDREN'S PLAGUE

POLIOMYELITIS, DISABILITY, AND TWENTIETH-CENTURY AMERICAN CULTURE

Richard J. Altenbaugh

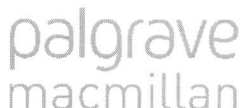

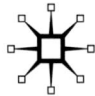

THE LAST CHILDREN'S PLAGUE
Copyright © Richard J. Altenbaugh, 2015.

All rights reserved.

First published in 2015 by PALGRAVE MACMILLAN® in the United States—a division of St. Martin's Press LLC, 175 Fifth Avenue, New York, NY 10010.

Where this book is distributed in the UK, Europe and the rest of the world, this is by Palgrave Macmillan, a division of Macmillan Publishers Limited, registered in England, company number 785998, of Houndmills, Basingstoke, Hampshire RG21 6XS.

Palgrave Macmillan is the global academic imprint of the above companies and has companies and representatives throughout the world.

Palgrave® and Macmillan® are registered trademarks in the United States, the United Kingdom, Europe and other countries.

ISBN: 978-1-137-52784-4

Library of Congress Cataloging-in-Publication Data

Altenbaugh, Richard J., 1948–
    The last children's plague : poliomyelitis, disability, and Twentieth-century American culture / by Richard J. Altenbaugh.
        pages cm
    Includes bibliographical references and index.
    ISBN 978-1-137-52784-4 (hardback : alk paper)   1. Poliomyelitis United States—History—20th century.   2. Poliomyelitis—Social aspects—United States—History—20th century.   I. Title.
    RC181.U5A48 2015
    362.19892'83500973—dc23
                                                        2015013415

A catalogue record of the book is available from the British Library.

Design by Amnet.

First edition: September 2015

Contents

List of Figures	vii
Foreword by Philip Gardner	ix
Acknowledgments	xiii
Introduction: Why Children, Disease, and Disability?	xvii
Abbreviations of Archives/Collections	xxix
1 The American Plague	1
2 Many Yellow Caskets	23
3 After Treatment	55
4 Wheelchair Gladiators	89
5 Home Sweet Home	123
6 The Cripples	159
7 Polio's Legacy	189
Notes and Sources	193
Bibliography	247
Index	263

List of Figures

Figure 1.1   Quarantine Poliomyelitis   16

Figure 2.1   Iron lung ward, 1955. Courtesy: March of Dimes   34

Figure 3.1   Anderson poster. Courtesy: March of Dimes   69

Figure 5.1   Acute Anterior Poliomyelitis (A Communicable
             Disease). Keep Out of this House   127

Foreword

Richard Altenbaugh is of my generation. Our early childhoods—his in the US, mine in the UK—in the baby-boom years following World War II were played out in contexts with many local differences, but also with profound commonalities. One of the most prominent of these was the dark shadow cast by the continuous fear of a devastating childhood disease from which there was no known protection. Polio is a word that is, in one way or another, etched into the collective memory of all those who lived through those years. But in the way of things, though the risk of polio disproportionately impacted the young, the fear of the disease and its catastrophic consequences fell most acutely on their parents, desperate but, in the years before the arrival of the Salk vaccine, ultimately helpless in their desire to safeguard their children.

I have known and admired Richard Altenbaugh and his work across two decades, since our first meeting at a history of education conference in Birmingham, UK, in 1995. It has been both a privilege and an inspiration to discuss his research with him over the intervening years, and particularly on his regular visits to the UK in the capacity of Visiting Fellow of St. Edmund's College in the University of Cambridge. It is a particular pleasure that some of the themes that are explored in Altenbaugh's highly significant new book were honed in the course of a series of memorable exchanges, formal and informal, both within St. Edmund's and at a number of departments across the university. The appearance of *The Last Children's Plague* will be much welcomed and warmly applauded by all of Richard's many friends and colleagues in Cambridge.

Simultaneously painstaking and compassionate, Altenbaugh's fine and highly original study makes clear that for those societies now mercifully free of polio, it is hard to grasp the scale and the depth of the dread that it once brought. For those who lived through the height of the disease but were untouched by it, childhood memories of polio will most likely be fleeting and indeterminate. It is only as we grow older, as a widening historical understanding begins to mingle with distant personal memory, that we are able to get a fuller measure of the times through which we lived as children. That is one of the reasons that *The Last Children's Plague* is such a revealing work. Here, history and memory resonate with one another in uncovering and evoking the past both as it was and as it continues to speak to the present.

A work such as this is borne along by narrative recollections from long ago, and in reading it, the book brought to mind with a new vibrancy a memory of my own, as a newly qualified young schoolteacher in the city of Bristol in the long, hot summer of 1976. A case of polio in a neighboring school—one of the last cases in the UK, as it turned out—was suddenly announced. The notification stirred the echoes of earlier, almost-forgotten memories from the 1950s and projected them anew into the circumstances of the present moment. Overnight, the mood of the local community was thrust back more than a quarter of a century, to 1950, when there had been 316 cases in the city, with 32 fatalities. The startling new outbreak dominated the front page of *The Bristol Evening Post* for a week, beginning with the frightening words, "Fears grew this afternoon that a girl who is in hospital with polio may have been in contact with people on a bus, at a garden party and at a bingo session." The juxtaposition of such mundane and routinely unthreatening activities of everyday life with the sudden eruption of an immediate and deadly threat to every aspect of that life was an existential shock. Fears that were thought to be long past were revived in an instant. Moves to trace the girl's contacts were put in place, and a full-scale vaccination program covering nine schools and twenty thousand people was completed within three days.

On the second day of the outbreak, under the headline, "Polio Peril That Never Fades," the newspaper reminded its readers, "Poliomyelitis, once one of the most dreaded diseases in the minds of caring parents, now only very occasionally surfaces." But it was precisely this fact, it continued, that "leads to complacency in the minds of parents that such fearful diseases as polio have been eradicated. This is certainly not the case." Thankfully, the outbreak was contained. The story slipped from the front page and was soon forgotten. Fear subsided. This in itself highlights an important lesson from *The Last Children's Plague*. Altenbaugh's work shows that the desire to push the memory of polio away, to consign it to the past, is a common one. His book stands as powerful and pertinent warning from history. The polio threat still has not been eradicated from the world.

The Last Children's Plague is, however, much more than a warning from the past. It is also a compelling account that places narratives of life at its heart and that celebrates them passionately. It is an intensely human work centering upon the lived experience of those whose lives were changed forever by their encounter with polio. This, then, is not simply a medical history. It is a people's history. It is about the places where suffering lives were lived and about the people with whom those lives were most intimately shared and upon whom they depended so entirely. Moreover, it is a story that, in its telling, calls not just for compassionate understanding but also for extensive expertise in many complex historical and methodological fields—the histories of childhood, of the family, of gender, of disability, of the classroom, of the hospital ward, and of memory itself. All are brought to bear here and drawn together into an overall narrative of immense range and richness. Richard Altenbaugh has met the challenge he has set himself in this project with all the intensity, sensitivity, and imagination for which it calls, together with the customary skill, insight, and wisdom that has characterized his many earlier publications as a leading educational and oral historian. Ultimately this is a book that opens us to one of humanity's most painful and poignant challenges—the cruel and unfathomable suffering of innocent children.

In reflecting upon the wealth of knowledge and insight afforded by the existing medical, institutional, and policy histories relating to the twentieth century's long battle against polio, Altenbaugh has pointed to a striking deficiency in the available record, prompting him to ask the question, profound in its simplicity, "But where are the patients?" We can be grateful that he has provided such a fulsome answer in this admirable and deeply moving book: the patients are here.

Philip Gardner
University of Cambridge

Acknowledgments

I owe so much to so many individuals and institutions that I do not know where to begin. I will try, in the hope that I do not omit any; if I do, I sincerely apologize. First, the idea for this study sprung from an informal conversation with Phil Gardner, over dinner and a bottle of wine. Polio had always occupied the fringes of my life. I was a first grader in the Pittsburgh Public Schools when Dr. Jonas E. Salk's nationwide vaccine tests succeeded. He quickly became a local hero. I also remembered standing in a line in my school's hallway as we all waited to be vaccinated. Moreover, I recall shuddering every Sunday as I heard contemporaries' metal braces clanking their way down the church aisles to the communion rail. In junior high school, I had an English teacher whose withered leg belied her attractiveness: We only saw her brace and cane. Finally, without a clear idea of why, in the late 1990s, all of these isolated incidences began to flood back into my memories. Whether it was because my two sons were growing up untouched by many of my childhood disease threats or because I was witnessing the deterioration of my own physical abilities because of age, I felt compelled to explore my past. Phil patiently listened as I rambled on about these experiences; I grew to very much appreciate his steady support over the years. Without him I would not have been able to spend the 1999, 2006, and 2011 Michaelmas terms at St. Edmund's, as a Visiting Fellow, researching, reading, writing, and attending history of medicine seminars at the University of Cambridge's renowned Department of History and Philosophy of Science. His many unselfish letters of support for grants provided much-needed subsidies. My colleagues at St. Edmund's provided the perfect environment for thinking, relaxing, and fellowship.

Second, I am indebted to friends and colleagues. Bruce C. Nelson over the decades helped me to mature as a historian through his probing questions, insightful criticisms, and demands to be an incisive and economical writer. In short, any craft I may have as a historian is very much due to his intellectual passion. Before his untimely death, he read many early papers and published articles related to this topic, providing rigorous criticism and offering excellent editing comments. I miss him. Laurie Moses Hines read early drafts of articles and chapters and wrote many letters to grant agencies. Susan Semel, after hearing one of my presentations on this topic, gave me much long-term moral support and encouragement. William Reese generously solicited this manuscript for Palgrave Macmillan; I was highly flattered by his invitation. There I encountered an enthusiastic Kristin Purdy, who shepherded it through the review and contract process. The production process could not have gone smoother.

My national and international colleagues offered wonderful forums to introduce my formative findings and thoughts at the annual meetings of the Canadian Historical Association, the Disability History Association, the European Conference for Educational Research, the International Conference for the Study of the History of Education, and the Medical Humanities Consortium and Medicine & Health group of the Social Science History Association. The invitation as a keynote speaker for the 2005 meeting of the British History of Education Society gave me the opportunity to seriously sharpen my historiographical thinking about this project. Early versions of some of my ideas were kindly published as "Polio, Disability, and American Public Schooling: A Historiographical Exploration" (*Educational Research and Perspectives* 31 [December 2004]: 137–55) and "Where Are the Disabled in the History of Education?" (*History of Education* 35 [November 2006]: 705–30). This intellectual process continued as the good folks at the Institute for Advanced Studies, University of Minnesota, in 2012 invited me to lecture and participate in an extremely helpful critique of a chapter.

Third, this project generated many conversations among my many physician friends. Their interest proved gratifying. Chief among them was Dr. John Schulhoff, who always displayed an intense interest in history. He pointed out episodes in medical history pertinent to this study and my understanding of the history of American medicine from a clinician's viewpoint.

Fourth, I received valuable aid from several institutions. Slippery Rock University provided a sabbatical to assist me during the 2006 fall semester and ample travel subsidies to attend conferences, present papers, and conduct research. And the Rockefeller Archive Center provided a much-needed grant to conduct research there.

Fifth, I cannot adequately express my gratitude for all of the genial and thoughtful assistance so many librarians and archivists have provided over the years at the American Philosophical Society, Bennington Library (University of Michigan), Carnegie Library of Pittsburgh, Chicago Public Library, New York Academy of Medicine, New York City Municipal Archives, New York City Public Library, Pennsylvania State Archives, Philadelphia's College of Physicians Archives, Pittsburgh Board of Education Archives (housed at the Heinz History Center), and University of Pittsburgh's School of Medicine Archives, and the incredible efforts of the good folks at Slippery Rock University's Bailey Interlibrary Loan Office to locate obscure articles and books. Several individuals stand out over the years. Ray White, director of the Watson Institute, always proved to be hospitable, patient, and accommodating as I pestered him with email queries and visits to conduct research. David Rose, at the March of Dimes Archives, likewise moved heaven and earth to facilitate my many requests over the years, and he proved to be a warm and helpful host when I visited that repository. He too read the complete manuscript, offering both substantive and stylistic comments. Finally, Edith Powell Chappell kindly presented me with a personalized copy of her coauthored book, *Black Oasis: Tuskegee's Fight Against Infantile Paralysis, 1941–1975*, which proved to be highly informative.

Most importantly, I am blessed with a wonderful family. Marianne, Ian, and Colin have always supported me without question or doubt. They provided terrific companionship and patience as they accompanied me on my forays to archives and conferences. Protocol Bluebonnet, our sweet and loving English cocker spaniel and a special family member, passed away as I wrote this book. After fifteen years of Bonnie sleeping under my desk, loyally keeping me company in my study, her absence proved unbearable; we simply could not live without another English cocker spaniel. Daisy entered our lives in 2009 as a naughty and curious puppy. She too now sleeps under my desk and, more importantly, brings me her precious toys, "persuading" me to take breaks from the tedium of writing. Thank you all!

Introduction

Why Children, Disease, and Disability?

In 1969, at two years of age, Justine Guckin caught poliomyelitis from a playmate who had received a live virus inoculation, otherwise known as the Sabin vaccine. She was vulnerable because she had earlier failed to receive the third injection of the Salk vaccine due to an ear infection. This had compromised her immune system, Guckin remarks: "When I came in contact with the other person who got vaccinated with the live vaccine I contracted it." Only fourteen years after Jonas E. Salk's successful national trial, her physician, as well as those at her local hospital in Newington, Connecticut, failed to recognize its symptoms.[1] Effective vaccines had quickly erased polio from the collective memory of Americans.

What, then, is poliomyelitis? In its simplest terms, it is a virus that quickly attacks the central nervous system. More often than not, it remains benign and asymptomatic, but it can occasionally cause flu-like traits; in its most virulent state, it results in permanent paralysis and infrequently in death. It is not a single virus but a family of three individual strains. In addition to the label poliomyelitis, this virus has been known as infantile paralysis, Heine-Medin's disease, debility of the lower extremities, and spinal paralytic paralysis, but polio remains the colloquial choice. Regardless of its name, it remains a maddeningly deceptive disease. It symptoms vary to this day, involving a low-grade fever and sore throat with full recovery within twenty-four hours. It also can induce temporary, or abortive, paralysis. Bulbar polio sparks the worst-case scenarios. This variation of the virus destroys nerve cells in the medulla oblongata, sometimes resulting in respiratory failure and often death. Each of the three variations can cause various degrees of illness and even paralysis; however, while all cause the disease, they differ in their degree of severity. Type I represents the most statistically common version and has been responsible for almost all epidemics. It can cause paralysis of the legs, arms, and sometimes diaphragm. Type II is a bit milder, but it can, on rare occasions, paralyze and kill its victims. Type III, the rarest form, is the most perilous: it leads to bulbar polio and, in turn, respiratory akinesis that usually causes death; this strain averages 6 percent of total infections. Of these,

90 percent die. However, during the 1946 Minneapolis epidemic, that rate multiplied several times. A University of Minnesota researcher, at that time, discovered that at least four types of bulbar polio existed. Children also could suffer from more than a single type of infantile paralysis, infected with one variant during one season and another during a second year, eventually contracting all three forms in their lifetimes. Post-polio expert Richard L. Bruno further delineates the high variations within this virus: These three types possess about fifty different strains that directly relate to polio's destructiveness, its "differing ability to multiply in [the] body, to get inside . . . neurons and damage them." Polioviruses thus "mutate inside people and can change their virulence." This explains why, as the twentieth century unfolded and the virus jumped from one person to another, it grew deadlier, "causing more paralysis and killing more people in 1950 than [it] did in 1920." Finally, this virus is extremely harmful to the human body. Johns Hopkins pathologist David Bodian, in the 1940s, estimated that it destroyed up to 50 percent of spinal cord motor neurons for those who became paralyzed, but even those who escaped still experienced some severe neuron damage; in all cases, this virus caused some degree of brain impairment.[2]

Its first symptoms occur within nine to twelve days after initial contact, while paralysis appears from eleven to seventeen days after exposure. Permanent paralysis affects less than 25 percent of patients, and more than 50 percent recover with no residual paralysis. The "greatest return of muscle function takes place within the first six to nine months after diagnosis, but improvement can continue for as long as two years."[3] And it is a painful disease. All other forms of paralysis destroy the sense of touch, but poliomyelitis intensifies it, as Anne Finger, who contracted this disease at age six in Utica, New York, during the 1950s, points out in her memoir: "The affected parts of the body may be more sensitive, nerves jangling and twittering, so that touch itself can become painful." This occurs because the "virus attacks the motor neurons, leaving nerves that carry sensation intact." Finally, throughout the first half of the twentieth century, mortality rates hovered between 5 and 10 percent.[4]

At the beginning of this century, this disease was hardly newsworthy. Reports of it were relegated to small and obscure articles hidden deep on the inside pages of newspapers (for those few of us who still read the print version). It seemed like a rare and exotic illness that only occurred in far-off continents. In June 2002, the World Health Organization (WHO) proudly announced that poliomyelitis had officially been wiped out in Europe. This virus lingered only in Africa and South Asia. A year later, WHO confidently predicted the end of polio by 2005. With only 235 cases reported during the first half of 2003, that organization expected to see 175 million additional children immunized by the end of that year. By 2011, WHO proclaimed India free of this disease. Its complete eradication appeared imminent. Nevertheless, in 2013, it suddenly reemerged in politically unstable northern Pakistan and war-torn Syria. A year later WHO noted, now in a nervous tone, that the poliovirus continued to spread, listing cases in Afghanistan,

Cameroon, Equatorial Guinea, Ethiopia, Israel, Nigeria, Pakistan, Somalia, and Syria. And once infected, no effective treatments exist.[5] Indeed, the scale of worldwide efforts to combat, and hopefully extinguish, this perplexing disease continues to boggle the mind.

However, few Americans remember, or even realize, that the worst epidemics occurred here. From the beginning of the twentieth century until 1955, with the introduction of the Salk vaccine, "polio enjoyed the infamous distinction of being the only remaining serious epidemic disease in the Western world."[6] *Time* magazine has ranked the 1916 epidemic as one of the "Top 10 Terrible Epidemics" the world has ever witnessed.[7] This disease proved to be especially deadly among young children ages five to nine until the 1930s, when it began to affect adolescents. Age therefore played a major role in morbidity rates. During New York City's 1916 outbreak, 80 percent of patients were aged four or younger. This figure slipped to 50 percent nationwide by 1931, 20 percent in 1944, and less than 20 percent in 1952.

> Although the percentage of five-to-nine-year-olds who got polio was a relatively constant 30 percent from 1916 to 1954, the percentage of polio patients older than ten increased from less than 10 percent in 1916 to about 55 percent in 1952. Between 1950 and 1955, just over half of polio patients admitted to one Massachusetts hospital were older than sixteen, and nearly a quarter were older than thirty. By 1955, 25 percent of polio patients were older than twenty.[8]

Infantile paralysis lurked in the shadows, a persistent threat of sudden illness, incapacitation, or even death: the reality of playing outside one sunny, warm summer day and the next day fighting for survival in a frightening hospital setting permeated with the pungent smells of alcohol, disinfectant, and ether, surrounded by strangers in starched white uniforms, isolated from friends and family. The lives of too many healthy youngsters, if they even survived the initial onset of the disease, experienced a profound transformation almost overnight: they turned into what became known as *crippled children*. Thus, a 1952 "national poll . . . found that polio was second only to the atomic bomb as the thing that Americans feared most."[9]

The polio epidemic and the crusade to eradicate it has become a classic American tale, conquering the "last of the great childhood plagues."[10] Franklin D. Roosevelt, disabled by it, became a legendary American president, elected to an unprecedented four terms. The March of Dimes pioneered organizational structures and fundraising efforts that are still used to this day in the philanthropic world. Salk rose to heroic levels in medical history because of his tireless efforts to develop a dead virus vaccine. What more can be said? This is precisely what I asked myself as I stumbled onto this historical literature. Nevertheless, as I initially immersed myself in secondary sources, the more I thought about it, the more I realized that the history of polio weaves together seemingly different experiential strands. This disease struck able-bodied children and too often caused them to become disabled in a relatively short period of time.[11] What were the social implications for such a rapid transformation? How did their parents respond? Siblings? Did they return to school? If so, did the relationships between educators and these students change?

These and many other questions drove me to pursue a different approach, drawing me into many other, but related, areas of history. Once again I found many gaps, and these raised additional questions. What effects did disease in general and disability in particular have on childhood? Infantile paralysis struck children, yet where were their voices in the scholarly narratives? Childhood history has greatly expanded and enriched its themes and contexts in recent decades. Historians have addressed children's rights, juvenile delinquency, poverty, truancy, and work, among other topics. They also have analyzed the impact of acculturation, adolescence, gender, emigration, poverty, race, rural living, slavery, and the urban environment.[12] However, the topic of childhood diseases has largely escaped the historian's pen, as medical historians Russell Viner and Janet Golden point out:

> It remains for historians to excavate the historical experiences of children's encounters with illness and suffering. And while this task poses particular methodological and theoretical challenges, it can no longer be ignored. Such investigations promise to yield not only a deeper understanding of how children experience illness, but to enrich our knowledge of what Roy Porter has called "sufferers' history," in which experience is primary, in which non-professionals are understood as the primary agents of care, and in which the intellectual agenda encompasses beliefs and conditions that medical historians have traditionally overlooked.[13]

When addressed, it disappears into a larger context. James Axtell alludes to the effect of diseases on child mortality rates during the colonial period; Susan E. Lederer presents the rare analysis of children as medical test subjects.[14] The former study is broadly focused on the dynamics of the colonial family, while the latter treats human experimentation in medical history. Moreover, as disability historian Paul K. Longmore stresses, "disability-specific histories" remain rare.[15] Except for Ernest Freeberg's biography of Laura Bridgeman, we know little about the personal side of children with disabilities. Historian Robert Dawidoff asserts that this "marginalization and misunderstanding" is all too common.[16] The polio story allows us to integrate these experiences into the mainstream.

The impact of diseases on the family's size, interpersonal relationships, roles, and educational mission has been significant but likewise overlooked. The American family has conveyed literacy, values, and work skills to its children, operating as an informal educational institution. During the colonial period, the New England Puritan family, church, and school maintained strong bonds as they worked together to *save* young souls. Meanwhile diphtheria, dysentery, and smallpox, among others, raged through those settlements, inflicting high child mortality rates. Many nineteenth-century families moved west across the continent to seek land and opportunities. This arduous journey exhausted children, who often walked the entire distance. With depleted food supplies and concomitant malnutrition as well as tainted drinking water, they easily fell ill. Wagon trains left many small graves in their wakes. By the early twentieth century, children had become emotional rather than economic assets, gradually removing them from the world of work. With children now more economically dependent, parents became the center of their universe; the household itself insulated them from threatening and at times lethal environments. How did illness reshape familial relationships in this close-knit world?[17] Family history certainly plays an integral part in the polio story.

Educational historians generally write the stories of able-bodied students and teachers in public or private, secular or religious school settings. This creates a narrow view of educational change; it also distorts educational experiences. What about the children who, for whatever reason, were not able-bodied? Was schooling the only source of formal, institutionalized education for them? Some forty years after the recommendations of Bernard Bailyn and Lawrence A. Cremin to broaden our definition of education, historians remain ever fixated on mainstream institutions (i.e., schools) and *normal* children.[18] Since then educational historians have only addressed individuals with disabilities as an afterthought, often relegating them to the history of special education. Even that overlooks the specific influences of disease on school policy and practice. First, this subfield generally categorizes emotional, intellectual, and physical needs as organic and, thereby, rarely accounts for students moving from being non-disabled to disabled. Second, it tends to ghettoize children with disabilities, isolating their experiences from the broader social context.[19] The restricted focus of *special education*—even the term itself—implies a school setting. This analysis, most importantly, overlooks the lives of students with disabilities themselves. They shaped culture and institutions in a variety of ways but remain hidden—an entire group of children has been overlooked as a result. Likewise the relatively new, rich field of the social history of the classroom insightfully delves into teacher-student interactions and relationships, discipline, daily classroom routines, instructors' lives, and students' experiences. However, it has yet to address the impact of disability on schooling in general and the classroom in particular.[20]

Even standard treatments of individuals with physical disabilities have oversimplified this experience. Relegated to a purely individual problem, it requires personal solutions through physical and mental rehabilitation and acceptance of a new life: adaptation.[21] Once we "shift from medical to sociocultural and political definitions of disability,"[22] we can move these individuals to the center of human experience by analyzing their interactions with peers, relationships with adults, and roles as students.

Finally, as medical historians Roger Cooter and John Pickstone boldly assert, "the history of medicine is the history of the twentieth century."[23] Medical historians, writing about the golden age of medicine, generally covering the period from the late nineteenth century through the first half of the twentieth century, recount the contributions of famous researchers, inventions of cutting-edge technologies, and the discoveries of new medications, among other topics. Rarely do they take into account patients' experiences while being treated within the health system and after being discharged. The impact of infantile paralysis on children, during hospitalization and subsequent physical rehabilitation, represents an integral part of the history of medicine.

Several fundamental questions have emerged from these numerous historical oversights: How can we illustrate developments in special education while ignoring the disabling effects of certain diseases on children? How can the history of medicine marginalize children, often the subjects of medical treatments? Poliomyelitis became a notorious childhood disease, but where are the patients?

The polio epidemic represented a mass childhood disease addressed by large-scale means, both organizationally and institutionally. This decades-long story demonstrates how the lines between hospitals, rehabilitation centers, home, and schools blurred. While hospitalized, young patients continued their lessons through tutors or in hospital classrooms. Physical therapy, which sometimes lasted years, included education in some form or another. When children came home, most parents arranged their houses like hospitals to accommodate them. Likewise, school administrators sent tutors and visiting teachers to continue their lessons. After returning to school, students with disabilities found few adaptations or relationships, yet most continued their education. No other disease has universally mobilized so many institutions in American society to treat and adapt to it; no other disease has redefined so many groups and organizations. These symbiotic relationships constitute the polio story. This part of the tale has not been told.

A disease, whether viral or bacterial in origin, is both a biological and a social experience. Historical analyses of disease transcend health issues, the tragic toll on lives, and medical breakthroughs and treatments; social reality cannot be ignored. Everyday lives and human institutions are affected as well as shaped by infectious outbreaks. This "social construction" encompasses the role of culture, both in the public and private realms. For instance, the polio experience proved to be highly gendered. The maternal parent, more than any other family member, loomed large in the care and treatment of her children. Moreover, young women paid a far heavier social and emotional price than their male counterparts, because disability defeminized them. A contagion therefore not only "invades" the individual's body, causing illness, suffering, and often death, but also influences society and transforms institutions.[24] This particular historical episode represents that rare convergence of a wide diversity of private and public groups and organizations: children, hospitals, media, parents, philanthropies, public school administrators and staff, and rehabilitation facilities.

Within this complex intersection of social, scientific, and educational forces, institutions served as social "mediators" in serious health matters, according to medical historians Charles E. Rosenberg and Janet Golden. The many and dynamic relationships between children, families, schools, and of course the medical community characterized its significance. Usually health facilities, such as hospitals and public and private sanitariums, operated as treatment centers and, failing that, provided custodial services.[25] Compulsory public education introduced an entirely new medical, institutional model: special education classes and schools, divorcing children with disabilities from their able-bodied classmates.

The organization of this book, therefore, does not follow a neat chronological sequence. Many polio narratives, whether intended or not, connote an odyssey. "To go from home to hospital is to make a journey," literary scholar Anne Hunsaker Hawkins explains. "However long or short that journey may be, the psychic distance is immense. The individual—now a patient—crosses a threshold into a strange otherworld of rituals and ordeals, an unknown territory that must be negotiated alone and, after, in pain and fear." The second leg of this voyage, the hospital itself, involves "liminal" attributes: "passivity, humility, and near nakedness, obedience, anonymity, and sometimes painful and invasive medical tests and procedures." Subsequent steps in this journey involve gradual "return to the world" through a "pilgrimage." It not only involves psychic dimensions but spatial ones as well. "Each literal move to a new room or place," Hawkins continues, "is accompanied by an existential movement out of the contracted world of illness and into a new and wider dimension." The culmination of this quest is the return to "health or life received . . . Or the sick person may bring back the gift of knowledge, that vision of a deeper meaning in life that serious illness or impending death sometimes confers upon the sick and that sometimes leads to profound personal changes."[26] While this may be a common ending point for typical illness pathographies, children with polio had yet one more portion of this trek. Many recovered from the initial infection, but would they survive the stain of disability?

This study analyzes the impact of this disease on children's personal lives, encompassing public health policies (Chapter 1) that too often transformed them into epidemic refugees; hospitalization (Chapter 2), involving physical and emotional trauma; philanthropic and organizational responses (Chapter 3), illustrating how the National Foundation for Infantile Paralysis fit into a larger context and its use of poster children in its fundraising campaigns; life during therapy (Chapter 4), revealing the reality of disability and the fashioning of ward culture; family life (Chapter 5), dissecting the many changes that shaped its members and functions; schooling (Chapter 6), placing disability at center stage, both academically and socially; and reviews the roles of individuals disabled by polio in leading the disability rights movement. These chapters piece together society's perception of disease and disability—the public world; another recreates the daily lives of these children—their personal realities. I argue that agency was prevalent within these institutions.

This is ultimately a story of disease and children. It ambitiously attempts to synthesize their diverse worlds through an interdisciplinary approach that incorporates the seemingly different lenses of education, disability, and medicine; at the same time, it not only stresses the tension between some of these institutions but also analyzes the roles of everyday people.[27] It builds this context through an in-depth social calculus and accounting of the multilayered textures of human experience. Published autobiographies, biographies, literature, memoirs, and oral histories help to reconstruct it. But these have to be approached with a healthy dose of intellectual skepticism as well as a concern for the macro and micro levels of human reality. Studies of disability encompass three historical perspectives, according to special education writer Elizabeth Bredberg. The first flows from institutional experiences, namely records that draw on medical treatment regimens as well as blueprints and drawings of equipment for people with disabilities. A second interpretation emerges from "vernacular" influences; that is, the broader culture consisting of folk traditions, broadcast through "literature, popular theatre, works of art, or proverb." An experiential analysis, the third type, provides valuable insights, but it too has its limitations. These draw on the personal lives of people with disabilities; yet, as in the case of individuals like Helen Keller, they can become simple "'inspirational' reading," ultimately distorting that experience. Bredberg hints at a potentially rich, synthetic approach, which I employ: "The risk of presentism, of interpreting the past in terms of contemporary values and practices, is substantially diminished as a historian becomes intimately acquainted with a particular setting in all its complexity and richness."[28]

Recollections produce valuable insights, humanizing the polio experience. During the fifty years of epidemics that swept the United States, "patient-centered medicine" did not exist. Then, as now, physicians treated diseases rather than tended to the "welfare of sick persons." Pathography, according to Hawkins, operates as a "form of autobiography or biography that describes personal experiences of illness, treatment, and sometimes death"; it endeavors, in short, to restore the "patient's voice to the medical enterprise." These insights recount "adventures," if you will, of "heroic . . . struggles of brave individuals confronting what appear to be insurmountable forces." The ill are thrust into alien institutions (i.e., hospitals), becoming "hostages" or "prisoners" who at first "'resist their captors and then try to appease them by good behavior.'" These "glimpses of what it is like to live in the absence of order and coherence" (i.e., our *normal* routines) can be "disquieting." Pathographies, Hawkins concludes, reveal the "attempts of individuals to orient themselves in the world of sickness." Through their eyes, we see their personal dramas unfold.[29] Doing this uncovers those unheard children's voices, as Viner and Golden assert:

> We can use these sources to reconstruct an external picture of the child in medical situations, studying the demographics of practice, the social geography of medical interactions, and the types of procedures children experienced or were denied. We can also draw conclusions about the social relations of children with their parents and doctors in both illness and health, and map how physicians redrew the child's body and life, bringing it under increasingly closer scrutiny.

This allows us to gain some sense of agency. "The voices and perceptions of children have had no champion," Viner and Golden continue. "Children have not been seen as historical actors but as subjects, largely because their choices and actions were highly constrained by their dependency, particularly in the case of infants and young children."[30] This concept of dependency is crucial in this study.

A deep sense of suffering is also revealed through these voices. This is too often overlooked in the study of diseases. Suffering transcends physical pain. It can be manifested through fear or uncertainty. Furthermore, suffering is not isolated to the patient. Others, like family members, become swept up in this experience. It likewise has serious social and cultural meanings, such as redefining femininity and masculinity, what is acceptable and what is not. A new status quo therefore emerges from illness. Finally, suffering is manifested through a sense of loss.[31]

Such qualitative sources, though, tend to be questioned or challenged because of their subjectivity or reliability. Jacqueline Foertsch, another literary scholar, keenly analyzes accounts portrayed through women's magazines, memoirs, novels, and newsletters in the post-World War II period, separating the "polio experience in its immeasurable variation and the polio story," one that seems too pat at times.[32] Oral histories in particular have been challenged because they rely on recollections of the past, filtered through a myriad of experiences. Historian Jerrold Hirsch raises another, often ignored, aspect. Existing accounts of the polio story, whether film or written versions, that rely on oral history only tell part of it. On the one hand, they stress public dread as each summer signaled another epidemic, on the other hand, they focus on the scientific struggle to find a cure, culminating with the development of Salk's vaccine. What is missing is that it "virtually silences survivors' accounts of being disabled in an ableist society." This creates a narrow view of that history, as Hirsch points out, because of the "absence of interviews that seek to capture the disability history of the survivors and the social construction of disability that they had to deal with in their culture."[33]

These do not function as memories in the ordinary sense for individuals affected by infantile paralysis. Certainly a "published narrative of an illness is not the illness itself, but it can become the experience of the illness." But this particular illness "is never really finished."[34] It remains a permanent reality, not anchored in the remote past but alive in the present. In addition to permanent disability, discoveries since the 1970s have uncovered another legacy: post-polio syndrome. American survivors "may still exceed 400,000," and many of them have developed new symptoms:

> (1) excessive fatigue and reduced endurance; (2) new joint and muscle pain; (3) progressive muscle weakness, not only in muscles previously affected, but also in muscles apparently unaffected by acute polio; (4) new or increased breathing difficulties, in some cases requiring the use of ventilatory devices; and (5) cold intolerance that contributes to muscle weakness and is accompanied by burning pain.

For a generation of physicians who had never seen this disease, they often misdiagnosed their patients' ailments, contributing to their frustration and possibly leading to depression. Dr. Richard Owen, who worked at the Sister Kenny Institute in Minneapolis, founded the Post-Polio Center in 1981. There he discovered poor cardiopulmonary fitness due to a lack of adequate muscular exercise or use. Subsequent research by others found that this virus had often struck surreptitiously, showing "little or no significant paralysis at the time of acute infection." Hospitals summarily discharged these patients. To make matters worse, we possess little scientific knowledge about the post-polio experience. New symptoms began about thirty years after the original onset of this disease. The cause otherwise remains an enigma, while effective treatment appears uncertain. The impact likewise continues to be unclear, with widely divergent estimates ranging from 20 to 80 percent of previous victims. The 1985 Mayo Clinic study calculated it at 22 percent; five years later, the Sister Kenny Institute reported a 41 percent rate. This virus continues to haunt and elude us.[35]

Polio transformed young lives and stumped the medical science community. We know about the latter's stellar success in developing effective vaccines. What we lack is historical insight into the former's emotional, physical, and social experiences—the other half of the story. Hawkins asserts that the "pathography written by the patient . . . can be seen as the logical counterpart" to formal medical history. "It would seem that they should be very similar, since both genres are concerned with the sickness and treatment of a specific individual. In fact, however, they are radically different in subject, purpose, structure, authorial persona, and tone." Why? Because "a pathography is an extended narrative situating the illness experience within the author's life and the meaning of that life."[36]

The recollections of individuals affected by polio reveal the severe physical pain that permeated each stage of this disease, from onset to diagnosis to treatment. They capture anger, frustration, and terror not only among children but also parents, neighbors, and medical professionals. Still, these *memories* too often tend to stress this as a personal or individual struggle, only rarely and generally alluding to an ambiguous collective experience. Only by reading between the lines and carefully discerning commonalities can social patterns be unearthed and agency uncovered. Infantile paralysis indeed proved to be a significant social (in addition to medical) phenomenon at many different levels.

My goal therefore is to locate the subjectivity of children's illnesses and disabilities within the larger context of the first half of the twentieth century. But this cannot be done by using individual records alone; rather, they must be seen as individual pieces of a jigsaw puzzle that, when combined, produce a larger and more meaningful picture. This process of assembling and synthesizing stories of illness fits into the notion of "narrative medicine," as termed by literary scholar Rita Charon. It gives us "patients' experiences of their bodies and their health." The primary point of this study is to enter, see, and interpret the world of illness from the collective use of the "patients' point of view" as much as possible. For Charon, "narrative medicine has come to understand that patients . . . enter whole—with their bodies, lives, families, beliefs, values, histories, hopes for the future—into sickness and healing, and their efforts to get better . . . cannot be fragmented away from the deepest parts of their lives."[37]

Abbreviations of Archives/Collections

American Philosophical Society, Philadelphia, PA   (APS)

Carnegie Library of Pittsburgh, Pennsylvania Room   (CLP)

Chicago Public Library, Municipal Reference Collection, Harold Washington Library Center   (CPL)

College of Physicians, Philadelphia, PA   (CP)

D. T. Watson Institute Archives, Pittsburgh, PA   (WIA)

Thomas Francis Papers, Bentley Historical Library, University of Michigan   (BHL)

Georgia Warm Springs   (GWS)

March of Dimes, White Plains, NY   (MOD)

Elizabeth Kenny Papers, Minnesota Historical Society, St. Paul, MN   (MHS)

New York Academy of Medicine   (NYAM)

New York City Department of Records and Information Services, Municipal Archives   (NYCMA)

Pennsylvania State Archives, Harrisburg, PA   (PSA)

Rockefeller Archive Center, Sleepy Hollow, NY   (RAC)

Roosevelt Warm Springs Institute for Rehabilitation   (RWSIR)

University of Pittsburgh, Health Science Library System   (UPITT)

Social Welfare History Archives, University of Minnesota   (SWHA)

Chapter 1

The American Plague[1]

*The New York epidemic is without doubt the
greatest scourge of poliomyelitis which
the United States has ever experienced.
It bids fair to be the most severe of its kind in the world.*

—John D. Robertson

Epidemics have always exacted a heavy toll on children. And cultural artifacts, like the poem "O Betsy Bell and Mary Gray," acknowledge them in unique ways. This Scottish children's nursery rhyme, often sung as a ballad, now obfuscates its origin. It is directly connected to the dreaded bubonic plague that struck Perth, Scotland, in 1645–1647, killing some three thousand people. Two friends, Betsy and Mary, the daughters of the Laird of Kinvaid and the Laird of Lednock, respectively, fled to the countryside to escape infection: "They bigget a bower on yon burn-brae/And theekit it o'er wi' rashes./They theekit it o'er wi' rashes green,/They theekit o'er wi' heather."[2] This represented a common response, since it exacted a ghastly toll in Europe's cities. "In 1630–31 Venice lost 30 percent of its people; in Genoa, plague and famine in 1656 led to the death of up to three quarters of the population . . . About one fifth of London's population perished in each of the plague outbreaks of 1563, 1603, 1625 and 1665, the death toll in 1665 approaching 80,000." In response, northern Italian cities created public health boards, originally composed of noblemen, that banned religious processions, destroyed dogs and cats, locked churches, regulated burials, and quarantined the sick, isolating them from the general population. The power to enforce these measures fell on the shoulders of local magistrates.[3] Betsy and Mary, in spite of their efforts to escape harm, became infected and died. That poem continues, "But the pest cam' frae the burrows-town,/And slew them baith thegither." They could not be buried in the churchyard, according to custom, and instead were interred "near the bank of the river Almond."[4] Betsy and Mary, even at death, had fallen prey to the age-old practice of containing diseases. That plague eventually abated, but children continued to pay a dear price due to a host of other diseases. High infant and child mortality rates branded Western culture for the next two centuries, especially in the United States.

By 1900, 18 percent of American children died before the age of five, one of the worst rates among comparable countries at that time. Deaths among children younger than fifteen were concentrated at the youngest ages: 88 percent among those four or younger and 59 percent of infants. "A 1908 survey of schoolchildren in New York found that 66 percent needed medical or surgical attention or better nourishment." Researchers Samuel H. Preston and Michael R. Haines, taking into account ethnicity, race, and class, found that a significantly higher number of children residing in urban areas suffered than their rural counterparts. They reason that "this influence reflects primarily the greater efficiency with which infectious diseases are spread in denser areas." American children died of bronchitis, cholera infantum, diarrhea, diphtheria, enteritis, influenza, measles, meningitis, pneumonia, scarlet fever, smallpox, tuberculosis, and whooping cough at alarming rates. Morbidity levels proved to be even higher. "Among the top 10 cities, the highest child death figures were found in the large eastern port cities of New York, Philadelphia, Boston, and Baltimore . . . Boston, with the highest child death rate among the largest 10 cities, had a mixed regard of providing public health in the form of good water and sewerage." Preston and Haines assign a great deal of weight to public health and sanitation measures in reducing child death rates in urban areas.[5]

Young African Americans suffered the highest morbidity and mortality rates, "both absolutely and in relation to whites." Before the age of five, the death rate was 58 percent higher, and in the urban North, in particular, 89 percent higher. Tuberculosis proved to be especially virulent. Poor diet, inadequate housing, the absence of health care, and lack of proper sanitation all exacted their toll. Because of poverty and de facto segregation, African American families generally lived in the unhealthiest parts of northern cities. High rates of adult illiteracy exacerbated this situation because parents lacked access to information about child care, health measures, and medical treatments. "Race was a caste-like status in 1900, and the degraded social and economic circumstance of blacks, who had virtually no chance of entering the mainstream of American life, is undoubtedly reflected in their exceptionally high mortality."[6] Even though a steady decline in child mortality rates marked the first half of the twentieth century, race continued to play a role well into the 1940s. Until that point nonwhites maintained about a 60 percent higher rate of death than whites from all causes among children between ages one and fourteen. The fifteen- to twenty-four-year-old group, however, began the century with a sharp difference, about a 200 percent gap during the early decades, but converged during the late 1940s. These disparities narrowed considerably for all ages but never quite equalized, even through the 1950s.[7]

But there appeared to be more to this social context: the American medical community remained moribund in its beliefs and practices. In spite of major breakthroughs by Louis Pasteur and Joseph Lister in the cause and prevention of infections, most American physicians during the last two decades of the nineteenth century continued to rely on miasma theory to explain the sources of illnesses and dictate treatments. Infectious odors from cesspools, open sewerage, and slaughterhouses, among others, they believed, "disrupted the body's balance, and doctors often attempted to restore its balance through purgatives, diuretics, and emetics." Many doctors too embraced social Darwinism, believing that some human beings had inferior physical constitutions that made them especially susceptible to infections. They asserted that the immoral lives and dirty living conditions of African Americans and southern Italian immigrants, for example, only supplemented their "inherited organic weakness." Although germ theory began to erode these views, many continued to cling to outdated notions during the early years of the twentieth century. Finally, physicians knew virtually nothing about children's disease, a major void in their rudimentary training. "In 1887, less than a half-dozen general hospitals in the U.S. had wards for infants." They simply considered "high death rates of infants and young children . . . to be an inevitable concomitant of this vulnerable stage of development."[8]

Mandatory school attendance unintentionally intensified the likelihood of childhood epidemics by promoting congestion. A legislative outcome of Progressive educational thought during the late nineteenth and early twentieth centuries, it certainly contributed to a better-educated population. Enrollment, attendance, and completion rates steadily increased after the Civil War. Elementary and secondary enrollment grew from 7.6 to 21.6 million between 1870 and 1920, from 65 to 78 percent of five- to seventeen-year-olds. The average number of days attended grew by 50 percent during that period, from 78 to 121. Finally, high school graduation rose from virtually zero to 231,000 during that fifty-year period.[9] Overcrowded, poorly ventilated, and unsanitary schools fed morbidity and mortality rates.

A turning point in both Europe and North America occurred during the second half of the 1800s. According to demographer Catherine Rollet's analysis, although infant death rates in general did not decline during this period, "it appears that mortality of children between ages of 1 and 5 dropped faster and more continuously than infant mortality throughout the nineteenth century." This occurred because a gradual transition began to unfold in Western culture regarding guardianship; that is, the child became less a "private 'good'" and more a "public 'good.'" This involved four periods that, of course, often overlapped as well as depended on the country involved. The first stage, about 1860 to 1870, saw childhood becoming a recognized stage of life. As a result, the public grew more aware of infant and child mortality, which became an important social issue, one that induced deeper emotional responses than before. The United States, though, lagged behind other Western countries because it rarely turned to public options. This produced spotty and irregular child health care, generally relegated to urban areas. The US Children's Bureau, a federal initiative, began operations in 1912 (and continued until 1969) to pursue research activities and programs for maternal and infant welfare. In 1921, Congress "adopted the first law governing the welfare of mothers and infants, the Maternity and Infancy Act, also known as the Sheppard-Towner Act. This Act guaranteed State funding for the development of health services for mothers and children." Congress failed to reauthorize it in 1929 due to the budget constraints of the Great Depression and to American Medical Association opposition, which saw it as a form of socialized medicine. The United States therefore only embarked on late and short-term public sector efforts to address children's health. The second period, sometime during the 1880s and 1890s, involved the impact of medical advances. New discoveries and technologies caused physicians and hospitals to address infant and child mortality as never before. Diphtheria antitoxin and smallpox inoculations became more widespread in Western countries. While the use of the *bacille bilié de Calmette-Guérin* (or BCG) vaccine in Europe impeded the spread of tuberculosis, the American medical community never adopted this preventative approach. Improved surgical techniques also generally reduced mortality rates. And public health institutions and mechanisms played larger roles in children's lives. In this case, proper nutrition became paramount. This involved more care about the purity of food, especially milk. Public health agencies also dispatched visiting nurses to the homes of sick children to offer assistance and oversee parental care. The third approach emerged around 1900 with special attention to the role of mothers in raising healthy children. Western nations had elevated child care to a science; since it was now a "serious task," they rationalized and systematized it. This effort began with care during the neonatal period, continued with "disease-free births," and culminated with teaching mothers about "infant care." In the United States, and growing out of feminist activism, "maternalism" supplanted existing "paternalism." Women now oversaw children's health, protection, and welfare, largely utilizing various public and private organizations. The fourth and final movement began sometime during the 1920s, when the effort to lower infant and child death rates began to be viewed within the context of civil rights. "It was no coincidence that measures to improve child health were taken at the same time as the State began to legally enforce universal primary school education. All segments of society began to embrace the concepts of health care, education, and social justice."[10] Largely reinforcing Rollet's interpretation, demographic historian George Alter concludes that no single element alone accounted for a profound decline in infant and child mortality rates in Canada and the United States. He instead points to multiple factors that individually produced incremental reductions in young children's deaths but collectively trimmed them over a long period of time.[11] Poliomyelitis proved to be a wildcard, however.

This disease has existed for centuries. It manifested itself endemically in a subclinical fashion, as researcher John R. Paul points out in his classic, *A History of Poliomyelitis*. This virus silently infected and quietly immunized infants, an ongoing process. However, sanitation practices to combat bacterial infections, commonly employed by communities during the late nineteenth and early twentieth centuries, ignited "pronounced changes in the behavior of poliomyelitis." As human immunity changed, this virus began to savagely assert itself.[12]

But it did not strike suddenly like a lightning bolt. Storm clouds had been growing steadily and inexorably darker with each passing year. Relatively small and scattered but certainly noticeable eruptions had been occurring. The earliest clinical description of polio appeared in a 1789 medical text. It began to shift from an endemic state to sporadic outbreaks during the late nineteenth and early twentieth centuries. Although scattered outbreaks had occurred in Europe, the first claim of a "real epidemic" of infantile paralysis in the United States took place in West Feliciana, Louisiana, in 1841 when between eight and ten children, all younger than two, fell ill. By the 1870s, the American medical community not only noted the seemingly growing presence of this disease in very young children but also began to address it at professional conferences and lectures.[13]

The media, too, began to take notice. On December 9, 1887, *The New York Times* casually observed, in a minor news item buried on page 8, that the New York Orthopedic Dispensary and Hospital had treated a total of 731 new patients, 98 of which (or 13 percent) had been diagnosed and treated for infantile paralysis. With the threat of more ubiquitous diseases on a grander scale, this small article treated this particular one in a prosaic fashion; it appeared relatively unknown, and therefore the *Times* naturally minimized it. Four years later, that paper reported that the same hospital had treated 144 patients disabled by poliomyelitis (7 percent of all new patients). No doubt, viewed in isolation, they certainly represented marginal rates. However, these figures only represented one hospital. Pieced together with subsequent cases, a string of precedents surreptitiously had begun to emerge. They appeared fitfully until 1896, upon which cases began to be reported each year. A front-page article posted the headline "New Poliomyelitis Cases" on August 7, 1899, reporting the number of infections and deaths in Brooklyn and Poughkeepsie, in an outbreak that continued until the middle of that month.[14] But newspaper coverage divorced these episodes from any previous ones. From 1907 in particular, reported cases surfaced revealing less scattered infections and in larger numbers; death rates for that period ranged between 5 and 10 percent. The *Times* reported additional flare-ups for several weeks in August and September 1907. It began with a front-page headline describing cases in Ridgway, Pennsylvania, and by September 12 the paper informed its readers that between three hundred and four hundred cases existed in New York City itself, and it accounted for others in New Jersey and Pennsylvania. Three years later, during those same months, this paper reported outbreaks in New York City and in much of New England, Indiana, Iowa, New Jersey, and Pennsylvania. While states did not require doctors to document this disease, Pennsylvania broke ranks, announcing it reportable, and from its data, it estimated a total of 658 "infant paralytics" from this most recent incident. Nevertheless, on April 21, 1912, the *Times* ran a piece titled "Less Infantile Paralysis," in which a relieved Surgeon General Rupert Blue identified 5,861 cases of infantile paralysis nationwide in

1910 but only 1,933 in 1911; the number of deaths declined as well, from 950 to 440. However, both he and the newspaper failed to acknowledge that the mortality rate had increased from 16 to 23 percent. Beginning in July and continuing through October, the paper pointed to incidences in that city as well as Buffalo and as far away as Alaska. Only irregular reports continued to appear in the *Times* between 1913 and 1916, due largely to the dominance of war news from Europe.[15]

Nevertheless, a pattern began to take shape. The frequency and intensity of outbreaks had been increasing for two decades. First, based on Swedish outbreaks, Haven Emerson, director of New York City's Department of Health from 1915 to 1917, noted that it tended to be a rural disease. The distribution of outbreaks there seemed to be widely scattered and aberrant, with low numbers of cases. Second, in the United States, as early as 1895, American physicians were aware of Europe's isolated cases. That year Charles S. Caverly, president of Vermont's State Board of Health, summarized the existing literature on this disease to the forty-sixth annual meeting of the American Medical Association in Baltimore, citing infections in Boston, Germany, France, and Sweden during the second half of the nineteenth century. All of them had been formally reported in American and German medical journals published between 1843 and 1895, including symptoms and pathology. Third, the outbreak with the highest profile in the United States occurred in Vermont in 1894, with 123 cases. Caverly at that time provided the first highly detailed clinical study, leading to his discovery of abortive infections; that is, non-paralytic polio. Children younger than age six constituted about 75 percent of those infected, including twice as many males as females. Some level of paralysis affected 110 of them; 50 fully recovered, 10 died, and the remaining 50 became permanently disabled. In spite of his study, this disease remained a mystery. Caverly's epidemiological evidence dismissed unsanitary conditions as a cause, noting that the cases appeared equally in rural areas and towns and that both poor and affluent children became infected. Fourth, numerous recorded domestic episodes occurred in Nebraska and New York City in 1907; Massachusetts in 1908; Nebraska and St. Paul, Minnesota, in 1909; California, Iowa, Pennsylvania, and Washington in 1910; California and Cincinnati in 1911; and Buffalo and California in 1912. Between 1910 and 1915, polio deaths in 25 states and Washington, DC, totaled 5,616. Rural cases outnumbered urban ones 3,159 to 2,457; overall, children four or younger made up more than half of them. Fifth, and even more germane, in the ten years prior to 1916, the New York Orthopedic Hospital treated an average of 75 cases a year, with the latter five years jumping to 99 per year, a 33 percent increase. A quiet pattern of growth was unfolding, according to this hospital's statistical reports. In 1907 alone, that city's health department confirmed 800 infections but estimated, because of poor reporting or faulty diagnoses, that they actually totaled 2,500. Individually these could be, and probably were, dismissed as scattered, anecdotal evidence, but in the aggregate a clear blueprint had emerged.[16] Taking into account the consistent escalation of national flare-ups as well as New York

City's rising number of cases (albeit with annual fluctuations), it appears that the 1916 epidemic should not have caught public health officials by complete surprise. From this point onward, though, infantile paralysis would no longer be ignored or marginalized by either the medical establishment or the media. The "Americanization" of polio had begun.[17]

That year polio not only often became front-page news but also dominated entire issues of the *Times*. The scale of that outbreak dwarfed any previous experiences and overtaxed New York City's health infrastructure, one so carefully constructed since the late 1800s. The first reported incident occurred on May 13, 1916, and the last one on October 31, 1916, amounting to 7,108 total cases with 1,654 deaths, a 25 percent mortality rate. The peak period occurred between July 1 and August 26. The week ending August 5, 1916, accounted for the worse seven-day period, with 1,206 infections and 374 deaths, for a 31 percent fatality rate.[18] The New York City Department of Health, hailed as the cutting-edge municipal public health agency in the country, frenetically sprung into action, but seemingly to no avail. These annual epidemics would continue to unfold during the next four decades, and they proved devastating to children.

With few exceptions, historians thus far have produced four specific genres in analyzing this modern epidemic: biography, hagiography, inspirational, and institutional. Individual heroism dominates, whether as renowned scientists or determined *cripples*. Philanthropies are hailed. These works certainly have contributed a great deal to our knowledge of this sometimes fatal disease that mainly counts children among its fatalities. That is all well and good, but this study argues that a more complex and nuanced set of experiences unfolded.

A Simple Tale?

I know that I tread a well-worn path. Polio's story has been portrayed in the award-winning 1958 Broadway play and 1960 movie "Sunrise at Campobello." It has also been the subject of children's books, journalistic accounts, personal recollections, and television documentaries.[19] And, of course, many historians, journalists, and researchers have preceded me. This latter body of literature as a whole provides rich analyses of this last great children's epidemic in the United States. Lacunae nevertheless exist. These accounts, with rare exceptions, generally follow a surprisingly pedestrian approach. Narratives generally commence with the 1916 nationwide epidemic, yet they dwell on New York City and march decade by decade to the 1950s, culminating with the nationwide field trial and mass vaccination campaign. The literature also carefully constructs a pantheon of heroes. Its celebratory tone tends to center on renowned individuals, like Franklin D. Roosevelt; institutions, such as the March of Dimes; as well as medical scientists, like Jonas E. Salk. Some have ably blended all three elements together. Nevertheless, these histories rarely include the public in general and parents and schoolchildren in particular—agency is all but forgotten.[20]

Four interpretative frameworks exist. Biographies of this disease[21] generally maintain a one-dimensional focus and a largely linear approach. This category relies on a descriptive narrative that comprehensively and chronologically presents the overall impact of polio on individuals, families, fundraising strategies, and research techniques and breakthroughs. A steady stream of this scholarship has been published for more than forty years.[22] Hagiography narrowly dwells on the medical pioneers who, with their contributions, provided pathbreaking treatments and ultimately a cure. Their perseverance and sacrifices benefited children affected by polio, their families, and ultimately society. Scholars tout their roles as the chief actors, if not saviors, rising above the tens of thousands of sufferers to single-handedly provide relief and eventually vanquish this disease. No other experience or actor holds more status. Jonas Salk, Albert Sabin, and Sister Elizabeth Kenny usually serve as the center of attention in these studies.[23] A number of works about polio history also focus on individuals who viewed their paralysis as an extraordinary life obstacle to overcome. Their universe allowed them neither to wallow in self-pity nor struggle for the rights of the disabled. In the world of the able-bodied, disability did not represent an option for them. Their success stories instill hope in others who face similar physical and social challenges, and they herald the triumph of the human spirit. This inspirational body of literature rests on the successes of individuals rather on the plight of the disabled majority. Biographies of Roosevelt and Wilma Rudolph exemplify this brand of history. In a few of these cases, strong religious beliefs inspired individuals to persevere.[24] "Fight Infantile Paralysis" long served as the rallying cry and motto of the National Foundation for Infantile Paralysis (NFIP). The final genre principally has an institutional focus, namely the NFIP and the March of Dimes, its popular fundraising tool.[25]

In sum, all of these histories, some of them award-winning works, maintain a limited scope in one way or another. They generally follow a chronological approach and rarely offer critical analyses. Two trends attempt to transcend this orthodoxy. The first is represented by a collection of autobiographies, memoirs, and oral histories. These provide powerful insights into personal struggles with this disease and its aftermath. At the same time, they present somewhat fragmented and isolated snapshots of a broader experience.[26] Daniel J. Wilson's commendable and valuable scholarly efforts, especially *Living with Polio: The Epidemic and Its Survivors*, epitomize the second direction, breaking new ground in this refreshing social history. He pursues a comprehensive agenda, describing and analyzing topics like the impact on families and the hospitalization ordeal. His scope too is broad, encompassing the young as well as adults. However, and unfortunately, children's voices are rare, and therapeutic, home, and schooling experiences are minimized.[27]

Although a solid foundation has been laid, this study diverges from the others by synthesizing individual recollections into a collective experience and analyzing them experientially, focusing on key points in people's lives. Roy Porter's 1985 seminal work, "The Patient's View," although criticizing a much broader historiographical landscape, certainly applies to polio's histories: "Medicalization theory harbors . . . the implication that the rise of medical power is in some sense eluctable and unilinear, the ghost train speeding down the old Whiggish mainline from magic to medicine."[28] But it is more than that: The history of polio is about children and their experiences as patients, with rehabilitation, rejoining their families, resuming their education, and grappling with disabilities. This conforms to Porter's clarion call. He confronts traditional historiography (i.e., the progress of medicine from the professional's perspective) and argues instead for "medical history from below." Porter asserts that not only were the patients and medical professionals involved in "medical events," but families and communities were as well. "In medicine's history, the initiatives have often come from, and power has frequently rested with, the sufferer, or with lay people in general, rather than with the individual physician or medical profession at large." Porter points to two specific oversights. First, he laments the lack of historical treatment of the family as a health-care institution: "We should never underestimate the key role of the family in sickness care." Second, as he continues, "Most maladies have not in fact been treated by the professional but by self- or community help."[29] Here "community" will be defined in its broadest sense. Illnesses and treatments encompassed almost all of the institutions that crossed the paths of these young sufferers. In short, what were the social patterns of poliomyelitis? This represents a far more difficult challenge and portends a richer outcome.

A Continuous Calamity

On Tuesday, July 5, 1916, a front-page *New York Times* headline exclaimed, "25 More Deaths from Paralysis." Infantile paralysis no longer languished on inside pages as it had for several days. Its apparent suddenness and scale now made it a prime topic, dominating front-page news for the next two days. Although this disease hit New York City the hardest in 1916, it also struck the rest of the United States with devastating results. Twenty-six states reported some 27,000 cases, claiming 6,000 deaths.[30] Little tangible scientific data about this disease existed; yet it was not new, as we have seen.

This epidemic—what historians commonly note as the first significant poliomyelitis episode—is best understood when placed within the context of early twentieth-century public health policy. Children became its focal point. As the physical, concrete embodiment of an unseen threat, they in turn became the objects of fear. Public health officials invoked regulations to restrict their movements, forcibly remove them from railway trains and automobiles, and require travel papers. Children became isolated, shunned, and hunted as a result of public fear and mandates.

New York City mayor John Mitchel hosted an emergency meeting on July 12, 1916, and formed a "special committee" to oversee newly reported cases, implement isolation actions, and coordinate a corps of physicians and nurses, thus mobilizing that city's vaunted health department. Simon Flexner, of the Rockefeller Institute for Medical Research (RIMR), and Alvah H. Doty, former health officer of the Port of New York, served as executive officers of the committee. In addition to Emerson, that meeting included local and national public health representatives, researchers, and clinicians, among them the renowned Joseph Goldberger. Flexner secured $50,000 from the Rockefeller Foundation to assist this effort. That foundation granted another $5,000 to subsidize the printing and distribution costs of an informational pamphlet on polio, informing the public on a mass scale.[31] This two-sided leaflet, *Infantile Paralysis (Poliomyelitis): Information for the Public,* served a twofold purpose. First, concerning prevention, it stressed the need for cleanliness, screened windows to keep flies out of houses, and a nutritious diet. It further cautioned people to avoid crowds and discouraged adults from kissing children. A second, quite intrusive objective existed. It encouraged neighbors to immediately report any cases of infection. This endorsement of surveillance destroyed family privacy at best and intensified fear and created divisiveness at worst. The health department likewise released the names and addresses of new cases and deaths to *The New York Times,* which the newspaper published daily throughout the epidemic.[32] When this committee adjourned after its second meeting on August 3, it had rendered the scaffolding for public and philanthropic responses to poliomyelitis for the next four decades.

City officials meanwhile appealed to the public for calm in a July 12 *New York Times* front-page story, "Paralysis Takes Lives of 32 More." Mayor Mitchel assured the public that all of the city's medical facilities and municipal services had been mobilized to combat this epidemic. He implored New Yorkers not to "panic" and "become overwrought" over this health crisis. A frustrated Emerson likewise attempted to assuage the fears of that city's inhabitants by putting this particular situation into perspective, referring to the previous year's measles outbreak that claimed six hundred to nine hundred cases each day, with a 20 to 50 percent mortality rate: "There were more lives lost and more permanent injuries from the epidemic of measles last year than will result from this outbreak of infantile paralysis."[33] These facts failed to calm the public.

As alarming reports trickled in from New York City during the spring of 1916, John D. Robertson, Chicago's commissioner of health, decided to travel there to conduct observations. He immediately recognized it as the "greatest scourge of poliomyelitis which the United States has ever experienced." When he returned, Chicago's health officials, as those elsewhere, resorted to the tried-and-true sanitation doctrine and age-old quarantine measures to contain this contagious disease. In the former case, they believed polio to be "more prevalent in rural communities than in cities and congested areas." This led them to hypothesize that milk shipped from outlying dairy farms represented a dangerous vector, a convenient and deadly mode of transportation that directly connected this virus to children. Robertson, on July 22, 1916, "by virtue of the police powers granted him in cases of emergency, issued an order that all milk and cream sold in the city of Chicago be pasteurized at the temperature of 145 degrees Fahrenheit and maintained at this temperature for a period of 25 minutes instead of 140 degrees Fahrenheit held for 20 minutes as required under normal conditions."

Based on these experiences, the following February, Robertson, working through the mayor's office, tried to anticipate the 1917 summer outbreak by creating the Association for the Prevention of Infantile Paralysis as a proactive force to control such outbreaks. It consisted of fifteen committees: Cooperation of Women's Clubs, Clean Up and Paint Up, Clean Milk, Housing Conditions, Gardens, After Care, Standardizing Diagnosis, Chicago Medical Society, Hospitalization, Medical Research, Fire Insurance, Life Insurance, Neighborhood Suburban Communities, Church, and of course Public Schools. The association operated as a bureaucratic infrastructure to mobilize and coordinate a variety of resources, "the idea being that some concerted plan of action should be adopted to prevent and control infantile paralysis in the entire territory in and around Chicago." Attendees endorsed two means of accomplishing this public health goal. The first involved stepped-up sanitation methods. Chicago's health officers maintained the axiom that a "clean city" was a "safe city." This time they focused, with certitude, on houseflies as the principal virus carrier and proceeded to "eradicate breeding places for flies." The city council passed an ordinance on March 17, 1917, requiring screens for doors and windows. It also ordered the containment of garbage in cans and reduction of horse manure in the streets; alleys and streets were ordered cleaned and oiled them in order to reduce and contain dust, another suspected vector. Its 1918 annual report exclaimed, "It is confidently believed that the city's clean-up movement . . . had much to do with mitigating the severity of the outbreak of the disease in Chicago." The second tactic focused on the confident assertion by Maximillian Herzog, chair of the Committee on Research at Cook County Hospital, that he and his research team would have a polio serum by the summer. In spite of his good intentions and ebullient attitude, the committee followed the former course of action.[34]

In 1917, Emerson wrote a comprehensive formal analysis, *The Epidemic of Poliomyelitis (Infantile Paralysis) in New York City in 1916*. Its tone appears to be sober, conveying a sense of a calm, systematic approach during that crisis with medical experts deliberating and the health department acting in a prudent manner; in short, it depicts researchers and public health officials acting as though they knew precisely what they were doing. This study markedly departs from contemporary reports that summer. Whether the latter may have reflected newspaper sensationalism, somewhat reactionary rhetoric and hasty, reflexive actions on the part of city authorities, or a little of both, the former offers a fascinating retrospective. This is especially the case with earlier outbreaks. During the 1916 epidemic, local, national, and international precedents appeared to be either ignored or, at best, referenced in the most superficial ways. This is not the case in Emerson's published 1917 report; he recognizes previous outbreaks as growing more frequent and serious, especially during the early years of the twentieth century. This seems to lead to a conclusion that some preparedness should have been in place. However,

Emerson dismisses this notion because of the lower number of deaths during those previous outbreaks; New York State only began to require mandatory reports of infantile paralysis in 1910, and possible misdiagnoses may have distorted the number of cases and fatalities. Sounding defensive, Emerson reaches for logical closure: "Only a thoroughly alert public and a forewarned profession could have prevented the delay in official knowledge of the threatening epidemic."[35] Emerson would not be alone.

Policy regarding polio epidemics simply remained a shot in the dark well into the 1960s. Thomas M. Rivers, a pioneer RIMR virologist and a key player in the President's Birthday Ball Commission and its successor, the National Foundation for Infantile Paralysis, reminisced, "As far as public health advice on what to do during a polio epidemic went in 1943, the [Foundation's Virus Research] Committee couldn't give any better advice than the course which was followed by Dr. Haven Emerson during the great polio epidemic of 1916 . . . Even knowing as much as we do about polio today . . . I still wouldn't know what to tell a public health officer to do during an epidemic." This was especially the case with decisions about schooling. "Many physicians in the city urged that the schools be kept shut, but Dr. Emerson laid his head on the chopping block and fought to open them. In the end he won out, the schools were opened, and to everyone's happy surprise the incidence of polio in the city began to decline." In some ways, Rivers speculates, public school attendance may actually have mitigated the outbreak: "Today, looking back, we can say that it was coming to that time of year when the incidence of polio would drop anyway. But what was probably more important was the fact that when children went to school they came under school discipline—they didn't run around putting their hands in each other's mouths, and were more careful in their personal hygiene going to and from the bathroom." The 1952 epidemic amounted to an astounding 57,000 reported infections. Public responses appeared familiar, shuttering movie theaters and summer camps. Parents literally imprisoned their children in their homes to isolate them from potential infection.[36] One epidemic even spawned a minor diplomatic imbroglio. Because of serious outbreaks in the Lone Star State, Mexico, beginning in 1949, denied Texans from crossing its border "without proof of being polio-free for at least three years."[37]

Public health policy did not work, resulting in a "continuous calamity."[38] Three distinct but not necessarily coordinated responses grew out of New York's 1916 epidemic, and municipal health departments from this point onward would replicate them. First, they simply implemented prevention and containment policies that they already had in place for other diseases dating back to Europe's bubonic plague. Second, they often resorted to tried-and-true approaches dictated by still-dominant sanitation beliefs in the hope of stemming the epidemic. Finally, they also attempted to learn as much as quickly as possible about this unknown disease, and for this they turned to scientific experts.

This virus struck all five boroughs, but Brooklyn claimed the highest morbidity and mortality rates. Health department figures reveal 8,928 total cases between June 1 and November 1; of these, 2,407 died. Fatalities hovered at 27 percent, with 83 percent of them aged five or younger. Native-born American children suffered the highest rate of infections and deaths. Commissioner Emerson further observed that the "negro is less susceptible to the disease than that the white" but the "general mortality and case fatality rates are higher for the negroes then for the whites." Finally, girls fared a little better than boys, with 43 and 57 percent, respectively.[39]

This epidemic seemed to be contained geographically, at least at the beginning. The Bureau of Contagious Diseases of Chicago's Department of Health reported no cases of infantile paralysis until 1910; then it recorded nineteen cases. This represented a mere .004 percent of the total number of 42,700 cases of all contagious diseases recorded in that city. In 1911 that city's health department recorded its first official polio outbreak, with 25 cases. This jumped the next year to 135. But only 36 cases occurred during each of the next four years. These statistics paled in comparison with those of the East Coast in general and New York City in particular. Mortality rates followed a similar pattern, with the highest occurring in the northeast: 44 out of 100,000 children with infantile paralysis died in New York City; 22 out of 100,000 in Boston; and 18, 12, and 2 for Philadelphia, Baltimore, and Chicago, respectively.[40]

New Jersey's health officers definitively connected local infections to the New York City outbreak. It began in northern New Jersey and relentlessly moved south as more and more terrified New York residents fled with their children to various beach resorts. This very much matched the pattern Ivan Wickman, a Swedish pediatrician and epidemiologist, found during Sweden's 1905 epidemic in Trästena, 160 miles southwest of Stockholm. A clear geographic pattern existed: He found that infections followed the main roads and railway lines. New Jersey represented a classic case of "expansion diffusion."[41]

After 1916, the number of cases in Chicago, America's second largest city, rose and fell each of the subsequent years, with a high of 551 in 1917 with 187 deaths, followed by 96 in 1918 with 27 deaths; this pattern of alternating highs and lows persisted throughout the 1920s, but the total number of cases never exceeded 148. At no time did that city's health department deem any of these as "severe epidemics," and most ill children remained at home for treatment, as well as to facilitate containment. Recorded outbreaks in 1923, 1924, and 1925 seemed to decline, leveling off at about 66 per year, but the proportion of boys and girls subtly began to shift. Starting in 1923, the percentage of boys who contracted this disease crept up to 58 percent. Moreover, the percentage of all infected children hospitalized jumped to an annual average of 85 percent. While Chicago remained "exceptionally free from acute anterior poliomyelitis in 1926" with only 28 cases, that total jumped the following year to 148 and then dropped to 25 and 28 in 1928 and 1929, respectively. The morbidity rate may have declined those two years, but the mortality rate sharply increased. This fluctuation in reported cases continued into the next decade, suddenly shooting up to 170 with 32 deaths in 1931 and plummeting to 49 and 9, respectively, in 1932. Chicago's board of health listed 113 cases and 6 deaths the following year. Between 1934 and 1938, it recorded an average of 155 cases and 15 deaths, for a 10 percent mortality rate, per year. This roller coaster ride continued. The highest number of cases occurred in 1937 with 355 cases and 35 deaths, while the lowest appeared the following year with 27 cases and one death. Virtually all of these fatalities occurred among European American male youths, with the overwhelming majority of them between the ages of five and fourteen.[42]

Although New York City accounted for 31 percent of cases nationwide in 1916, poliomyelitis did not strike urban areas alone. Rural settings remained vulnerable as well, but not consistently, perhaps due to the lack of accurate reporting methods. Michigan's secretary of the State Board of Health in 1916 confirmed outbreaks not only in Detroit and Flint but also many, if not more, in that state's farmlands. And four years later, that state confirmed that the majority of documented cases that year had occurred outside of cities. This virus exacted a tragic toll on rural children, because these isolated areas lacked the resources for many families to secure medical help and did not have the public health infrastructure to even host a visiting nurse. Well into the 1940s, one Arkansas family found itself in that exact situation. The parents' only son contracted polio as a baby. Because of his subsequent paralysis, he "crawled about on the floor much as a crab would scuttle across the bed of an ocean" until his early teens, when the Arkansas Infantile Paralysis Foundation learned about him and purchased a wheelchair. He never attended school and thus remained illiterate; rather, he spent much of his time outside—if the weather permitted—sitting under the trees, talking to various animals, and whittling.[43] In sum, during any given year, the poliovirus reached epidemic proportions in some locales but not in others. No simple or clear spatial pattern emerged.

Poliomyelitis showed no clear morbidity pattern nationwide between 1916 and 1946. During that thirty-year period, only two years exceeded 25,000 reported cases. This would all change following World War II with the appearance of the baby boomers. Some 42,000 cases were recorded in 1949 alone, with 57,000 in 1952.[44] Nevertheless, as historian Daniel J. Wilson points out, the 1916 epidemic continued to rank as the worst: "The polio rate that year was 41.1 per 100,000 population, the worst in American history. However, the total number of cases, 27,000, was substantially fewer than the 57,000 in 1952. Because the population of the United States had increased substantially since 1916, the polio rate in 1952 was only 37.2 per 100,000."[45] The age cohort would expand as well. Children from infancy to age five suffered the most, averaging 72 percent of the total cases from 1916 to 1918. With each passing decade, infections would strike older children and eventually young adults. By 1940, it mostly attacked five-to-nine-year-olds. Between 1944 and 1955, those younger than five held relatively steady at about 26 percent, five-to-nine-year-olds dropped from 32 to 25 percent, ages ten to fourteen from 21 to 15 percent, and ages fifteen to nineteen from

11 to 9 percent, but cases involving those age twenty and older increased from 11 to 25 percent. Finally, race at first seemed to matter but not gender. European American youngsters represented virtually 100 percent of the 1916 cases, split evenly among boys and girls.[46] This too would change.

What made infantile paralysis especially unique was its lingering effects, remaining highly visible, sometimes permanent. While life quickly resumed following the 1918 influenza epidemic, with the reopening of churches, restaurants, stores, and theaters, poliomyelitis differed. It evoked deep emotions and constructed an enduring reality. "When other epidemics had run their course the survivors recuperated and the dead were buried and forgotten." But polio's impact proved to be far less ephemeral. It largely infected children, intensifying sympathy toward these helpless and innocent victims; they could remain paralyzed throughout their lives, requiring constant, long-term care and treatment, as well as demanding and expensive assistance from their caregivers.[47] Moreover, with little or no understanding of its cause and even less certainty of how it spread, this disease resurrected the age-old community reactions of sanctuary or social ostracism. This virus not only exacted a priceless physical toll on its young victims and their families, but it transformed their social world too. For many Americans, it became nothing less than the "modern plague" for children.[48]

Epidemic Refugees

Diseases produce contested spaces. Quarantines of cities, if not entire states, to restrict the movement of people did not work. Developments in early twentieth-century mass transportation intensified the speed of migration and concomitantly contagious diseases. Road, railway, and water travel networks certainly provided logical choke points for public health officials to use to curtail that movement. Yet these efforts resulted in uneven outcomes. Connecticut, New Jersey, and Pennsylvania shared borders with New York State and suffered substantial infectious rates. Chicago's municipal authorities employed the same tactic, and it seemed to work. However, the distance, not the approach, may explain its success; that is, proximity represented the main variable in that virus's distribution in 1916. Or maybe not.

Two different types of containment exist. The first, a *spatial barrier*, involves isolating an infected individual or community (i.e., quarantine); this method has been embedded in Western culture for centuries, and New York City's health officials executed it in 1916. A second type, *defensive isolation*, "entails the building of a spatial barrier around a disease-free area." Thirteenth-century Italian cities introduced this response. They "posted gatemen to identify potential sources of infection from visitors to the city." Port cities, like Venice, instituted a waiting period of thirty days for visitors as a defense against the plague in 1377.[49] Although many towns and states implemented a similar approach in 1916, Chicago's authorities carried out a highly ambitious effort. In either case, such a social policy "has the power to isolate those labeled 'diseased.'" Such containment policies stigmatize

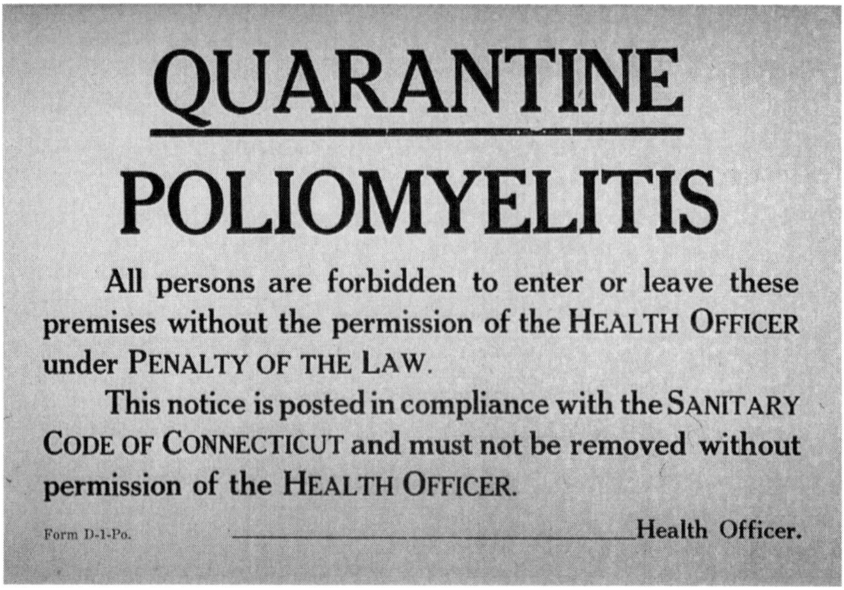

> # QUARANTINE
> ## POLIOMYELITIS
> All persons are forbidden to enter or leave these premises without the permission of the HEALTH OFFICER under PENALTY OF THE LAW.
>
> This notice is posted in compliance with the SANITARY CODE OF CONNECTICUT and must not be removed without permission of the HEALTH OFFICER.
>
> Form D-1-Po. _____Health Officer.

Figure 1.1 Quarantine Poliomyelitis.

groups suspected of carrying a contagion, becoming a real (or physical) as well as an imagined (or social) threat. And children became prime targets during the 1916 polio epidemic.[50]

Many terrified New Yorkers decided to either flee that city with their children or send them away in order to avoid contamination. Removing infants and young children from city environs during summer months represented a routine practice. During the 1880s and 1890s, officials in Philadelphia's health department, as a matter of policy, arranged for poor children to cross the Delaware River into New Jersey to avoid "summer diarrhea" and generally improve their health, ultimately reducing death rates.[51]

However, escaping New York City's 1916 polio epidemic did not always prove easy. An eight-page pamphlet titled *Circular of Information Regarding Procedure in Poliomyelitis: Information for Field Workers* reveals how public health administrators reverted to the age-old use of quarantines. Inspectors visited all reported cases, posted multiple placards on all designated houses and tenements, dated and initialed them, and followed up by meeting with building janitors to ensure that those warning posters remained undisturbed. These officials, if they deemed it necessary, could ultimately summon an ambulance to remove ill children from the premises. That department also sent its own nurses to visit every documented case. During subsequent daily visits, they instructed the family regarding quarantine regulations and about "home cleanliness, personal hygiene, [and] the danger of infection by flies." They also met with building custodians to reinforce isolation rules. These proved to be draconian. Patients would be segregated for eight weeks from the "onset of the disease." All children younger than sixteen had to be isolated for at least two weeks after the "termination by death, removal or recovery." These measures applied to trips outside of the city and state as well. Travelers had to present a "certificate of good health" at "transportation terminals." These could only be obtained from city and U.S. Public Health Service officials. Equally stringent regulations applied to those individuals reentering the city. Any infected or exposed children who were city residents could only return by "private conveyance" in order to minimize exposure to the general population. The sanitary police enforced these segregation restrictions on a daily basis, reporting any violations, which resulted in fines and even criminal charges. Health authorities had thus instituted a dual quarantine: They isolated those already sick in their homes or hospitals within the city and simultaneously restricted out-migration to regionally contain the epidemic.[52]

Inhabitants of outlying communities, themselves equally frightened, often resorted to extreme measures to repel those desperate refugees, to insulate themselves from the contagion that outsiders might be carrying with them. Volunteer inspectors in Huntington, Long Island, visited every home, searching for children who had escaped from the city proper and, finding many, immediately restricted them to those residences, essentially placing them under house arrest. In another Long Island case, wealthy summer residents of Rockaway Peninsula donated land and funds to erect an emergency medical facility to house children stricken with polio. It had been hastily constructed within a week using portable garages and outhouses for the staff. Sensing opposition, they hired twenty detectives to protect it. Permanent local townspeople feared that the influx of so many infected individuals would spread this pathogen to their community. They attended a town council meeting to air their grievances and loudly boo proponents. Highly dissatisfied with the council's decision, they spilled out of that gathering to take matters into their own hands. Some six hundred protestors wielding rakes and torches surrounded the newly constructed facility and threatened to burn it down, conjuring up the frightening cinema image of terrified villagers attacking Dr. Frankenstein's laboratory; in this case, sick children served as the monsters. The *Times* described the tense scene: "The deputy sheriffs threatened to shoot any one who attempted to take a patient into the hospital, and the detectives threatened to shoot any one who attempted to approach the building without permission." Finally, in yet another case, Westchester communities launched motorboat patrols along the Hudson River shore to intercept any escaping New Yorkers.[53]

Adjacent states too implemented blockades or created major obstacles to discourage frightened New Yorkers. Pennsylvania state officials deployed medical inspectors to guard the roads, blocking terrified migrants attempting to escape New York City by crossing the state line; civil authorities in Paterson, New Jersey, likewise denied entry to desperate New Yorkers; and in New Haven, Connecticut, health authorities barred all New York children younger than fifteen from entering that city. To make matters worse, fleeing New York City did not ensure safety. Marian Hamlin, a nine-year-old whose parents had escaped from Brooklyn with her and her two-year-old sister, died shortly after arriving in Newfane, New York, in Niagara County; her sister became ill as well.[54]

A backlash occurred. On the one hand, after thirteen Connecticut communities banned New York City children younger than sixteen, Charles E. Banks, of the U.S. Public Health Service, threatened them against such "unreasonable" exclusionary practices. Banks sent a letter reprimanding health officers and refused to extend any assistance by that agency. He had already served notice on one New Jersey town; it quickly withdrew its policy. On the other hand, in a letter to the *Times* editor, the health officer of Bethel, Connecticut, H. Frank Moore, chastised his New York City colleagues for labeling Connecticut's citizens as overzealous because they barred New Yorkers from entering their towns. Moore cleverly turned the accusation on its head: "We still wonder why New Yorkers are fleeing by thousands, if the danger is so insignificant. Such action would seem to indicate that there is some 'hysteria' even in New York." He also dismissed the vain public relations efforts of New York's health officials who expressed optimism in order to calm that city's residents even as polio infections and deaths grew.[55]

In Chicago, Robertson implemented a callous public health program aimed directly at children. That city's health department closed kindergartens and forbade children from mingling in crowds. It further implemented a remarkable, large-scale cordoning policy. Chicago's health officials dispatched fifty "school health officers," ordinarily on vacation during the summer months, to outlying stations to intercept westbound trains. There they "inspected all the children on the train and obtained their names and addresses with their departure points and destinations. Children coming from New York directly," the health department's summary report later boasted, "were held by the health officer at the station until the office of the bureau of medical inspection could be communicated with and assurance obtained that the child did not come from infected premises." They examined 16,906 children in August alone. That city's department of health conducted the same search routine on boats docking at Lake Michigan wharves. Chicago, in effect, had been sealed to prevent potentially infected individuals from entering. And health officers with this personal information could now keep "suspects . . . under surveillance." That health department published updates in 140 foreign and English newspapers in 1916, displayed warning posters in streetcars, and hosted informational meetings at seventeen public schools. The most serious outbreaks did not occur until late August and early September. Health commissioner Robertson decided to open the schools on the scheduled starting date but delay the beginning of kindergarten. But every child entering the building had to produce a health certificate from a personal physician or submit to being examined by the school health officer. As an "additional check," each child underwent another medical inspection, as the commissioner's report described: "The school doctor and nurse go into each room of their schools and take a position by the window where they have good light and the pupils in the room walk by in a single file; as they pass the doctor he examines their hands and arms for evidence of contagious disease; the child opens his mouth so the doctor can see the throat and also retracts the lower eyelid so the conjunctiva can be observed." His report touted these actions as part of what it regarded as a "progressive, up-to-date" public health program, in an enlightened era of medical care. Chicago's health department proudly credited these efforts for that city's low morbidity and mortality rates that year, with 264 documented cases of infantile paralysis; of these, 34 died.[56]

Meanwhile, the 1916 epidemic taxed the resources of New Jersey's state department of health. It received reports of 3,973 cases at a rate of 134.8 infections per 100,000, "the highest case incidence which has been observed in any state during the epidemic." It attempted to contain this disease in New York City and northern New Jersey as much as possible through use of U.S. Public Health Service agents, who guarded the New York-New Jersey border. Even New Jersey's efforts appeared to be a Sisyphean task: its borders contained "seventeen bridges, twenty-three ferries, sixteen steamboat lines not ferries, forty-two roads and nineteen railroads and trolley lines which enter the state at various points." Nevertheless, forty health department inspectors managed to examine 46,519 children younger than sixteen, turning away 3,747 because they either lacked an approved certificate or had none at all. That department's summary report cast serious doubt on the effectiveness of this quarantine policy, since adults who might have been carriers encountered no restrictions whatsoever. Furthermore, inspectors found this effort to be useless, since in some instances they found children already paralyzed wielding an approved certificate. In the end, the New Jersey health department saw it more as a psychological tool to assure the public that it was doing all it could to limit morbidity. In addition, Pennsylvania's commissioner of health implemented a similar policy, but it followed a double standard, allowing that state's children to travel freely to New Jersey but demanding health certificates for those entering from New Jersey.[57]

For four decades, parents, lacking any firm knowledge about this scourge, resorted to a variety of strategies to protect their children. Mothers made their children wear white gloves or pouches filled with alum when they went out. During the 1916 New York City epidemic, many Italian immigrants closed their windows, in the sweltering heat, to prevent the contagion from entering their apartments and infecting their children. Public health nurses sabotaged this when they intruded, throwing open all of the windows for fresh air as part of their gospel of sanitation. Another response grew both organically and spontaneously out of that epidemic, openly defying public health containment regulations. Families, especially affluent ones, fled to the "clean country" with the "swift natural water, the salt sea, the sparkling lakes, the good air, the high mountains"[58] or sent their children there. This developed into a common practice as waves of outbreaks broke out, becoming embedded in American culture through popular literature.

Chaim Potok's novel *In the Beginning* depicts the annual outflow of young refugees to summer sanctuaries. In this coming-of-age novel set in the Bronx largely during the interwar period, sickly Davey Lurie, the main character, and his younger brother race away with their parents every August "somewhere near tall mountains far away from the city . . . My father," Davey narrates, "called it going to the country. We went to escape from . . . polio that made people very sick and sometimes paralyzed or killed them. 'The Angel of Death is doing his job again,' my father would say, and he and my mother would pack quickly and we would go off in a car to the white cottage and the forest."[59] Although it seemed to work in Potok's character study, this tactic failed to be foolproof in reality. Infantile paralysis often struck children in the pristine environment of the mountains or along the windswept beaches of the eastern seashore. As one frustrated parent wrote in 1938, "It is simply—always with us . . . It is simply *here*."[60]

The 1916 polio episode readily revealed serious weaknesses in public health policies that attempted to contain this disease. In spite of attempts to scrub the environment, restrict the movement of people, and examine countless schoolchildren, that polio epidemic continued unabated.[61] New York City's quarantine would represent the largest in human history, both numerically and geographically. Until the twentieth century, public health administrators certainly faced enforcement obstacles, yet nothing undermined discharging their duties more than new modes of travel. These officials remained seemingly oblivious to the "collapse of geographic space" in the early twentieth-century United States. Railways and automobiles caused exponential increases in average travel distance. These changing travel patterns had profoundly expanded the spatial boundaries of diseases. Relatively cheap mass transportation networks and new technologies allowed people to move far and fast with a minimum of resources and with comparative ease. Anxious refugees using trains, as we saw in Chicago, could be caught to some extent; however, automobiles introduced virtual anarchy. Train stations could be reasonably monitored but not all main and secondary roads. With modern modes of conveyance, diseases could not be feasibly contained. Nevertheless, these officials invoked harsh measures, holding children solely responsible. They demanded their papers at railroad stations, state lines, and wharves. They sometimes submitted them to physical examinations on the spot and occasionally sent them back to their homes. They treated American children as unwanted refugees in their own country.[62]

Children's lives became highly regulated. New York City's 1916 epidemic interfered with every facet of their realities. From public health authorities invading their homes to forcible separation from their parents, from play and entertainment to travel, they found themselves banished, hunted, and reviled. Children became the other, beings to be avoided. They represented the physical, concrete embodiment of an invisible threat. In spite of a massive attempt by a variety of medical and police officers to vigorously hunt them down, the epidemic remained largely unabated—a failed health policy that made each child into an object of fear and trepidation.[63]

Polio's story is deeply embedded in broader twentieth-century American social history. This disease sparked the introduction of a sophisticated and institutionalized philanthropic effort, altered the medical world, reshaped families, challenged the public schools, and ultimately redefined disability. American culture likewise shaped every aspect of this disease. The development of mass media, the explosion of cheap and accessible transportation, the emergence of modern medical science, and the maturation of public schooling led to a variety of responses to this disease. Finally, initial infection marked the beginning of a medical and social journey for children, one filled with physical pain and emotional trauma.

Chapter 2

Many Yellow Caskets

I didn't know what they were going to do.
I didn't know what they were going to feed us,
or what they were going to let us do—stand or sit,
or let us see our mothers . . .

—An eleven-year-old boy

One summer day in 1947, ten-year-old Mary Ann Hoffman, growing up in rural North Dakota, complained to her parents that she did not feel well:

> I had been out to the barn, roller skating up in the hay loft . . . [M]y muscles ached. I had a terrible headache and a temperature, so my mother told me to lie down . . . Sometime that week, our family doctor came out to the house to examine me. He thought that I had rheumatic fever. I also remember that he looked in my throat and said, "Those tonsils need to come out. As soon as you get over this, we'll put you in the hospital and take them out." Well, I've still got those tonsils. They were all right, but I wasn't![1]

Hoffman had poliomyelitis; her recollection is typical. The onset of this virus involved three distinct scenarios, representing a universal experience. A nose and throat infection and high fever, as well as the likelihood of diarrhea and vomiting, marked the first. The victim felt somewhat ill but seemed able to pursue a typical daily routine. The symptoms grew worse in the second case, with weakened or paralyzed limbs. This, more often than not, proved temporary and is usually referred to as abortive paralysis. The third and worst experience involved permanent paralysis. Breathing stopped if it spread to the diaphragm and respiratory system. Until 1930, this too often meant death.[2]

This disease forever changed the realities of tens of thousands of children. In some cases, they fought for their very lives. Torn from their families, they had to cope alone with strangers caring for them. Pain became their new and enduring companion. Death no longer remained an abstraction. Their futures now followed a different trajectory than those of most of their peers. They helplessly and inevitably moved through various institutions, adapting to them as well as shaping them.

"I REMEMBER HEARING CHILDREN CRYING."

For many, life with infantile paralysis began with an anxious trip. Robert Gurney fell ill at age seventeen in 1940. The ambulance arrived at his home to transport him to the hospital, and as the attendants picked him up, he recalls, "my mother said the pain was so great that I passed out and became unconscious." They covered his face with a rubber sheet because they feared infection, a common notion at that time. Michael W. R. Davis, a seventh-grader at the time, notes that "none of the commercial outfits would transport a contagious polio patient." Since both of his parents were World War I veterans, the local American Legion sent an ambulance to take him to the hospital. Hearses were sometimes used to transport children because of an ambulance shortage. Philip Lewin, an orthopedist at Northwestern University, writes in his 1941 medical textbook, *Infantile Paralysis: Anterior Poliomyelitis*, "Too many hospitals . . . refuse to accept cases of acute poliomyelitis." When Mia Farrow fell ill in 1954, her parents phoned her pediatrician, who made a house call at her Los Angeles residence and conducted a spinal tap. After confirming that she had contracted polio, he carried her to the waiting ambulance and ordered her parents to burn everything in her bedroom. This simple action marked a crucial turning point in her life: "I was nine when my childhood ended."[3]

These epidemics overwhelmed local hospitals. Kentucky's 1944 outbreak caused severe bed and staff shortages. Ill children swamped both Kosair Crippled Children's Hospital and the General Hospital in Louisville. The American Red Cross and the National Foundation for Infantile Paralysis (NFIP) sent additional equipment and personnel to offer some relief. During the North Carolina epidemic of 1944–1945, ambulances arrived at the Hickory emergency treatment facility from Charlotte. When doctors opened those vehicles' doors, they discovered that many of the children had died during the trip. A nurse who worked at Pittsburgh's Municipal Hospital graphically describes how she felt crushed by this onslaught: "One year the ambulances literally lined up outside the place . . . It was an atmosphere of grief, terror, and helpless rage. It was horrible. I remember a high school boy weeping because he was completely paralyzed and couldn't move a hand to kill himself."[4]

Once at the hospital, confusion reigned and isolation occurred immediately. Until the nineteenth century, various epidemics forced infected individuals into often "hastily erected" buildings known as "pest houses" to segregate them from the rest of the population. Special hospitals dedicated to containing patients with contagious diseases replaced them by the late nineteenth and early twentieth centuries; most large American cities hosted one by 1908. In Cleveland, it was the City Hospital for Contagious Diseases, connected to the main hospital by an underground tunnel. Opened in 1910, it expanded in 1922 to accommodate two hundred patients. During that city's most severe period of polio epidemics, between 1949 and 1955, it devoted two entire floors to infected children. The average stay at Gillette State Hospital for Crippled Children, in St. Paul, Minnesota, in the 1930s amounted to 189 days.[5]

Initial hospitalization divided the family; parents and their sick children followed two divergent paths. "The admissions process might be thought of as a ritual separating the patient from his or her previous identity . . . This depersonalization was carried out as well in the fashionable practice of referring to each new admission by the number of his or her bed; this not only symbolized . . . efficiency . . . but discouraged the 'inappropriate' familiarity that sometimes developed between nurses and patients."[6] At Los Angeles General Hospital, the medical staff took Mia Farrow from her parents without any ceremony and wheeled her into an elevator:

> I screamed all the way upstairs to a big room where there were curtained cubicles and lots of children on gurneys, all screaming just like me. A nurse wearing a mask over her nose and mouth hissed, "Be *quiet*, you're only making things worse for everybody," but I was beyond terror, I threw up. Everything hurt—my back, neck, legs, and chest; it even hurt to breathe.

She only saw her parents three times a week for twenty minutes each, and only through a glass window.[7] Anne Finger's initial experience seems dreamlike: "Eerie gowned figures. A glass wall."[8] That partition separated parents from their children relegated to the isolation ward. Parental separation only represented one part of this trauma. Older children faced another, potentially more horrifying reality: they were all too aware that "disability was certain and death was likely."[9] For all children, the unknown loomed large.

They had entered an alien world. This building proved to be intimidating with its dark, stern exterior and spare, clinical interior, containing terrifying glass syringes with long, gleaming needles and steaming autoclaves to sterilize exotic and menacing stainless steel instruments. Hospitals had depressingly drab-colored walls, painted with institutional brown or olive green. The unpleasant and combined odors of disinfectant and alcohol struck them as attendants quickly wheeled their gurneys through stark hallways, adding to their apprehension. Furthermore, these children knew no one.

The entire experience proved bewildering for adults and children alike as strangers encountered each other. Parents had to entrust their children to physicians they may have just met in the corridor, and then only briefly. They also sought information from nurses who too were unknown to them and changed with different shifts. And staff empathy appeared to be in short supply. Professional demeanor trumped any emotion on the medical side of the personal equation. While the medical community as a whole had little, but at least some, knowledge about the physical impact of infantile paralysis, it knew absolutely nothing about the psychological trauma. It even endorsed complete isolation of children to protect them from the "hovering of an anxious mother." This, according to nurses' manuals, "would help the children make a 'better adjustment' to their illness." Their superiors ordered them to only give terse reports, using such terms as "good," or "fairly good," or "serious." Their training taught them that an emotional parent was "psychologically immature."[10]

These professionals, as theorist Rita Charon expresses it, had "no idea, most of the time, of the depth and the hold of the fear and rage that illness" brought. Isolated children meanwhile lay in pain as this virus controlled their bodies. Lost among other sick and dying children, whom they did not know, they waited while adults dressed in stiffly starched white uniforms rushed around as new patients arrived and others' conditions worsened. "Many patients," Charon continues, felt "abandoned by their doctors, dismissed in their suffering . . . or objectified by impersonal care."[11]

They were marked. While in the isolation wards, "children lay on beds, or in oversized cribs, with signs above them stating in big letters POLIO. They were put in pajamas with big red dots on their backs to warn of contagion."[12] Michael Davis had been admitted to Louisville's Kosair Crippled Children's Hospital in 1944. He "was placed in the middle of three beds in a room on the sun-hot west side." A glass-lined wall existed so nurses could observe the patients in that room. "Weak and lying flat on my back in an iron bedstead with this mattress over thick board, all I could see . . . were the white-masked faces of attendants moving back and forth, and the ceiling. My feet were firmly placed against an upright board across the foot of the bed to keep my foot muscles and hamstrings from shriveling."[13] Their abrupt introduction into this chilling and impersonal environment compounded their emotional distress, almost dwarfing their physical discomfort. As one eleven-year-old boy articulated it, "I didn't know what they were going to do. I didn't know what they were going to feed us, or what they were going to let us do—stand or sit, or let us see our mothers."[14] Quarantine had quickly and brutally ruptured emotional ties with parents, friends, and school, the key components of their universe. This proved to be traumatic for Carol Boyer: "I remember it was awful being left alone without my mom. I just cried and cried and cried. I remember hearing children crying." A cacophony of choking, gasping, screaming, and yelling children flooded the isolation unit.[15] The solitary confinement of infected individuals proved to be totally useless, "even after it was shown during the 1940s that patients' stools could remain loaded with the virus for several weeks." Fear trumped reason, and emotional trauma compounded the illness experience.[16]

Relationships could not be sustained in this fluid context. At Pittsburgh's Municipal Hospital, a few adolescent boys and girls attempted to carry on romantic dalliances in spite of being segregated by wards. Bill Kirkpatrick and his four paralyzed male roommates discovered an equal number of young women residing directly across the hallway from their room. Once "they felt strong enough and brave enough," they would call "out names, make introductions, then talk, tease, laugh, and flirt, growing . . . fond of one another based on the sounds of their voices alone." Over the next two weeks, Bill grew particularly close to one of the girls but then was sent to the D. T. Watson Home for Crippled Children for rehabilitation. Smitten by the mere sound of her voice, he wrote her a letter, only to have it returned with the word "deceased" written on it.[17]

Acute Care

Children's clinical experiences unfolded in four distinct and sequential stages, covering a plethora of emotions. First, the physicians' initial examinations involved spinal taps with three-inch-long needles, a terrifying and painful medical procedure. Second, once diagnosed, the medical staff isolated infected children, a lonely and traumatic experience that detached them from any real human contact. This spanned anywhere between two and seven days. Third, following that, doctors prescribed a regimen of orthopedic care, involving splinting, casting, physical therapy, and, if necessary, braces. All of these, whether separate or in some combination, inflicted relentless anguish. Fourth, young patients adapted to the hospital environment, usually manifested through returning to some semblance of a regular routine.[18]

Children affected by this virus never forgot the initial awareness and shock of losing control of their bodies. Robert W. Lovett, an orthopedic surgeon at Boston's Children's Hospital and a Harvard Medical School professor, noted in his 1917 monograph, *The Treatment of Infantile Paralysis*, that paralysis appeared to progress; for instance, beginning in the legs, it "gradually extends upward."[19] Hugh Gregory Gallagher vividly and eloquently recalls those chilling moments as he awoke one spring morning in 1952 in his bedroom:

> The actual paralyzing process began, first with the toes of my left leg. I am not sure how I came to notice that the toes of my left foot would no longer wiggle . . . Soon, in a matter of minutes, the foot and ankle were powerless.
>
> The paralysis gradually worked its way up my left leg . . . Once the paralysis had worked its way up to my left hip, it seemed to stop. I half expected that it would momentarily go away—as though the leg had simply "fallen asleep" for a second or two. The whole paralytic process had taken not much more than half an hour.

Within a similarly short time frame, the same thing happened to his right leg.[20] In 1949, the parents of twelve-year-old Peg Kehret rushed her to the hospital in Austin, Minnesota, because she had been diagnosed with infantile paralysis but had not developed any paralysis. She fell asleep there and a little while later awoke thirsty. She had no idea that she was now paralyzed, and she vividly describes that realization as well as the panic associated with it: "I tried to reach the water, my right arm did not move. I tried again. Nothing happened. I tried with the left arm. Nothing. I tried to bend my knees so I could roll on my side, but my legs were two logs . . . I was too weak even to lift my head off of the pillow." She screamed for the nurse. Seeing her condition, the nurse called the attending physician. He proceeded to examine her. "Each time the doctor asked me to move a part of my body and I could not move it, my terror increased." Her parents' absence only intensified her alarm: "I wanted my Mother and Dad. I wanted to be well. I wanted to go home."[21]

Infantile paralysis ravaged young bodies. As nerve damage quickly advanced, children suffered from extreme spinal pain that grew in intensity and radiated throughout their bodies. Older ones lost dozens of pounds within the first couple of weeks and became emaciated. Charles L. Mee's weight, for example, fell from 160 to 90 pounds. Their flaccid muscles and sallow skin caused a skeleton-like appearance. Searing and unrelenting pain flooded their extremities. They became delirious from the endless discomfort and high fever, and they suffered from sleep deprivation, as Mee describes: "Polio caused encephalitis, an inflammation of the brain." Their muscles shrank and stiffened as their limbs became contorted. With bulbar polio, reflexive muscle control dissipated or disappeared altogether. This had numerous consequences, as Kehret recounts: "It was hard to swallow my own saliva. Food was more than I could manage . . . Because of my fever, it was important for me to drink lots of liquid . . . I was thirsty. I sucked a mouthful through the straw . . . I sputtered and choked. The choking made it hard to get my breath, and that frightened me . . . After that, I didn't want to drink . . . I was afraid of choking." The inability to swallow—and concomitant fear of swallowing—compounded matters. Children's physical and emotional conditions further deteriorated with dehydration, the lack of proper nutrition, and inhaling less oxygen. Bowel and urinary failure led to the insertion of catheter tubes and a regimen of enemas. The former procedure, according to Davis, added to their agony. "Without recalling the kind of pain I know that the ensuing catheterization—there were no numbing local anesthetics to apply in those days—was even worse than the racks of the muscular spasms and headaches."[22] Impacted bowels occasionally required a nurse using her rubber-covered finger to dig out fecal matter. For Gallagher, the entire hospital ordeal destroyed any privacy or intimacy: he had "lost all sense of property rights over his body." After weeks in isolation, Gallagher's notion of self had been reduced to a dysfunctional body: "My [impacted] bowels were still causing me pain and anxiety; my lungs still needed constant aspiration. The catheter, which passed through the urethra of my penis, had to be changed frequently; my urethra was sliced to bloody ribbons. Crystals, which had formed upon the catheter, developed into kidney and bladder stones, and my urinary tract was infected."[23] Not only did the virus invade the body, but physicians and nurses who fought this disease had to violate it with instruments, causing humiliation, additional pain, and a loss of dignity for young children. Nighttime proved to be the most difficult time, as one nurse observes: "There are frequent fits of crying bordering on hysteria, and extreme nervous tension resulting in insomnia." Children gagged on their own mucus. Bedsores and the threat of bacterial infection added further complications—prior to antibiotics, this condition could be fatal. Care, therefore, was complex. It took at least five nurses, who closely choreographed their movements, to simply turn a paralyzed patient in bed.[24]

Respiratory failure always lurked as a threat. As paralysis spread into the upper body and neck, the simple act of breathing grew ever more difficult. Gallagher reconstructs that terror: "I lay there, concentrating upon each breath. Each breath became a conscious decision, an exhausting labor, less and less satisfying, ever more tiring."[25] Physicians could draw on only two weapons in their medical arsenal, a tracheotomy and an artificial respirator, as we will see.

Death relentlessly prowled hospital wards. Simon Flexner's 1916 graphic, clinical description revealed the last throes of its victims:

> When death does occur it is not the result, as in many infections, of a process of poisoning that robs the patient of strength and consciousness before its imminence, but is caused solely by paralysis of the respiratory function, sometimes with merciful suddenness, but often with painful slowness, without in any degree obscuring the consciousness of the suffocating victim until just before the end is reached. No more terrible tragedy can be witnessed.[26]

The isolation ward, for eleven-year-old Leonard Kriegel, "was a place of passing toward death, we assumed, although we rarely mentioned that possibility even to each other."[27] Many children saw their roommates die. One ten-year-old girl recalls how she watched a younger patient die in front of her: "She was sitting on the bed and she was gasping trying to breathe . . . I remember her turning dark and falling over. She was dead then."[28] Farrow describes another such night for a two-year-old girl in her ward: "The lights went on and the curtains were pulled around her crib, and doctors and nurses all crowded into that corner in a hurry, talking loudly. I pulled the covers over my head . . . The next morning the crib was empty.[29] Moreover, being cognizant of the possibility of imminent death, aware even of dying itself, remains a unique human quality that many of these children knew. Like all of those who faced it, Gallagher's struggle wore him down: "I was literally 'burnt out' . . . My state became almost serene." However, unlike younger children, nineteen-year-old Gallagher possessed a conscious awareness of his condition: "Things, details, lost their importance before the overwhelming big question, which was simplicity itself: stop or go, yes or no, live or die. I finally decided to live." But this decision did not occur as an epiphany. It represented an accumulation of incremental delays: "It was never an affirmative decision. It was a negative one: I do not choose to die, not yet. This not-yet business was . . . a minute-to-minute matter, until the minutes became hours, the hours became days—until gradually, the question receded from my present consciousness."[30] Because of the delicate balance between life and death, because of their unstable condition, many young patients received the last rites.

The death of children, as we have seen, represented a fact of life in the United States. During the colonial period, child "illness and death were apparently accepted in a passive attitude of Christian resignation." Even into the nineteenth century, parents "appeared to regard serious illness as inevitable."[31] With the "transformation in the cultural meaning of childhood," shifting from an economic asset to a "new exaltation of children's sentimental worth," death assumed a new mantle during the late nineteenth and early twentieth centuries. "If child life was sacred, child death became an intolerable sacrilege, provoking not only parental sorrow but social bereavement."[32] The emergence of mourners' manuals, elaborate grave markers, and funeral art symbolized this cultural shift. By the mid-nineteenth century, for middle-class families, children's coffins began to morph into caskets. The casket became an object to place something cherished, a public demonstration of the depth of parental sorrow. "It closes with a lock and key, not sinister screws and screwdrivers. It is not made of wood but of metal."[33] They could not do enough to eulogize their dead children. During the twentieth century, unlike ever before, the "death of a young child became the most painful and least tolerable of all deaths."[34] Until the 1950s, most families hosted wakes at their homes. Small caskets sat in living rooms where friends, neighbors, and relatives paid their respects, though some fearful of contamination avoided such visits. The penultimate moment arrived when parents stood at the gravesite, tearfully watching that little coffin slowly being lowered into the ground. They could retain few keepsakes, since local health authorities, still clinging to zymotic theories of infection, often ordered them to burn all of their dead children's clothes and toys, obliterating virtually all physical traces of their existence.

Even if a child avoided death, poliomyelitis left many with an indelible imprint; social ostracism sometimes began with health professionals. And race always compounded this. African Americans faced medical segregation since the antebellum period. The staff at the Philadelphia Almshouse in 1846 relegated them to the attic, while in other locales they received care only in the basements of those institutions. Regional attitudes especially skewed the delivery of medical services in the segregated South. Few incidences of major polio epidemics had occurred there until the 1940s. Not surprisingly, Georgia, Mississippi, and South Carolina restricted access to acute-care treatment. During the 1930s, the University of Texas Medical Branch opened two facilities: the eighty-six-bed Children's Hospital, fifty of which were devoted to polio patients, and the "Negro Hospital" to "accommodate ninety-two patients. Special services included a small ward for crippled African-American children." Texas health clinics had "Colored Days" and "White Days" well into the 1940s. Staff members at these rehabilitation centers even forbade blacks from eating in their cafeterias and using their restrooms.[35] In other parts of the South, they had to endure segregated waiting rooms, only being called after the last white patient was seen. If they were admitted at all, hospital administrators consigned them to beds located in basements, with their parents providing nursing care.[36] In Dallas, the Texas Scottish Rite Hospital for Crippled Children, opened in 1923, represented a scarce alternative, since it admitted all children. Houston's Jefferson Davis Hospital also had integrated polio wards. Bobby Johnson recalls the nonchalant relationships that developed: "There was a black kid named Marvin and we became pretty good friends. I had never known a black person before other than just seeing people . . . We would hang around each other's bed because that was all you had—your bed and your wheelchair."[37] Their lives had only become intertwined because of a disease. But this proved atypical. North Carolina later integrated its hospital wards because public health officials there deferred to NFIP personnel. Even this failed to become a universal practice, since members of local NFIP chapters "usually complied with segregationist traditions in their communities."

Few options existed. Isolated treatment centers only began to emerge in the early 1940s, especially with the inauguration of the Tuskegee Institute's Infantile Paralysis Center for Negroes. In 1944, "the Davidson County National Foundation chapter in Nashville, Tennessee, donated '$11,000 worth of physiotherapy equipment to Hubbard Hospital,' a black medical facility that was managed by Meharry Medical College administrators." This of course followed Tuskegee's example. "It would ultimately take education and economic incentives," historian Stephen E. Mawdsley asserts, "to motivate widespread integration of polio wards in the South by the late 1940s and early 1950s."

Although de facto segregation dominated neighborhoods in much of the North, Midwest, and West, racially integrated wards prevailed for a pragmatic reason: specialized care and equipment proved too expensive to duplicate at separate locations. Such was the case at St. Paul's Gillette State Hospital for Crippled Children. Jerry McNellis remembers his African American roommate with fondness; he helped Jerry with his reading skills by taking turns reading to each other for hours every day. Hospital wards, in fact, often became great levelers, as dozens of children from different social, economic, ethnic, and racial backgrounds occupied beds in the same room.[38]

Furthermore, fears of this disease literally and immediately transformed many of these sick children into outcasts, regardless of race. Ambulance drivers and attendants typically covered children with rubber sheets to contain any suspected contagion. Covering a body with a bed sheet from head to toe, to be sure, connoted death. This message proved to be a shock for these young patients. Even some otherwise well-meaning hospital personnel reflexively avoided newly admitted children who had been diagnosed with infantile paralysis. "Doctors seldom touched patients, and when they did, it was with gloved hands. Some did not even enter the rooms of children with polio but stood in the doorway or waved through a glass partition." During the 1949 epidemic in San Angelo, Texas, a pediatrician at Shannon Hospital, terrified of contracting this virus, refused to conduct spinal taps on sick children. Nurses rarely lingered in isolation wards. Many others simply refused polio-patient duty. As a child left a containment area, the hospital staff, fearful of further contagion and reverting to the long-discredited zymotic theory, burned all of the patient's clothes, flowers, get-well cards, souvenirs, toys, and beloved teddy bears. Much of this behavior could be attributed to being poorly trained, as Carmelita Calderwood, clinical instructor in orthopedic nursing at Denver's Children's Hospital, observed during Colorado's 1939 epidemic.[39]

Fear, though, occasionally found some basis in reality. The Los Angeles County Hospital itself became off limits during that city's 1934 epidemic, characterized by a large number of young adult infections with a mild nonparalytic strain. Nurses and interns grew terrified, with one or two becoming infected daily, eventually totaling 198 cases. Nurses suffered more than twice the rate as the general population, while interns experienced about a 20 percent higher figure. That hospital soon gained the reputation as a pest house. Nurses and interns became pariahs. Attending physicians halted daily rounds, opting instead to consulting with the staff by telephone. With such mass hysteria, no one invited those nurses and interns to private residences for simple socializing when off duty.[40]

During such epidemics, while at the same time harboring the fear of becoming infected, medical professionals pushed themselves through extreme fatigue. Nurses worked over twelve hours a day with no days off. Exhaustion and stress took their toll. This often led to short tempers and outbursts, some of them directed at their young patients. A paralyzed Kehret awoke in the middle of the night in excruciating pain. She screamed for the nurse, who responded immediately. However, the nurse refused to accede to her plea to be rolled over in order to ease her extreme discomfort. "'I just turned you, not ten minutes ago,' she scolded. 'I'm not turning you again already. You'll get turned every thirty minutes, the same as every other patient in this ward.'" The nurse then stomped out, leaving Kehret terrified and angry at the same time. She was totally dependent on this person, but she also wanted to retaliate. Her only consolation came as a result of her parents filing a complaint. Kehret never saw that nurse again.[41] Student nurses, with no seniority and regardless of their own anxieties about this disease, had to accept assignments to the polio ward. World War II epidemics caused special problems. Branches of the armed forces leased hospitals, causing a severe shortage of hospital beds for young patients. Likewise, medical personnel became scarce because of military duty. Adaptations involved an increased use of medical interns and assigning nurses to multiple hospitals through the duration of these epidemics. During the 1955 Massachusetts epidemic with about four thousand cases, William Tisdale, a second-year resident, recalls interminable twelve-hour shifts: "We were exhausted, depressed by what we'd seen." A University of Minnesota physician articulates the anxieties of all medical professionals: "It was like being in combat. You have to be on the ball and ready to go all the time. You were tired, exhausted, and frightened at the same time. We didn't want to get polio ourselves. We were all concerned as heck about it because we'd bring it home . . . You couldn't avoid it. Because you were covered with saliva, you'd bring it with you."[42] By the 1950s, nurse shortages were common for two primary reasons. First, care proved to be extremely demanding, as we have seen, and consequently required more training, time, and pressure. Yet these nurses received the same salaries as those with regular duties. Working in the isolation ward was therefore not an attractive job. Second, "many nurses who were mothers avoided working with polio patients, fearing they might infect their own children."[43] This virus profoundly changed the lives of medical health professionals, parents, and most importantly the children they treated.

Cyanosis

Diane Odell, who spent fifty-eight years in a seven-foot, 750-pound tank respirator, otherwise known as an iron lung or steel cocoon, died at her home in Jackson, Tennessee, on May 28, 2008, at age sixty-one. A power outage had occurred, and the emergency generator failed to operate. Family members even resorted to a second backup system: the manual pump attached to the respirator. It too did not work, and tragically she suffocated to death.[44] Those who survived the initial onset of the poliovirus often lived fragile lives, temporarily or permanently dependent on an artificial means to breathe. The iron lung became a stark icon of this disease as paralysis crept into patients' diaphragms.

Before the inception of these machines, through the 1920s, children who contracted virulent polio strains accounted for many deaths because of respiratory failure. These rates could be as high as 50 percent during some epidemics. A tracheotomy offered the only approach to maintain breathing. This basic procedure involved the surgeon making an incision in a patient's throat to allow air to pass freely and directly into the esophagus and lungs. This proved to be traumatic for young children, as Gallagher tells of his experience:

> No one warned me that surgery was to be performed . . . I was much too sick to be moved to a surgery theater, and so, the operation was performed at bedside . . . I was too sick . . . for anesthetics . . . Very bright and hot lights were brought into my room, and my memory is one of dazzling brilliance.
>
> The doctor wore glasses. He worked feverishly and held his head close to his work. This meant that his eyeglasses served as a mirror for me. In the bright light, clearly reflected, I could watch his hand as he slit my throat . . . My nose and mouth, struggling to gulp air and force it into my lungs, suddenly were left gasping . . . I had an acute and overwhelming sense of suffocation, as my mouth and nostrils were now powerless to assist in obtaining air.[45]

One study estimated that tracheotomies had to be used in 20 percent of all cases to assist respiration. The signs and symptoms requiring this procedure involved "irregular shallow or periodically apneic respiration or both; exhaustion, agitation, restlessness, or apprehension; progression of bulbar involvement with increasing dysphagia and the presence of suffusion and cyanosis."[46] Such paralysis spawned the use of artificial respirators.

Philip Drinker, a Harvard University engineer, invented in 1929 what became known as the iron lung. This large, unwieldy contraption proved to be a lifesaver, and clinicians grew increasingly dependent on it, using it early in the "failure of the respiratory musculature"; it was not to be relied upon as a last resort. Drs. Earl C. Elkins and K. C. Wakim, in a 1947 article, insisted that it should be employed "before the symptoms of a serious lack of oxygen become obvious. This is logical," they explained, "not only because the anoxia will produce damage to nerve cells but because the overexertion of the weakened respiratory muscles increases fatigue and at this stage of the disease may increase paralysis."[47] However, as medical historian David J. Rothman points out, it was "useful against only one form of polio, intercostal paralysis, but not against a second form, bulbar polio." The latter virus strain "irreversibly damaged the nerve cells in the breathing center of the brain and these nerves would not regenerate over time." Intercostal muscles, on the other hand, could partially or fully recover. Physicians knowing this physiological fact still placed "dying and gasping patients" in them. "Recognizing that the intervention was futile, but hoping against hope, they tried it anyway—and in the process built up an association, both statistical and anecdotal, between high levels of mortality and the use of the iron lung." In all, 10 percent of patients relied on them to breathe.[48]

This pioneering medical technology led to ethical questions during severe epidemics. In some cases, especially during the early 1930s, too few of these machines existed to meet the demand. Physicians faced difficult decisions: Who should be treated? And concomitantly, who should be condemned to die? Even then, studies conducted in 1931 and 1932 concluded that the

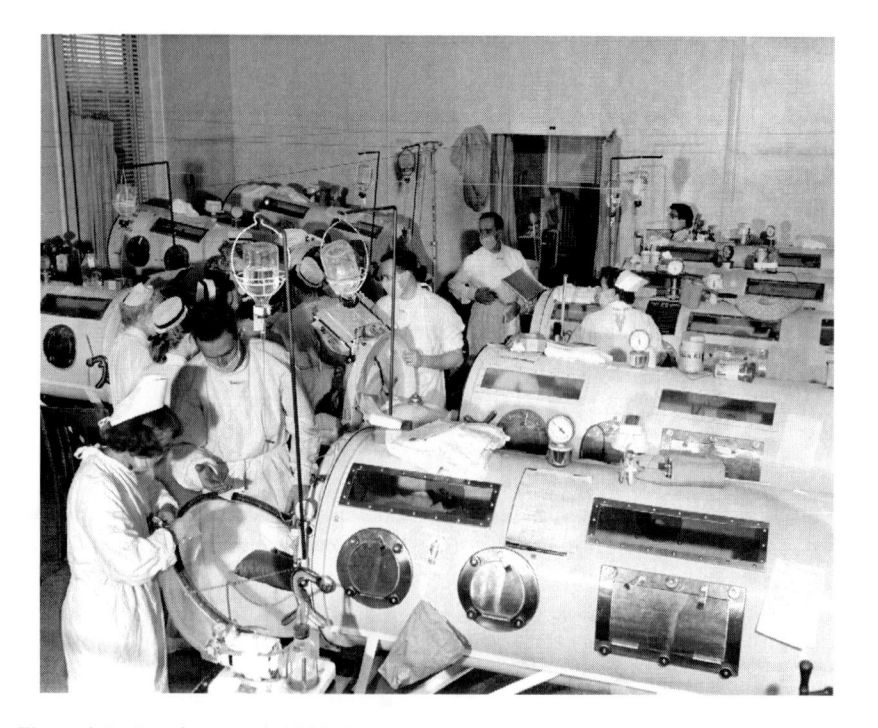

Figure 2.1 Iron lung ward, 1955. Courtesy: March of Dimes.

mortality rate for iron lung patients ranged between 60 and 75 percent. By 1939, the number of tank respirators had increased to seven hundred nationwide. During the 1948 Los Angeles epidemic, physicians assigned one-tenth of 2,900 cases to them. Sixty-five percent of patients during the major epidemic years, between 1949 and 1954, were children; some 1,500 of them had to be inserted into respirators nationwide.[49] About five hundred medical institutions claimed to have an iron lung: "55 percent of these hospitals had only one respirator patient. Eighty percent had three or less."[50]

An additional challenge arose over when to utilize iron lungs with patients. At first, during the 1930s, physicians tended to employ them too late, usually as cyanosis, dyspnea, and tachycardia set in, too often with very poor results. By the mid-1950s, after many years of trial and error, they experienced much better outcomes with early use, resulting in morality rates dropping from 50 to less than 20 percent.[51]

From a clinical standpoint, the medical staff inserted patients into these long metal cylinders, with an interior measuring 66 inches in length and 22 inches in diameter that contained a mattress and an opening for the head. These usually adult-sized machines dwarfed children who were placed in them, a terrifying feeling. Thirteen-year-old Regina Woods describes a typical hectic scene: iron lung machines flooded the hospital's hallways, lined up along the walls "like so many yellow caskets." A leather or rubber collar sealed the patient's entire body in a completely airtight compartment. The Collins respirator used rubber bellows attached to the bottom of the tank, while the Emerson version relied on a leather diaphragm at the end of the tank. Both had five rubber arm portals and one bedpan door. Nurses used screw caps mounted on top to permit the insertion of intravenous tubes. Each respirator had a mirror angled over the patient's head to provide a field of vision, albeit limited. One respirator at Boston Children's Hospital, which Lewin illustrates in his 1941 medical text, could accommodate multiple patients. It occupied a small room with four patients, two stacked on top of two others. A floor-to-ceiling steel partition, with the usual airtight collars, sealed patients' heads outside of this huge machine. Physicians and nurses could thus enter the pressurized part of the room to attend to their patients, bypassing the need for portals.[52]

Care proved to be demanding, complex, and dangerous. Individual nurses needed special training to work with artificial respirators; they had to attend to the patient as well as "manage the machine," requiring "technical competence, speed, and skill."[53] Inserting a young child into an iron lung required a team to closely choreograph their actions to reduce pain and prevent injuries as well as ease patient anxiety. Wearing surgical masks—adding to the impersonal hospital atmosphere—they removed occupants for baths and linen changes, while patients remained positioned in the collar to facilitate quick reinsertion if respiratory arrest occurred. This required especially keen teamwork because of a two-minute time limit. In severe cases, children remained in their respirators while two nurses stationed themselves at both sides, using the portals to wash them and change their sheets. Although this machine proved to be a lifesaver, it also created its own unique set of hazards, as Robert M. Eiben, a pediatrician at Cleveland's Hospital for Contagious Diseases states: "The loss of an effective cough and the postural influences on the drainage of the respiratory tree could result in segments of malfunctioning lung, ultimately to atelectasis (collapse of a portion of lung) or bronchopneumonia."[54] Nursing teams had to constantly shift the patient's body position to prevent pneumonia as well as reduce skin irritations, although some models could rotate and tilt to obtain the same effect. Children suffered from constipation, either from the loss of muscle control or from reclining and being sedentary; nurses relieved this through enemas, which involved the awkward use of funnels and rectal tubes. The medical staff also often had to catheterize respirator patients; otherwise, the bedpan port had to be opened and closed quickly to maintain stable air pressure. This device also had a headrest that reclined sufficiently to fully expose the neck; this kept air passages clear as well as facilitated tracheotomies in serious cases. Finally, physicians and nurses, as a general rule, attempted to maintain a respiratory rate of 14 to 18 breaths per minute. This required close monitoring and adjustments to recalibrate the machine. Worse yet, it was not an exact science. "Charts (nomograms) and tables," Dr. Thomas M. Daniel explains, "allowed us to judge settings for average persons of given heights and weights." Properly adjusting the rhythm of an iron lung, though, required guessing in some cases. "Ventilation not only controls blood oxygen," Daniel adds, "but also blood carbon dioxide, a waste product excreted by the lungs, and pH, the body's acidity. Abnormalities in these two aspects of respiration produce rapid, and potentially lethal, physiological changes for which the first clue is often a change in mental states. But how does one judge the thinking of a terrified child?"[55] Ernest Greenberg, an anesthesiologist during the early 1950s in Westchester County, New York, recalls "We . . . had nurses suctioning these patients around the clock. Patients in iron lungs would have pooling of secretions because they could not swallow. These secretions would cause laryngeal spasm. They would become cyanotic, very blue, and then it was an emergency intubation." By the 1950s, physicians relied on a bronchoscopy, inserting a tube down the patient's throat, to suction any suffocating mucus and restore breathing. It was an agonizing procedure that had to be conducted every few days.[56]

Residing in an artificial respirator proved to be a fragile experience, characterized by complete helplessness. With their lives hanging by a thread, these young patients, while able to breathe, found that this mechanical device added to their discomfort and pain. Thunderstorms were especially terrifying because of potential electrical failures. These of course could interrupt the iron lung's operations and cause suffocation. Their lives hung in the balance, a delicate existence highly dependent on crude technology. Such power blackouts meant that the medical staff had to operate the respirators by hand, sometimes for hours. During the 1949 epidemic in San Angelo, Texas, Shannon Hospital's staff created a flying squadron of volunteers who rushed to respiratory ward stations at the sound of an alarm, ready to operate the awkward hand pumps, sticking to a prescribed rotation to avoid exhaustion. Juanita Howell, a nurse in Mississippi during the 1946 epidemic, vividly recalls that everyone, including custodians and gardeners, manually cranked the iron lungs to ensure that all of the patients could continue to breathe. Colds and bedsores represented additional serious threats before the discovery of antibiotics. The former further complicated breathing and could lead to pneumonia, usually resulting in death, while the latter proved extremely uncomfortable, were susceptible to infections, and took months to heal. Finally, muscle atrophy of patients' respiratory tissue sometimes spelled permanent dependence.[57]

Those confined to iron lungs suffered substantial sense deprivation. They usually could not speak, because of the lack of muscle control in their throats. Gallagher likens it to incarceration or worse:

> There are prisoners in small and windowless prison cells, but they usually have a small grillwork in their cell door. Through this, they are able to look directly at their corridor, at their jailer, man to man, eye to eye. With their vision, they may roam their cells, which has become their world, inspecting minutely the details of the floor, the walls, the fixtures; they retain proprietary ownership of their bodies. They are able to clean, care, and pleasure themselves; the iron lung patient has no such freedoms. His world is his field of vision, and this is dictated by the mirror and its angle and the direction in which the lung is placed.[58]

Devoid of physical contact, children at this stage of the infection had absolutely no control over their bodies, totally dependent on a mammoth, clanking machine to keep them alive and a small, angled mirror to maintain limited contact with the world. Some patients became psychotic, resulting in "'iron lung hallucinations,' usually imagining that they were traveling by aeroplane or train."[59]

Even the mere presence of this long steel cylinder evoked dread. Peg Kehret's condition deteriorated to the point that she awoke to find one sitting next to her hospital bed. She felt instant shock. It "loomed . . . hoses hanging like tentacles—a gray octopus ready to swallow me at any moment. As I imagined my future in an iron lung, tears of despair rolled down my cheeks, I could not raise my hand to wipe them away, and they ran into my ears."[60] Dr. Eiben corroborates this from a clinician's viewpoint. "It is unlikely that there was ever a polio patient who was not fearful of the 'iron lung,' an unfortunate term of obscure origin for the tank respirator. A number of patients acknowledged that they thought going into the tank respirator meant almost certain death and others equated the machine with a coffin in which they would be buried."[61] Parents felt the same way. Horrified to see their child in one, mothers and fathers usually suppressed their feelings and acted nonchalant for the benefit of young and vulnerable patients, gushing seemingly casual comments such as, "Oh, look at the funny house you're in." Mothers, as painful as it was for them, tried to appear cheerful for their children during visitations following isolation, engaging them in play.[62] However, an emotional maelstrom and severe stress lurked just below the surface.

Some children grew physically dependent on and emotionally addicted to this mechanical respirator. Within days of entering a hospital in Louisville, Kentucky, doctors placed thirteen-year-old Regina Woods into an iron lung. This represented the first relief she had experienced in days: "Such comfort! I was no longer struggling to breathe and the whole thing seemed simply wonderful . . . I did not know that these changes signaled a worsening of my condition and were viewed by my family with great alarm." She remained in it as days passed into weeks. Nurses attempted to remove her from the bulky contraption, substituting a portable one; it failed. This instilled an even deeper sense of dread in her: "From that day onward, I was filled with fear about leaving the lung." This anxiety intensified when the nurses once again tried to ease her out of it. After she lost consciousness on every attempt, experiencing extremely high blood pressure, enduring severe seizures, and coping with delirium, they gave up, but only after her parents put a stop to it: "This was only one of many instances in which my family, who had practically lived in the hospital, had intervened to protect me. There has never been any doubt in my mind as to why I survived when so many did not." This episode left her highly fearful and insecure: She needed her iron lung. Regina never fully recovered, and she spent the rest of her life experiencing only thirty to forty minutes a day without the aid of an iron lung or portable breathing device. Permanently weaning patients out of the iron lung proved to be a most difficult task, both physically and emotionally. The respirator symbolized security, life itself, not unlike a mechanical womb.[63] "Iron lung patients," historian Daniel J. Wilson concludes, "went almost full circle in their feelings about the machine that so dominated their lives. Once their breathing had become significantly impaired, their initial dread of the big yellow and green tanks sitting ominously in the hall awaiting new prisoners quickly gave way to appreciative dependence."[64]

The medical staff too found the sight of these huge steel respirators unsettling and the pressure of maintaining them stressful. A newly assigned nurse became terrified when she encountered them for the first time: "When I saw an iron lung in operation as I went on duty that night I was ready to run in the opposite direction. The isolation ward was filled to capacity."[65] To make matters worse, overworked medical professionals did not always show compassion. In one instance, while in a respirator, Woods did not like the way she and others were being treated by some staff members. A nurse who disliked a male patient punished him: she "moved his ham radio, the one thing left to him from his pre-polio life, so that he could not reach it." Woods, summarizing her medical treatment, says, "We were treated worse than animals, and there were frequent displays of unbelievable ignorance and cruelty."[66] In another case, because Marilynne Rogers cried from the painful abrasions she suffered from the iron lung's neck collar, a nurse punished her by turning off the machine and leaving the room. Rogers fainted because of asphyxiation; fortunately, other nurses intervened and restarted the machine.[67]

The National Foundation for Infantile Paralysis addressed the growing need for artificial respirators, particularly in the face of severe epidemics in the post-World War II period. Expertise represented one problem. "By the 1940s, along with the Red Cross, the Foundation held regular training sessions for nurses in the care of polio patients, especially those in iron lungs."[68] Supply presented a serious logistics challenge. "A 1949 survey conducted by the NFIP reported the existence of 448 respirator patients throughout the country. Almost four hundred of these patients were dispersed among 160 hospitals, 80 percent of which could handle no more than three respirator patients at a time." The following year it established fifteen poliomyelitis respiratory centers that stretched from New York to California, from Michigan to Texas. Dr. Eiben served as director of the Cleveland Center. The Southwestern Poliomyelitis Respiratory Center, affiliated with Baylor University College of Medicine and Jefferson Davis Hospital, opened in Houston on June 23, 1950. Patients arrived there from five states: Arkansas, Louisiana, New Mexico, Oklahoma, and Texas.[69]

This innovative and aggressive approach grouped respirator patients together, "side-by-side in highly equipped rooms while a specially trained medical team provided intense, around-the-clock supervision. A nurse was assigned to every two iron lungs in order to provide optimum, personalized attention to each patient."[70] According to one account, they sat "head to toe in a chaos of machinery, cables, thunderous bellows, extra lungs out in the corridor, nurses scurrying about, anxious families, visitors tripping over the cables, doctors dealing with crisis after crisis of choking, seizures, heart failure." Another observer likened it to a "medical pest house, complete with the stink."[71] Nevertheless, their structure and purpose represented the forerunners of modern intensive-care units, and more importantly the overall concept proved to be an unqualified success: "The average rehabilitation period in respiratory centers dwindled from twelve months or more to seven months. The subsequent cost decreased from about $20,000 to $7,000 per patient."[72]

Respirators continued to be refined through the 1950s, although the original Drinker or tank type continued in use. First, dome respirators added a clear plastic capsule that fit over an iron-lung patient's head, permitting them to continue breathing if they needed to be bathed, given therapy, or provided some other service. Second, a chesperator was a "turtle-like plastic shell that fit firmly over the chest" while patients remained in their hospital beds.[73] Third, the Respir-aid Rocking Bed, introduced in 1947, slowly oscillated up and down in order to use gravity to force air into the patient's lungs. Doctors began to substitute them for iron lungs in order to give older patients more freedom. While visiting the Watson Home for Crippled Children, located near Pittsburgh, to observe polio treatments, Charlotte Baron, a public health nurse from Toledo, Ohio, overheard Dr. Jessie Wright's casual comment on the need for an electrically powered oscillating bed. Baron shared this concept with her brother, who, along with two engineers, built a prototype. Wright, a renowned physical therapist and Watson's medical director, endorsed it after seeing it in action during its first clinical trial at Pittsburgh's Municipal Hospital. These iron bed frames swayed every few seconds, much like a seesaw, causing patients' diaphragms to move up and down, through gravity, to compress and release their lungs. Their feet rested on sponge rubber footboards, while a bar with two rubber grips held their shoulders in place. When patients' feet touched the bottom of the tilt, they inhaled, and when they moved backward, they exhaled.[74]

These experiences etched dark and enduring memories for many children. Boyer describes witnessing dozens of people confined to iron lungs, neatly lined up in the hospital: "I thought they didn't have bodies. I was afraid of what was happening to these people." This haunted her for a year, even after returning home. "I used to have nightmares, and they lasted for quite some time . . . [T]here were two very short men with long white coats down in my parents' basement, and they were going to put me in this ringer-type of machine . . . and mangle my legs . . . [I]t never dawned on me 'til I was older that it had been the iron lung."[75] Other children developed a strong fear of being buried alive. Even those who succeeded in avoiding these contraptions retained unpleasant memories. Michael Davis recalls hearing the clanking noises of iron lungs in another hospital room. "Only once did any of the machines cease their wheezing, during my third night in the ward when we were aroused by doctors and nurses across the hall. Subsequently we were told a twelve-year-old girl had died in the lung."[76]

The use of respirators did not preclude a tracheotomy. When patients experienced breathing problems even while in an iron lung, doctors had to act decisively. These children, by way of the iron lung's angled mirror mounted above their heads, in the wee hours of the night, watched in horror as frantic physicians made incisions in their throats and inserted breathing tubes, allowing air to pass directly to the lungs. In these situations, doctors avoided using anesthetics and sedatives, because of damaged nervous systems. This certainly resolved an immediate threat but introduced yet another procedure, one more demanding and delicate, as Dr. Eiben notes:

> The tracheotomized patient was particularly vulnerable to pulmonary complications. The respiratory tree was open to the environment, the ability to change the patient's position became impossible. The initiation of a regimen of intermittent deep breathing proved of great value in preventing atelectasis in patients confined to a respirator. This was achieved by exhausting air through a porthole by applying suction from a flanged hose of a vacuum cleaner during the inspiratory cycle of the tank.[77]

Even when tracheotomies worked, the nightmare of suddenly witnessing one's throat being cut endured. But they did not always succeed. As anesthesiologist Greenberg cryptically notes, the medical staff typically felt helpless: "A small child, about five years old . . . turned cyanotic. Intubated him, transported to the operating room for tracheostomy and later died. It was a stressful day . . . It really bothered me terribly for many weeks to see a small child that I was involved with that I could do nothing about."[78]

Witnessing children experiencing respiratory failure traumatized staff members. As a Harvard medical student completing his clinical experience at Haynes Memorial Infectious Disease Hospital, Daniel found himself in the center of Boston's polio epidemic. Jeffrey, a teenage boy, was admitted one night in August 1954, experiencing serious breathing problems. The staff promptly placed him in an iron lung. But Jeffrey could not coordinate his breathing with the respirator's rhythm. The attendants then resorted to an experimental machine that sent electrical shocks through his neck to stimulate his diaphragm. Daniel reconstructs their desperate efforts to keep Jeffrey alive: "I took my turn that long night, along with . . . interns and residents. Our fingers held the electrode on his neck, our eyes watched his chest, and we kept it up as best we could before yielding to fatigue and turning the electrode over to the next person. We continued during the following day, now with more help as others came to work. I went home that next night . . . When I returned to the hospital early the following morning, Jeffrey was dead."[79]

Immediate Post-Acute Treatment

Although the majority of cases did not result in permanent paralysis, it represented a visible and dramatic outcome. It struck suddenly, with onset usually (but not always) occurring between 48 and 72 hours. For the 1916 epidemic, Chicago's Department of Health statistically pinned down the affected areas: 82 percent legs, 11 percent face, and 11 percent arms. By 1940, according to the U.S. Children's Bureau data, infantile paralysis accounted for 19 percent of children with disabilities—the leading cause—while other national estimates were as high as 24 percent. Moreover, the rate varied widely between states, from 6 to 38 percent. Many physicians believed that paralysis could be corrected, and following critical care but while the patient was still hospitalized, they began to attack it.[80]

Samuel D. Gross, of Jefferson Medical College in Philadelphia, and Mary Putnam Jacobi, of the Women's Medical College of New York, proposed the first recorded treatments in the 1870s. They suggested, among other things, using counterirritants and electricity to stimulate atrophied muscles as well as applying a "red-hot iron" to the back in order to create a draining ulcer, providing the means to extract the virus. Physical therapy involved muscle massages, mercury ointment rubs, and slapping the affected area with a cold, wet towel until the skin glowed red.[81]

By the early twentieth century, remedies changed based on the newest medical findings and techniques. Lovett proved highly influential through his speeches, his articles, and his 1917 publication, *The Treatment of Infantile Paralysis*. His dictums became medical mantras for decades. These new remedies began after the body temperature returned to normal, although some residual muscle sensitivity usually continued for three to six weeks. First, limb or body immobilization involved applying splints or casts. Orthopedists prescribed the former when the patient's muscle sensitivity remained too great, though the latter represented the preferred approach. Second, heat treatments, using infrared lamps or hot packs, began at this stage.[82]

Immobilization

Ostensibly to minimize the impact of paralysis, this treatment dominated through the 1930s. It entailed splints or plaster casts to lock the affected part of the body in a stable, normal position or posture. Initial immobilization lasted eight weeks, and with some limb improvement, it continued another eight weeks. This could continue for six to eight months, with intermittent testing every eight weeks. Doctors believed that prescribing such long bouts of inactivity for children would prevent or minimize deformities; that is, immobilization was meant to ensure physical symmetry. Such a treatment sometimes involved an overhead frame equipped with ropes and pulleys. This also meant intense attention and care by nurses because of pressure sores and potential "circulatory impairment." Finally, it proved to be excruciatingly painful for children while muscular atrophy exacted a devastating toll.[83] Nevertheless, this medical approach virtually became a fetish. During the 1934 Los Angeles epidemic, physicians immobilized 46 percent of patients with a Bradford frame, which provided support and stretched the upper torso, and splinted 74 percent in plaster casts for long-term treatment.[84]

Splinting occurred during and immediately following the acute period and involved apparatus made of iron, steel, and wood. Two pieces of a Thomas caliper splint, "made of heavy iron wire one-quarter inch or more in diameter," as Lovett described it, "run up on the outside and inside of the leg . . . and are joined together at the top just below the gluteal fold by a posterior iron band which is curved and padded." This "appliance" locked the knee into a straight position. The fitting of a sole plate, holding the foot at a right angle to the floor, prevented mild cases of drop foot. Knee contraction also had to be addressed at this point.[85] For slight paralysis, orthopedists placed affected joints in certain positions to ensure a return of function, or at least to preserve as much flexibility as possible. In the case of the neck, this involved using a roll of cloth placed under it, as the patient reclined in bed, or a cotton collar wrapped around it. Or they put folded blankets, pillows, or sandbags under the feet or knees to restrict movement. They also used fabric restraints as a "temporary substitute for plaster and metal splints." This was especially the case when they tied children's legs or wrists to their bedposts, locking them in place.[86]

Stubborn or severe paralysis caused orthopedists to resort to plaster casts, and different types were used. A "bivalved cast," or plaster shell, allowed half of a limb to be exposed (thereby allowing the physician access to that limb) but maintained the "physiological rest position for paralyzed muscles by means of protective supports." Straightening the ankle joint, for example, involved encasing the entire leg in a plaster cast, thus forcing it into position. Mild scoliosis conditions, for Lovett, could be addressed through the simple strategy of a canvas corset. In worse cases, "mild forcible correction" required the patient to be placed, face down, on a frame and using straps to exert pressure on the curved spine. Following this straightening process, physicians covered the patient, while still strapped to the frame, in a plaster cast for up to six months. Immobilization, in sum, involved splints, corsets, and body casts, using force to reposition a limb.[87]

Physicians regularly adjusted these casts to prevent "contraction deformities."[88] Susan Richards Shreve graphically relates how they routinely conducted an adjustment procedure on her roommate Caroline. A medical team breezed into their room with a toolbox and immediately turned her, in a full body cast, on her back.

> "We're going to tighten the screws here, Caroline," the first doctor said, indicating the metal contraption attached to her legs . . . "it's going to hurt."
> The doctor began working the plaster with his wrench.
> "Tell me when," he said, turning. "Now?" he asked.
> Caroline shook her head.
> "Now?" He had turned the wrench a little more. "Caroline?"
> Her face suddenly hardened as if she'd locked her jaw.
> "There," the doctor said. "High pain tolerance, Caroline. It takes a lot of self-control not to scream."
> He patted her head.
> Then they turned her over on her stomach, spread the sheet over her back, and opened the curtains.

They departed as abruptly as they had entered, leaving Caroline, whose face was "bone-white," to sort out her agony.[89] Immobilization seldom fulfilled the expectations of physicians and patients. It was simply wrongheaded, if not downright torturous. In 1971, Dr. John R. Paul reflected that decades of immobilization "did more harm than good."[90]

The Maverick

Early and prolonged immobilization seems to have run its course by the late 1930s. In many ways it intensified disabilities, since it resulted in the atrophy of unharmed muscles, ultimately affecting them much like nerve damage would. Fifty-nine-year-old Sister Elizabeth Kenny, with her twenty-three-year-old adopted daughter, docked in San Francisco on April 16, 1940, and introduced what appeared to be a viable alternative. Her timing could not have been more propitious. "Kenny's techniques . . . addressed a widespread dissatisfaction with polio therapy, and her dramatic results with patients who had been paralyzed for many years as well as with acute patients impressed everyone." She proved to be a divisive force, though. In both Australia and the United States, as a female crusader, she confronted male medical orthodoxy; as an opportunist, she courted politicians; and as a messianic figure, the general public, especially parents, willingly embraced her therapy with great hope and expectations.[91]

Born in 1880, Kenny received her training at a private hospital, never attending a nursing school. She served in Australia's outback, caring for minor injuries and illnesses, and this was where she first encountered an infantile paralysis case in 1911, with a sick two-year-old girl. Isolated in bush country, Kenny improvised by boiling woolen blanket strips, wringing them dry, and wrapping them around the girl's twisted limbs. This relaxed her tiny patient, allowing Kenny to move them without any undue force. The young girl recovered. World War I interrupted Kenny's civilian work; she served aboard troop transports, where she earned the title of "Sister," a formal title for nurses. She returned to treating polio patients after the war and, through her aggressive nature and drive, by 1936 had established clinics, with the backing of the Queensland government, in Brisbane, Sydney, Townsville, and Toowoomba. In addition to this political support, the public adored her and rushed their ill children to her for treatment. She became known as the "new Australian Florence Nightingale." Her role as a mere nurse, lack of formal training, and especially her steadfast insistence that she was right and doctors were wrong, combined to infuriate the medical community. The Queensland Royal Commission issued a scathing condemnation on January 1, 1938, based on 47 cases. This report, which reinforced reliance on splints and immobilization, stressed that her claims of success outstripped reality. World War II ended her quixotic quest as doctors and nurses joined the military, draining her clinics of personnel. With the situation looking hopeless, her small coterie of medical allies urged her to migrate to America, which was still at peace. One of these supporters had earlier visited the Mayo Clinic and wrote a letter of introduction for her, while another contacted the NFIP's Basil O'Connor. Her itinerary seemed to be set.[92]

News of her Australian efforts preceded her, and American reporters greeted her at the wharf. She immediately set out across the continent by train to New York City to meet with O'Connor. On the way, she visited polio wards in Los Angeles and Denver, observing the widespread use of splinting, plaster casts, and general immobilization. She met O'Connor on May 1, 1940, for three hours at his office. He offered no moral or financial support. She went next to Chicago to appeal to the American Medical Association (AMA), where Howard Carter, secretary of that organization's Council of Physical Therapy, likewise snubbed her. Such rebuffs would prove commonplace, because, as Kenny recalls, her ideas clashed with traditional medical beliefs:

> Where medicine saw strong normal muscles pulling against weak affected ones, I saw tightened, shortened structures which needed to be relaxed, in order to release the brake put upon the activity of the normal or unaffected muscles. Where medicine saw loose, flaccid paralyzed muscle, I saw one whose activity was, in some way, cast aside in order not to exaggerate the pain caused by the tightening or shortening of the affected opponents. I also saw, in most cases, that great disturbance had occurred in the coordinated movements of both areas.

She left Chicago to visit the Mayo Clinic in Rochester, Minnesota. There Kenny met with Melvin Henderson, who introduced her to Wallace H. Cole in the Twin Cities.[93] This proved to be a turning point.

Cole began his career as an orthopedic surgeon in 1914 at the State Hospital for Indigent Crippled and Deformed Children in St. Paul (later the Gillette State Hospital). During World War I, he served as a captain in the U.S. Army Medical Corps and became a part of what became known as the Goldthwait Unit, a specialized group of twenty American orthopedic surgeons treating wounded soldiers in Britain and France. Because of this intense experience, the "members of the Goldthwait Unit went on to dominate American orthopedics for the next thirty years." Although serving as assistant surgeon-in-chief at the Gillette State Hospital for Crippled Children, he accepted the position of chief surgeon at the new Twin Cities Shriner's Hospital for Crippled Children, and in 1929, he became professor of orthopedics and chair of the division of orthopedic surgery at the University of Minnesota.[94] Cole, growing somewhat dissatisfied with existing polio treatments, invited Kenny to examine some children at Gillette. "At the Gillette State Hospital, renowned as one of the few state-funded orthopedic hospitals in the country, Kenny saw familiar conditions." She found the same at the Shriner's and St. Paul's Children's hospitals; that is, casts, frames, and splints.[95] Impressed with her approach, Cole consented to allow her to remove splints and casts from several children and apply her hot pack therapy. She appeared successful.

Cole, along with Miland E. Knapp, head of that university's new physical therapy department, endorsed Kenny's method. With this institutional connection, Cole and Harold Diehl, the medical school's dean, telephoned O'Connor; based on this august recommendation, O'Connor promised March of Dimes support to the school to assess Kenny's method for a six-month period, mainly subsidizing her living expenses. John F. Pohl, an orthopedist, permitted Kenny to treat one of his patients, eighteen-year-old Henry Haverstock, Jr., who became her very first American patient. He had just returned from Warm Springs, Georgia, after months of treatment with limited results. Because of her therapy, he could move one leg after a week, walking out of that hospital on half-crutches within months. This impressed his father, a well-placed attorney. "Kenny's work with Haverstock was also a turning point in her relationship with the city's business establishment."[96]

Cole, Knapp, and Pohl quickly became Kenny acolytes. She began to lecture at university and city hospitals. Cole and Knapp also allocated 14 beds at the Minneapolis General Hospital in order to conduct formal observations, part of the evaluation of her approach. She had free rein in what became known as the Kenny ward. However, she complained publicly about the amount and irregularity of NFIP support. She even wrote to President Franklin D. Roosevelt on a couple of occasions, expressing her dissatisfaction with the NFIP's paltry subsidy. "Annoyed at Kenny's audacity at approaching Roosevelt directly, O'Connor contacted Cole, whom he saw as her formal supervisor." Cole informed Kenny, in turn, that the fault resided with him, since he had not completed all of the necessary grant forms. Minnesota experienced a mild epidemic that year, and Kenny only had the opportunity to treat twenty-four patients, an inadequate number to conduct a reliable statistical assessment. "Cole and Knapp wanted to retain her as both teacher and clinician . . . [and] asked the NFIP to allow her to stay during another polio season so that doctors, nurses, and physical therapists could become better acquainted with her methods." O'Connor agreed to a six-month extension. In February 1942, Basil O'Connor and Donald W. Gudakunst, the foundation's medical director from 1938 to 1945, visited Minneapolis. Consulting with university officials, they "formally institutionalized" the teaching of Kenny's methods. "Drawing on the model of postgraduate courses already in place at the university, the new program was directed by Knapp and financed by the NFIP. There were one-week courses for doctors, four-month courses for physical therapists, and six-month courses for nurses." Also as part of this formal recognition, O'Connor commissioned a manual, *The Kenny Method of Treatment for Infantile Paralysis* (1942), coauthored by Cole, Knapp, and Pohl.[97]

Kenny, a nurse, refused to defer to physicians, often antagonizing them. Seventeen-year-old Robert Gurney, completely paralyzed, "was among the very first acute patients to be treated by Kenny" at the Minneapolis General Hospital. He recalls his first impression of her, an imposing figure, both charismatic and formidable: "She was one big woman, and oh man! She carried herself like a queen. Her size sure didn't bother her at all." He, like all patients, had experienced persistent torment that felt "like you had a cramp, but multiplying the pain 100 times." Kenny soaked strips she had cut from a wool blanket in scalding-hot water, wrung them out, and completely wrapped Gurney in them. "They changed the hot packs every half an hour or 45 minutes the first couple of days." She then covered him with a rubber sheet to prevent the extreme heat from dissipating. For the first time since the onset of infantile paralysis, his pain-wracked body felt some relief. But Kenny met resistance from his doctor. Gurney vividly describes the incident when this physician entered his room with leg splints and arm splints:

> He put them on me and said, "These will help you."
> I asked how they could help, and he said, 'Well, that's all we know to do."
> I asked about Sister Kenny, and he told me, "They said I should work with her, but you're my patient, so I am going to do what I think is right."
> [B]ut when Sister Kenny came back that afternoon, she just stood there and took a look. Then she said to the head floor nurse, "Get me a pair of scissors," and she cut off those splints and threw them on the floor in the corner of the room. And then she said, "You don't need these; who gave them to you?"
> I told her that my doctor did, and she just smiled and said, "Well, he's just a young doctor; I'll have a talk with him."
> And that was the last I saw of those splints.

Gurney faced a rigorous daily regimen: breakfast at 7:00 AM and hot packs at 8:00 AM, followed by therapy involving "an exercise bath" as well as additional active exercises under the care of a physical therapist. After eleven months of this relentless routine, he walked out of the hospital with a limp while only using a cane.[98] Kenny further shocked many physicians by removing patients from iron lungs to restore their breathing through the use of hot packs on their upper trunks and necks. Many of them recovered. In her 1955 autobiography, Kenny unabashedly claimed, "The little children entrusted to my care were more limber when they left the contagion ward then they were before they contracted the disease."[99]

Stretching represented another component of the Kenny method, an equally excruciating reality. Seventeen-year-old Ray Gullickson experienced this firsthand. He acquired the virus while living in rural Wisconsin and transferred to the Fort Snelling Post, in the Minneapolis-St. Paul area, in order to receive the Kenny treatment. Gullickson had experienced uneven leg growth because of this disease: "My right leg was about two and one-half inches shorter than the left, and my back muscles were so tight that it was like having a 'charley horse' cramp that persisted, day and night, without relief." This treatment phase involved several staff members, as he vividly relates:

> They put me, face down, near one end of the treatment table. My upper body was resting on the pad, and my legs were both dangling over the end. One attendant, who was a huge guy of about six foot four inches tall, stood on one side of the table, leaned over, grabbed the edge and held the upper part of my body with his elbows. Another attendant got on the other side, reached across, and held my lower trunk firmly against the table. The Kenny therapist sat on the floor under the table and grasped my right leg, which was dangling over the edge with the healthy one . . . [T]here was no relief until minutes later, when they finished the treatment . . . Sister Kenny compared the length of my two legs. She said, "We *have it*; they're within a quarter of an inch!"[100]

But such improvements came at a painful cost. Kehret recalls the hamstring stretches: "I couldn't kick or pull away from [the therapist's] hands. My mouth was my only defense, and I used it shrieking and crying"[101]

Kenny's therapeutic approach appeared to produce positive outcomes, and it became the dominant treatment, but the concept driving it remained faulty. It diverged from empirical and widely accepted knowledge of nerve damage and instead focused on retraining muscles. The core of the controversy that surrounded her was that without any clinical evidence, she believed that the "poliovirus only temporarily disrupted pathways between nerve and muscles, not destroyed them." Not only was she a dull lecturer, but also her theoretical explanation undergirding her therapeutic approach proved to be incomprehensible. This rubbed many medical professionals the wrong way because it lacked any evidence, but this opposition failed to intimidate her; she soon expanded her treatments, which seemed to reinforce her successes. Her bluntness further alienated the medical community. She nevertheless gained grudging legitimacy for her technique. The American Congress of Physical Therapy honored her in 1942, while the AMA, based on research studies, approved "her work but without her theory." That same year, none other than George Draper, a highly respected polio expert who had served as Roosevelt's physician, noted Kenny's therapeutic advances in a letter to

The New York Times. She dined with O'Connor and Roosevelt at the White House. The NFIP featured a display of the Kenny method at the AMA's 1942 annual meeting in Atlantic City, New Jersey, and began to subsidize patients' treatments if doctors prescribed them, including direct payments to the University of Minnesota. That same year, she implemented a training program for what she termed "Kenny Technicians," and the foundation provided funds for nurses who wanted to spend a week there, studying her methods.[102]

Students enrolled in Kenny's two-year course for registered nurses completed classes through that university's Department of Nursing Education, culminating with a one-year course of study in physical therapy at the Mayo Clinic. At commencement they received a certificate that designated them as specialists qualified to treat patients with the Kenny approach as well as teach it to others. "By December 1943, this university alone had trained 358 doctors and 484 therapists and nurses; by mid-1944, 900 nurses and therapists had been trained." The NFIP responded by subsidizing five additional teaching centers at Stanford and Northwestern universities, Pittsburgh's D. T. Watson School of Physical Therapy, and, of course, the Georgia Warm Springs Foundation. Others followed in Illinois, Indiana, and New York City. The NFIP's New Jersey chapter cosponsored a training program for doctors, nurses, and registered physiotherapists, the first on the East Coast. Kenny, according to *New York Times* coverage, attended the formal dedication and expressed her delight with the facilities and equipment. Those registered for this program attended lectures at New York University (NYU), conducted through its School of Education and College of Medicine, and completed their clinical work at the Jersey City Medical Center. Kenny delivered the inaugural lecture on February 4, 1943, to 24 physical therapists who had been chosen from 500 applicants.[103]

Kenny's popularity with the American public grew to match that of Eleanor Roosevelt. The popular press, such as *Life* magazine and *Reader's Digest*, and medical publications, like *The American Journal of Nursing* and *The New England Journal of Medicine*, extensively covered her method. *The American Weekly* compared her to Clara Barton, Madame Curie, and Florence Nightingale. John Pohl translated her amateurish writings into mainstream medical terminology, resulting in the publication of her first textbook in 1943, *The Kenny Concept of Infantile Paralysis and Its Treatment*. That same year, the University of Rochester and New York University bestowed honorary degrees on Kenny in recognition of her work in treating infantile paralysis patients. Although the 1946 film *Sister Kenny* fizzled at the box office, it nonetheless made her a celebrity. Even before it went into production, she had won the support of professional athletes, newspaper moguls and writers, and business leaders, as well as many Hollywood stars, including Bing Crosby, Cary Grant, Basil Rathbone, Kate Smith, and Rosalind Russell, who portrayed Kenny in the movie.[104]

Kenny also earned the respect of a wide spectrum of African Americans by treating patients and training a small number of nurses. Moreover, Kenny

Foundation officials in 1949 named the new polio wing at the Jersey City Medical Center after Jackie Robinson, the first African American to play major league baseball. Finally, African American fundraisers and celebrities, like Dizzy Gillespie and Sarah Vaughn, subsidized much of the costs for that facility.[105]

Many medical facilities adopted the Kenny treatment. While recovering in Louisville's Kosair Hospital during the 1944 Kentucky epidemic, Michael Davis remembers the relentless heat; daytime temperatures soared between 90 and 100 degrees Fahrenheit, and the absence of air conditioning only intensified the hot packs. Patients undergoing this therapy received layer after of layer of them. Nurses at Shannon Hospital in San Angelo, Texas, gave children toys in order to distract their attention prior to applying excruciatingly painful hot packs. This gesture did nothing to offset their anguish. In fact it became a Pavlovian exercise, since they began to cry as soon as they saw these playthings that signaled what was about to follow. Hospital smells thus included the heavy stench of wet wool. Many individuals disabled by polio continue to associate this odor with that disease decades later, as Davis points out: "For me, since the summer of 1944, this wet wool smell has been the smell of polio."[106] Kenny traveled throughout the United States to examine children in medical settings under the watchful eyes of physicians, residents, interns, nurses, parents, and the general public. This included staff at Washington's Doctors Hospital and Indiana University Hospital. Her presentation usually consisted of a casual dismissal of orthodox treatments and a demonstration of her approach. Hoosier Richard Owen, at age fourteen, felt extremely embarrassed as they wheeled him into a large observation room on one of these occasions: "As she examined me, they were taking pictures right and left, and I was very fearful that I was going to appear in the newspaper wearing very little clothing. Her vision of treatment clothing was a tiny loin cloth."[107]

Nevertheless, Kenny became a controversial figure. Her claims too often exceeded reality. Henry R. McCarroll, an orthopedist at the Washington University School of Medicine (in St. Louis), challenged the accolades and early reports of her highly touted technique at the meeting of the American Public Health Association held in St. Louis. He leveled his most intense criticism at its miraculous claims:

> If the sponsors for the Kenny treatment would merely state that they have a relatively simple method of therapy which offers more comfort, greater freedom, and relief of muscle spasm if and when it is present, there would be no argument. When they go beyond this, however, and tell us they are able to control the after-effects of this disease and the degree of residual involvement (crippling after-effects) which these patients show, there is room for disagreement . . . [N]ot all of these patients get well.
>
> The answer to our problems in this disease is not possible in the field of physical therapy. The control of poliomyelitis can only be accomplished through prevention of the destruction in the spinal cord. Tinkering with the muscles themselves after this destruction of the ganglion cells has taken place can never restore their function.[108]

The outcomes, put simply, had been wildly exaggerated. Anne Finger, disabled by this virus, likewise sarcastically adds in retrospect, "Many of Sister Kenny's patients were left with significant impairments, even if this fact tended to be left out of publicity about her, where it seemed that her patients all but leaped up from their hospital beds and pirouetted across the floor."[109] Physical therapists funded by the NFIP traveled to Minnesota to study and analyze Kenney's methods. They too found "many of the claims not to yield better results than those already used by physical therapists, although the heat wraps reduced the pain and muscle reeducation came to the forefront."[110]

Kenny also continued to maintain a stormy relationship with the March of Dimes. O'Connor, who had at first patronized her at his office in 1940, officially and publicly endorsed her method in early December of 1941, based on her successes in Minneapolis. Gudakunst defended her therapy to physicians. In 1943, she even served as the guest of honor at the annual President's Birthday Ball. The NFIP published a pamphlet, "The Story of the Kenny Method," in 1944 that provided a short history of Kenny's method and her personal life, replete with photographs of her treating children and visiting with Roosevelt. As Kenny's method spread, however, she feared that she was losing control of it. The fact that it remained unpatented did not help. Many variations of it began to emerge, much to her displeasure. She repeatedly berated O'Connor about what she perceived as shoddy, short courses funded by the NFIP; she insisted instead on two-year programs. Not only was the Kenny method excruciatingly painful to begin with, but if misused, it also could cause serious injuries, as one young patient recalls: "The physical therapist took the hot pack out of the boiling water and pinned it to my hand so I couldn't pull away. My hand was badly burned and became infected."[111]

Kenny openly complained about these ill-trained practitioners, and Minneapolis city politicians and the business community responded by establishing a permanent center, with 65 beds, to treat and properly train Kenny technicians in a two-year course of study. It was dedicated as the Elizabeth Kenny Institute on December 17, 1942, and incorporated in September of the following year. Nine-year-old Marilynne Rogers remembers the lonely and grueling existence of Kenny's therapeutic treatments. The institute permitted parents to visit their children for only two hours each Sunday, an emotionally traumatic separation for such young victims. Rogers spent two years there, only seeing her family for those fleeting visits on Sundays. Between those respites, Rogers recalls, the treatment relentlessly continued, consisting of "steamed wool clothes wrapped around my upper arms, shoulders, back, chest, legs, and feet. The clothes were then wrapped in plastic to keep the heat in. I think I had those twice a day, and they were very hot." Then came the therapy, Rogers continues, "stretching for 10 minutes twice a day to keep our bodies mobile and prevent the tendency to tighten up. Tightening up causes deformation." Finally, at times, nurses substituted layers of hot wax. This proved inexplicable to Rogers, because it pulled out children's hair: "I remember a lot of the kids screamed over that."[112]

Although Mayor Marvin L. Kline, senior executive of its board, ran the Kenny Institute out of the Board of Public Welfare, it proved to be an expensive proposition for that city. In July 1944, he applied to the NFIP for an $840,000 grant, spread over three years, to continue Kenny technician training and "to establish a clinical research center at the Institute." O'Connor stalled initially; he had grown completely exasperated trying to work with Kenny as it was and wanted to avoid any closer associations with her. Not only did sharp personality differences exist between these two strong-willed individuals, but they also argued over policy matters. O'Connor eventually engaged an outside evaluation team from the National Research Council (NRC) to visit that facility and make a recommendation. The NRC sent a five-member committee on September 25 to commence its review. They met with Cole, Dean Diehl, Henry Haverstock Sr., Mayor Kline, Knapp, and Pohl, visited the facility, and watched Kenny demonstrate her methods. They found the institute's laboratory space inadequate. More importantly, "proponents seemed unable to explain how laboratory evidence would be integrated with clinical observation." Kenny's criticisms of the NFIP and O'Connor as well as her own antipathy toward additional research seriously undermined that grant's viability.[113]

O'Connor's grant rejection led to the establishment of the Kenny Foundation in March 1945. The Kenny-NFIP split was irreparable. The Kenny Foundation, in direct competition with the NFIP, embarked on its own national fundraising effort, with crooner and movie star Bing Crosby serving as honorary chair, and the foundation assumed responsibility for all of the Kenny clinics. Kenny's title "Sister" created confusion, causing many Roman Catholics to mistakenly support her for religious reasons. Crosby, a well-known Catholic, cemented this misperception. This initial campaign proved "vicious." Many state and local NFIP volunteers defected to the Kenny camp.[114] Its techniques, with pictures of young children disabled by poliomyelitis, celebrity endorsements, and Kenny's birthday as the annual kickoff, appeared remarkably similar to those of the March of Dimes. Kenny even resorted to staging major campaigns in New York City. Whether intentional or not, she seemed to be taunting O'Connor; she certainly eviscerated him in the press. Spokespersons for both organizations sniped at each other through the media. Kenny referred to her rival money-raiser as the "'O'Connor Foundation,' saying it was spending millions of dollars that belongs to the people to teach an obsolete theory." This inaugural campaign did not meet its goal of $5 million, raising only $516,000.[115]

The March of Dimes, however, continued to pay for patient care at the Kenny Institute in 1946 and 1947. A Kenny Foundation spokesperson publicly denied it. O'Connor also disclosed that the NFIP had "invested $653,852 to disseminate Kenny methods."[116] He otherwise remained mum.

More importantly, the NFIP had hired Harry Weaver as its research director in 1945, marking a shift in its agenda. "Weaver, and O'Connor, increasingly saw prevention, and not a therapist's magic hands, as the way to fight the poliovirus on its home ground." In addition to scattered breakthroughs, the NFIP began to study various strains of the poliovirus in 1947, the first step in developing a vaccine. The University of Pittsburgh's Jonas E. Salk became one of those investigators.[117] Kenny attended the Second International Poliomyelitis Conference in Denmark in September 1951, where Salk formally announced the results of the typing task, but the imminent possibility of a polio vaccine dominated the informal buzz at that meeting. She surely must have seen the writing on the wall. Suffering from Parkinson's disease, she returned to Australia after that trip; she would not witness the ultimate outcome of this research. Kenny succumbed to a stroke on November 16, 1952, and died less than two weeks later. That summer Salk quietly began to test a newly developed serum on children. This, however, did not diminish Kenny's contributions. She helped to revive the moribund field of physical therapy in the United States. This, along with the demands of veterans disabled by war, and with Howard Rusk's leadership, brought physical therapy to the forefront. In 1961, the federal government's Office of Vocational Rehabilitation recognized Rusk's Institute of Physical Medicine and Rehabilitation at NYU and the Kenny Institute, at the University of Minnesota, as the two leading centers for research and training purposes.[118]

Finally, therapists employed a few other post-acute treatment techniques to overcome, or at least minimize, paralysis. First, muscle training, which attempted to prevent atrophy, involved light and limited therapy through non-weight-bearing exercises; in short, the therapist supervised voluntary muscle motions. Second, underwater exercises—implemented "as soon as the acute pain and sensitiveness have disappeared," Lewin insisted, "possibly at the end of the seventh or the fourteenth day"—involved exercising in a stainless-steel tub of heated water, whether in a sixteen-inch-deep Hubbard tank or a four-foot-deep Pope tank. Third, the application of external dry heat increased blood circulation and offered patients some relief from the pain. Either light or heavy massage, conducted by trained personnel, usually followed. All of these treatments could take place in patients' homes, if they returned there soon after hospital quarantine. Visiting orthopedic nurses demonstrated physical therapy methods to parents such as warm tub baths, stretching limbs, hygiene, and diet. They also taught parents to use ironing boards or wood planks as stretchers. They covered lessons in the Kenny method as well.[119]

On the whole, the effectiveness of immediate post-acute care appeared good, according to data collected in 1941. The Harvard Infantile Paralysis Committee established that without aftercare, "the functional recovery of muscles is in ratio of 1 to 1. When parent or other untrained person administers the heat, massage and exercises, the return is 3 to 1; and when trained physical therapists give the child continuous care, the chance of recovery rises to 6 to 1." Another study found that children older than eight progressed much quicker than those three and younger. Lewin also pointed out that there "appeared to be but little difference in the progress of patients receiving rest, massage, and supervised motion who were adequately cared for in homes, and those who were hospitalized and given the same type of treatment." Thus, immediate, rather than delayed, physical therapy resulted in greater improvement.[120]

THE END OF CHILDHOOD

Suddenly wrenched from their families, entombed in terrifying large metal contraptions, facing death, enduring the sustained discomfort of immobilization and therapy, experiencing paralysis, and battling emotional depression, children with polio found their worlds transformed in every way. Hospitalization unleashed a host of emotions. Separation from their families elicited a great deal of stress, while the loss of motor functions intensified their insecurities. "The total situation," psychiatrist L. McCarty Fairchild wrote in 1952, "is one in which a tremendous amount of anxiety is thrust upon the patient in a short period of time. The resulting psychological picture frequently resembles the reaction to catastrophe." Collectively, children generally panicked at this stage. They seldom wanted to be alone, frequently requesting a staff member's presence. Staff responded by rejecting these pleas, seeing them as characteristic of a "spoiled" child; they simply refused to reinforce such behavior. However, such responses often backfired, causing more problems. This "failure to meet the initial dependency needs of the patient increases anxiety, dependency, and hostility," Fairchild explains. "Patients become angry when their needs are not fulfilled. This hostility is directed toward those failing to meet the patient's needs as he feels them. Patients already realistically dependent manifest this increase in anxiety and hostility by increasing their dependency demands." Patient enmity therefore grew from a secondary cause (the medical staff) rather than from the primary cause (the disease itself).[121]

Like most children affected by this virus, Marilynne Rogers's childhood ended with its onset. A normally active child who took dancing lessons and had many friends, she found that this had all disappeared: "When I came home from the hospital, my old friends would come over to visit, but we just didn't have much in common. They seemed really childish to me. I guess I had left my childhood years behind and was an adult emotionally. I had dealt with issues like life and death, and I no longer had anything in common with my friends . . . I just made new friends who were usually adults."[122] Many children infected by poliomyelitis experienced fragmented (if not isolated) and lonely lives, from the time they entered the ambulance until they returned to their homes; for others, it even stretched beyond that.

This disease sparked a process of isolating bodies, a process that assumed public, physical, and medical manifestations. Social consequences, however, overshadowed all of it. Neighborhood quarantine policies, spatially detaching the ill from the healthy, initiated it. Hospitalization followed, literally ripping children from their parents. This series of separations continued with rehabilitation during which these children could assess, with their own eyes, who was progressing and who was not. Sometimes, depending on hospital policy, genderizing bodies occurred with boys' and girls' wards. In all cases, the racialization of bodies remained intact, segregating African American and European American children. At the conclusion of the hospitalization process, these children endured the final act of separation: the different worlds of the disabled and the able-bodied. Therefore, children who contracted poliovirus ever so gradually withdrew from their former lives; as if moving ever outward through concentric circles, they followed a series of changes that steadily and completely severed them from their pre-polio selves. Even when they cheated death, they often perished socially.

Chapter 3

After Treatment

Oh Lord: Restore me to that state of mind and body in which I was, when you created me.

—Polio child's prayer

The *New York Times* boldly announced the commencement of the "anti-paralysis war" on July 11, 1916. Until that point, hospitals simply released their charges—no plan existed for subsequent treatment. The New York City epidemic, however, had introduced an unprecedented scale of sudden disability among young children that immediately overwhelmed public agencies as well as private ones. Aftercare in general did not seem important prior to 1916. Only prompt medical procedures or therapy prevented these children, the *Times* further reported, from "being crippled for life." The challenges of polio aftercare had rudely awakened American society. The initial response was scattered and loosely coordinated. In the decades to come, philanthropic and organizational responses to physical disability reached a magnitude unmatched in American history. Following initial diagnosis and quarantine, physicians sent many children to convalescent departments within hospitals or separate institutions, where they faced a rigorous regimen of physical activity or additional medical remedies. Others were sent home, where their mothers supervised their convalescence.[1]

A Medical Emergency

The New York City health department, the "public health vanguard for the nation," had long worked informally with charitable organizations, exchanging information about those infected and about aid provided. These benevolent societies especially focused on children with physical disabilities, with the earliest efforts growing out of tuberculosis. Polio epidemics intensified this effort "to identify, track, and guide crippled children to services." Business and fraternal groups, as medical historians Amy L. Fairchild, Ronald Bayer, and James Colgrove point out, "emerged as the leaders of the movement to assist 'crippled children'" following World War I. Restoring children to their "full economic potential" drove these efforts; they desperately wanted to eliminate social dependence.[2]

Some of that city's boroughs pursued their own efforts. On July 9, 1916, *The New York Times* reported that Louis C. Ager, who headed Brooklyn's aftercare program, solicited donations totaling $774 to subsidize follow-up attention. In the same article, the *Times* described the formation of the Committee on Crippled Children of the Brooklyn Bureau of Charities, which would attempt to address the needs of children who had been released by hospitals. Two months later, Ager pleaded in an open letter to that newspaper for contributions to the Kingston Avenue Hospital to subsidize the treatment and purchase of equipment, such as small chairs with trays, for children disabled by infantile paralysis.[3]

By the end of July, New York City's health officials took additional action. Health Commissioner Haven Emerson undertook a twofold policy. The first provided information. In a notice titled "Information for Parents of Children Recovered from Poliomyelitis," he offered advice about subsequent treatment to prevent "deformity" and included a list of hospitals that provided aftercare treatments.[4] In early September under Emerson's direction, the health department sent another circular to parents, just before their children were discharged from the hospital, giving them instructions about care: "With proper care this deformity will be greatly lessened. With neglect it will tend to increase. You are strongly advised to consult your family physician . . . or to visit the nearest one of the orthopedic dispensaries in the city given on the inclosed [sic] list. In any case, place your child under proper supervision for at least a year, as this tends to lessen permanent disability; neglect may increase deformity." He recommended three facilities: the Hospital of the New York Society for the Relief of Ruptured and Crippled, the New York Orthopedic Hospital, and the Hospital for Deformities and Joint Disease. As the health department's Donald A Baxter pointed out in the *Times*, they provided surgical procedures that relieved children from "lifelong deformity or crippling."[5] Other than this advice, the health department required no parental compliance and offered no assistance, relying on altruism and settlement house personnel.

Second, again relying on informal and voluntary means, Emerson, through the auspices of the department of health, began to solicit public donations to purchase "braces and supports . . . for the hundreds of children soon to be discharged from hospitals as recovered, but crippled." He estimated a total outlay of $15,000, with each case averaging $15.[6] The Guggenheim family generously gave $500. More modest donations continued to roll in, ranging from $2 to $100. Money sent to *The New York Globe* and *The New York Times* from their readers was turned over to the department of health. City officials increased their estimate for care and braces for "poliomyelitis convalescents" to $100,000 on January 1, 1917. Even more would be required after that date. By mid-September, contributions to the health department's brace fund grew to $40,000. Contributors included individuals but also businesses, like *The New York Tribune* and *The New York Times*. The latter listed the names of those who gave money and toys to the brace fund.[7]

Private organizations and philanthropies emerged as leaders in the aftercare movement, albeit largely through loosely managed efforts; it appears that institutional overlap and replication were prevalent. Lillian D. Wald, the head social worker of Manhattan's Henry Street Settlement, pleaded for aftercare facilities on July 20, 1916, meeting with polio expert Simon Flexner of the Rockefeller Institute for Medical Research (RIMR) and Emerson. Public officials, she pointed out, had been focused on the epidemic and preventative measures, but they had not considered the need for convalescent care. That settlement house was already sending orthopedic nurses to treat discharged children in their Bronx and Manhattan homes. Mrs. Averill Harriman donated $1,250 to Henry Street to subsidize the employment of an aftercare nurse. Other such gifts allowed the settlement to hire two more nurses. These health-care workers found complete disarray in families that had to care for children with paralysis. The children's weight alone often prohibited their mothers from moving or transporting them. Moreover, parents knew nothing about designated dispensaries where treatment was available. One donor gave that settlement house a car to facilitate transportation. The East Side Settlement House supplied braces, nurses, and "special medical care." By late August the sheer number of paralyzed children and the intensity and variety of their disabilities proved to be overwhelming. The Day Home and School for Crippled Children appealed for $10,000 to equip its facility with the apparatus necessary to care for children paralyzed by polio. Chaos reigned, with little or no coordination between various charities and the health department. The Children's Brace Fund for Victims of Infantile Paralysis was distinct from the Department of Health's campaign to provide apparatuses. On August 10, Mrs. W. W. Hoppin, Jr., treasurer of the Opposite House, wrote a letter to the editor explaining the need for the *Times* to promote public contributions to the Children's Brace Fund in order to help the "little cripples," in lieu of public rallies now banned by the health department to reduce infection rates. In October the Woman's American Supply League announced that the first motor ambulance of its "Militia of Mercy" would convey children disabled by this disease from their homes to hospitals where they would receive after-treatment. Meanwhile, in yet another initiative, several orthopedists agreed to contribute their services to "the needy" while charitable organizations continued to mobilize.[8]

This frenetic activity and confusion was not lost on key stakeholders. Jerome D. Greene, the Rockefeller Foundation's secretary, organized a one-day conference of leading orthopedists on August 5, 1916, at his office to effect some coherence. The foundation sponsored this conference because it had received numerous appeals from charitable organizations seeking aftercare support. It needed to tap expertise before it embarked on such ventures. That meeting included Greene; Wickliffe Rose, director-general of the

International Health Board; Flexner; Emerson; Dr. Linsley Williams, state deputy commissioner of health; fourteen orthopedic physicians and administrators from that city's hospitals; and five physicians from across the country but predominately from the East Coast, including Robert W. Lovett, professor of orthopedics at Harvard University, chief surgeon at Boston's Hospital for Crippled and Deformed Children, and a leading polio expert. The foundation appointed an advisory committee of orthopedic surgeons to oversee fund allocations. It also underwrote the New York City Committee on Aftercare of Infantile Paralysis Cases so that it could treat 2,000 children a year at an estimated cost of $37 a case.[9]

This committee gathered statistics about those infected, disseminated information about this virus, and arranged assistance for poor families. It divided New York City into districts, systematically grouping aftercare cases within them. It sponsored instructional activities as well, at a cost of $75,000 a year. The aftercare committee also secured a sanitarium in Stephney, Connecticut, where many of New York City's young patients were sent to recover; this represented a temporary solution, however. In one apparently well-executed effort, that committee used Henry Street's visiting nurses to check on paralyzed children recovering at their homes. They would ensure some degree of medical oversight as well as educate parents about aftercare. That settlement house already had 108 nurses in the field and would hire at least 10 more in subsequent weeks. This cooperation appeared rare, though. When New York's mayor, John Mitchel, sought advice about the feasibility of "establishing a colony of convalescents in the Jacob Riis Park or on other suburban property belonging to the city" to centralize care, Thomas J. Riley, chair of the Committee on Aftercare, bluntly disagreed and recommended instead that children remain with their families while the city made provisions to treat these children "either in its own municipal hospitals or in private institutions."[10] The term "colony," of course, connotes a location of outcasts, to be avoided, isolated, or discarded. Whether this attitude overtly drove Riley's opposition remains unknown, but it certainly appears to be implicit. The sheer number and presence of children with physical disabilities, in addition to being a medical challenge, began to grow into a social and political problem.

The Committee on Aftercare secured about $186,000 from "other sources for braces, treatment, and transportation." One of its approaches involved sending a general appeal letter during the Christmas holiday to tap into that season of giving. It relied on an emotional message comparing these children with "Tiny Tim," accompanied with photographs of them appearing at bottom of the letter. This became a consistent part of that organization's letterhead, first appearing in early 1918. This tactic, in many ways, foreshadowed the poster child used decades later by the National Foundation for Infantile Paralysis (NFIP). In 1919, the aftercare committee issued its general appeal letter but enclosed a contribution card and a pre-addressed envelope. The reverse side of that card now featured a picture of a child in braces being held upright by his sister, with a caption reading, "I'm teaching

Jimmie to walk again with his new braces." This, of course, exploited readers' feelings of pity in hopes of extracting cash donations—again, the prototypical poster child campaign.

In November 1916 Jerome Greene wrote Lillian Wald, saying that the Rockefeller Foundation wanted various agencies, after initially mobilizing them, to closely coordinate their aftercare efforts. An internal directive from John D. Rockefeller Jr. to Greene on August 21 had precipitated the Greene-Wald correspondence. In it Rockefeller reaffirmed his enthusiastic support of the aftercare initiative but, at the same time, stressed the foundation's limited role. It would merely act to advise and nurture the Committee on Aftercare; otherwise, it assumed no responsibility for it.[11] The Rockefeller Foundation contributed an additional $41,000 but made plans to withdraw its support by the early months of 1919, hoping that other agencies would assume responsibility.[12]

After-treatment issues loomed ever larger as outbreaks continued unabated and thousands of survivors emerged with physical disabilities. New York City's "premier charitable organizations" maintained a long and effective track record in combating childhood illness, like tuberculosis.[13] The 1916 polio epidemic likewise produced some initial private philanthropic responses; to a great extent, the Rockefeller Foundation symbolized the prototype. During and immediately after that outbreak, it embarked on three initiatives: public health measures, research efforts, and aftercare. First, as we saw, it subsidized the mayor's blue-ribbon emergency committee that consisted of Flexner, Doty, Emerson, and Goldberger. It tracked any reported cases and their families, and it oversaw isolation of those infected. Second, Flexner set up research facilities at the Rockefeller Institute. Third, the Rockefeller Foundation donated funds to aftercare charities, dedicating a total of $147,300 to public health efforts to control poliomyelitis epidemics in the New York City area, finance research, and assist charities in aftercare efforts. The latter alone absorbed $81,300 of the total: $41,800 to the city's Committee on Aftercare, $21,000 to the State Charities Aid Association, and $12,000 to the Brooklyn Bureau of Charities.[14] However, this represented a temporary, local endeavor; no permanent and well-financed private or public institutional support existed for the treatment of children disabled by infantile paralysis. Still, whether local or national, such disease campaigns were not new to American culture.

The Role of Philanthropy

Charities and their nonprofit organizations conducted prevention programs, subsidized treatments, and funded medical research. This would not occur with poliomyelitis until the advent of the Georgia Warm Springs Foundation in 1927, succeeded by the President's Birthday Ball Committee (PBBC) in 1934, and ultimately four years later by the NFIP. Its famous progeny, the March of Dimes, pioneered a public relations campaign that, to this day, many charities emulate. Its contribution to the eradication of this disease is without a doubt significant, but its methods did not prove to be entirely unique. Other disease campaigns, during the late nineteenth and early twentieth centuries, prefigured the foundation's sophisticated use of public relations methods.

The appearance of germ theory stimulated the development of foundations focused on specific diseases, like the National Tuberculosis Association. This disease caused 15 percent of all deaths in urban areas during the early twentieth century. In 1890 Robert Koch, a German medical researcher, announced that he had discovered the tubercle bacillus and a means of treatment, touching off the tuberculosis education campaign. Likewise, the idea to create and sell a special stamp to generate donations for the care of tubercular children originated in Denmark. In the United States, that movement grew and matured during the late nineteenth and early twentieth centuries. The Pennsylvania Society for the Prevention of Tuberculosis, a pioneering organization, was founded in 1892. Such voluntary medical associations evolved when Emily Bissell developed a one-cent Christmas stamp, or seal, to raise funds for a tuberculosis hospital in Delaware. This officially inaugurated the Christmas Seal campaign that continues to this day, and the Pennsylvania Society for the Prevention of Tuberculosis used this to forge mass education and fundraising techniques to fight the disease. "Christmas Seals, which were first sold in December 1907, captured the public's interest, broadened the Society's constituency, and fattened its treasury. Between 1908 and 1911, its income more than doubled, allowing annual expenditures of $9,947 by March 1911." The society also targeted churches, the press, and public schools to spread information. The latter program began in 1909 using traveling exhibits and other educational activities. Nevertheless, no

> method of public persuasion reached a greater audience than did the Christmas Seal campaign. In 1911 . . . more than eight hundred businesses—drug stores, cigar stores, department stores, and restaurants—participated in selling the stamps, while nearly every streetcar in Philadelphia carried an advertisement for them . . . By attaching the little stamps to their letters and packages, users learned about the campaign, publicized it, and felt good about helping others, especially at Christmas.[15]

Other, similar state efforts followed, culminating with the establishment of the National Association for the Study and Prevention of Tuberculosis in 1904; this organization shortened its name fourteen years later to the National Tuberculosis Association (NTA)—now the American Lung Association. The "anti-TB societies mounted the first truly mass health education campaign directed at a single disease." The campaign stressed printed media as well as visual; medical historian Nancy Tomes labels this as "popular health education." This association and its affiliates promoted anti-tuberculosis messages through billboards, films, newspaper articles, pamphlets, parades and pageants, popular lectures, posters, and traveling exhibits. For the first time, pictures of infected children became a symbol to exploit for fundraising purposes. These appeals legitimated research through emerging laboratory science. Prevention efforts promoted sanitary practices, such as by condemning the sharing of communion cups, outlawing public spitting, outlining housekeeping guidelines, and publicizing tuberculosis symptoms. Personal hygiene received special attention: Men had to shave their beards and mustaches, where it was believed that tuberculosis bacteria lurked; handshaking and kissing, as general social greetings, had to be avoided to reduce the spread of this contagion. African Americans, immigrants, and the poor served as scapegoats, the source of tuberculosis contagion.[16] The NTA also sponsored mass diagnoses. Tuberculosis checkups swept the nation using mobile units, like X-ray buses and trucks, to conduct examinations of individuals right in their neighborhoods. In many instances, these X-ray units stopped at schools to test the students en masse; such was the case in Wilmington, Delaware. Eventually, in 1947, the Division of Tuberculosis Control of the U.S. Public Health Service gave grants to cities and states for "tuberculosis control programs, and mobile chest radiology teams."[17] The anti-tuberculosis crusade in many ways foreshadowed the public relations strategies employed by the March of Dimes.

Diphtheria serves as yet another example. "Diphtheria toxin caused a thick, gray coating on the back of the throat that made it difficult for children to swallow or breathe." Suffocation could result. "The toxin also traveled to the heart, causing heart failure, and to the nervous system, causing paralysis."[18] In 1894, Emil von Behring and Carl Fraenkel, along with Shibasaburo Kitasato at the University of Berlin, coupled with the experiments of Emile Roux and Louis Martin at the Pasteur Institute in Paris, developed the notion of an antitoxin for the prevention and treatment of tetanus and diphtheria. In the United States by the 1920s, "prophylactic injections against diphtheria joined smallpox vaccination as the second immunizing procedure to be widely used by the general public." The Milbank Memorial Fund played a major role in this development. Founded in 1905 by Albert G. Milbank and devoted to education, health causes, and general social welfare, it donated $5,000 to a New York statewide diphtheria campaign in 1926. In so doing, it provided the "essential element in the administrative apparatus that brought toxin-antitoxin to the people through clinics and trained medical and nursing personnel." Although health officials used the "newest techniques of mass persuasion—newspaper advertisements, billboards, motion pictures, staged publicity events, colorful placards, using emotional appeals to parental duty and sentiment—[to] motivate the public," it all "proved ephemeral, requiring constant reinforcement that was expensive and time consuming."[19] This foreshadowed the polio vaccine campaigns of the late 1950s and early 1960s, appealing to a then-apathetic public as the frequency and intensity of these epidemics plummeted. Nevertheless, in the short run, New York City's diphtheria campaign appeared to be a success. That city's health department created mobile centers that circulated throughout poor communities, inaugurated health mobiles, and opened temporary clinics at public beaches and in local hospitals. "By the end of 1929 a total of 292,000 children were immunized with toxin-antitoxin, and the diphtheria rate fell from 6.75 per 100,000 in 1928 to 2.75 per 100,000 by the end of the year. The bulk of immunizations were given by the health department, and only 30 percent by private physicians." In sum, a continuum of health crusades promoted the growth of large and private nonprofit organizations.[20]

An institutional response to poliomyelitis, therefore, did not emerge in a vacuum. It certainly began with the Warm Springs, Georgia, treatment center, but separate developments converged to create that facility. Hydrotherapy itself was not new or even innovative. Germans had long practiced the partaking of mineral waters or sitting in heated springs to absorb the healing powers of nature. It spread to the rest of Europe, in the form of spas or resorts, and grew especially popular in the United States by the 1840s. In 1911 physicians and therapists began to prescribe it for children with orthopedic disabilities. At Gonzales, Texas, Warm Springs, a "spring of hot mineralized water flowed into a large circular tank on the grounds and into the swimming pool." In the case of infantile paralysis, water made bodies buoyant, allowing children to move, at least partially. The water's pressure and warmth also increased blood circulation to their paralyzed limbs. The Southern spa model proved to be the most influential. Usually located in a rural setting, it "offered only one hotel, fronting a park with surrounding cabins, in which clientele spent the summer partaking the waters." Walkways connected the cabins. This was precisely what Franklin D. Roosevelt discovered in Georgia.[21]

That complex also fit into a long tradition of isolated retreats where ill individuals sought treatments or cures for various diseases. Among these were sanatoriums based, again, on German models. They became increasingly popular in the United States during the late 1800s to nurse tuberculosis patients. The Adirondack Cottage at Saranac Lake, founded in 1885 by New York City physician Edward L. Trudeau, became the best known. It operated as a private institution and thus catered to affluent consumptives. In 1898, Massachusetts opened the first state-sponsored, open-air sanatorium. After years of planning and lobbying, the Pennsylvania Society for the Prevention of Tuberculosis secured an initial subsidy from Harrisburg, the state capital, to open a free hospital for patients at Lawrence F. Flick's White Haven, in the Lehigh River Valley, in 1901. Flick, a Philadelphia physician who had tuberculosis himself, had organized that society six years earlier. The maintenance of this facility, however, depended solely on donations from wealthy contributors.[22] Unlike private and fully and partially state-subsidized medical treatment institutions for consumptives, Georgia Warm Springs only relied on philanthropic sources to provide free therapy for individuals disabled by infantile paralysis.

This virus had disabled former assistant secretary of the navy and vice presidential candidate Roosevelt in 1921; he discovered the therapeutic benefits of Warm Springs three years later in Meriwether County, Georgia. It had a population of 26,000, mostly impoverished African Americans. There Roosevelt believed that he could swim his way back to health in the hot springs, and he convinced others as well. He purchased it for $200,000 on April 29, 1926, ignoring the concerns of his wife, Eleanor, and defying the advice of his law partner, Basil O'Connor. He poured his heart and soul into that facility, purchasing additional property adjacent to it for expansion. With New York architect Henry Toombs, Roosevelt designed a campus-like setting. He also oversaw the construction of a new cottage for himself and adapted all aspects of this dwelling, raising the toilet and bathtub, for example, to make them easily accessible. After winning the 1932 presidential election, Roosevelt's cottage became known as the Little White House. O'Connor formally filed for nonprofit status with the New York State Board of Charities, creating the Georgia Warm Springs Foundation, and appointed a board of trustees to oversee its operations. The Patients' Aid Fund, a largely informal operation, generated a modest revenue stream to cover the costs of those who could not afford to pay for their stay. Roosevelt effusively pushed the institutionalization process, which quickly unfolded, and won legitimacy for the facility from the medical community when the American Orthopedic Association endorsed it in January 1927. Warm Springs had developed from a regional, dilapidated, and outdated nineteenth-century spa to a twentieth-century, world-renowned center for the treatment of individuals disabled by infantile paralysis, the first in the United States.[23] O'Connor, raised in Boston, followed a wholly different path than that of the wealthy Roosevelt. He had worked his way through Dartmouth College and Harvard Law School to become a successful New York City corporate attorney. He invited Roosevelt as a law partner in 1924. After becoming New York's governor in 1928, Roosevelt relinquished supervision of Warm Springs to O'Connor, who continued to improve both the facility and care, overseeing the construction of an indoor swimming pool and a new main building. Roosevelt sought initial funds through philanthropic donations. Contributors included Edsel Ford. John D. Rockefeller Jr. alone gave a total of $65,000 from 1928 to 1933. The Great Depression, however, exacted a heavy toll on donations, and for all intents and purposes, Warm Springs was broke by 1933. This forced O'Connor to shape a formal, national fundraising campaign. He recruited public relations experts from New York to devise a keynote fundraising event. They decided that a national celebration of the new president's birthday provided the perfect opportunity and sponsored a musical benefit at New York City's Carnegie Hall, collecting $25,000. This spawned the National Committee for the Birthday Ball for the President, a celebration held every January using the luxurious Waldorf Astoria Hotel in New York City as its national headquarters. The inaugural national event took place on January 30, 1934, held in venues ranging from the Waldorf Astoria to one-room country schoolhouses throughout the country. It raised over one million dollars from "4,376 communities that had held 6000 separate celebrations." During its first year it allocated $100,000 to research. This successful annual event solidified Warm Springs's future, allowing treatment centers to be opened throughout the country. The second Birthday Ball proved to be even more successful, with 70 percent of all proceeds remaining with the local communities that had participated. Barn dances, hay rides, horseshoe contests, ski jumping events, and spelling bees represented many of the rural examples, while auctions, boxing matches, costume and formal balls, and dog and horse shows typified urban activities. Of all of the activities celebrated nationwide, none could top the annual black-tie affair at the Waldorf Astoria. In 1938, it occupied six ballrooms, with a renowned orchestra performing in each, and featured a cake over six feet in diameter. Noted donors, like Mrs. John D. Rockefeller Jr., famous musicians, Hollywood actors and actresses, and star athletes added to the glamor. In addition to ensuring treatment subsidies, this national charity developed a scientific arm, the Research Commission, led by Paul de Kruif, to begin to develop a cure. Nevertheless, the Birthday Ball Commission became a political liability: The bounds between private charity and public office blurred, with the White House staff and postmasters nationwide working on the annual campaign.[24]

March of Dimes

In an official statement dated September 23, 1937, Roosevelt introduced the National Foundation for Infantile Paralysis, sketched its scope, and declared that he would not longer be directly affiliated with any more fundraising activities, citing political reasons. In a second announcement, dated November 8, 1937, he traced how the President's Birthday Ball event and Georgia Warm Springs Foundation would be absorbed into the new organization. That same month Eddie Cantor, a popular singer and Hollywood star, coined the name "March of Dimes" for the foundation's massive fundraising campaign. Appealing for a mere dime enabled everyone to participate. This fueled a remarkable populist phenomenon, with ordinary individuals plunking their pocket change into March of Dimes cans at cinemas and retail stores, or giving money during nationwide door-to-door campaigns. Collections at movie theaters alone amounted to $8 million in 1945, representing 44 percent of the foundation's gross revenue. It also relied on popular media outlets to rally public participation. The foundation systematically tapped into people's emotions by holding press conferences and staging photographic opportunities with children disabled by polio. The message was simple: on the one hand, they were to be pitied; on the other hand, they could be saved. This effort also tapped fear: "From 1949, American cinemas were invaded by *The Crippler*, a twenty-minute melodrama"; that is, polio threatened everyone.[25]

The cover of 1938 issue of the *President's Birthday Magazine* depicts a broad-shouldered Roosevelt seated at a desk in the lower left-hand corner. He conveys the impression of a strong leader as he holds a pen in his right hand, intently staring into the distance. An extremely attractive and elegant woman with dark hair occupies most of the cover, but primarily the top right corner. She wears a dignified but nonetheless revealing satin gown as she parts a curtain with her left hand, peering down at Roosevelt. Four beautiful, wide-eyed children stand at the lower right corner, arranged in a pyramid. Two look directly at the reader, while one stares off to the left, and the fourth, who appears to be the oldest, holds a crutch as she looks admiringly at Roosevelt. A fifth child, in the lower left corner, stands at the president's elbow and, like him, stares off into the distance. All five of the children are girls. This cover was a replica of a full-sized painting, titled *The Dawn of the National Foundation*, by Howard Chandler Christy, an illustrator renowned for his patriotic World War I poster *Fight or Buy Bonds* (1917). Ms. Elise Ford modeled as the woman, while Christy used his granddaughter and four neighborhood girls as the other subjects. Christy's illustrations were scattered throughout this issue, with the same woman appearing as a winged angel. In all of them, Christy portrays Roosevelt as possessing great strength with his square jaw and broad shoulders. This was not new, though. Christy had painted another illustration for Roosevelt in 1935 with what appears to be Lady Liberty, enveloped in the stars and stripes, with her arms extended, each hand on the shoulder of a beautiful and healthy child. Reminiscent of war propaganda posters, these illustrations as a whole contained innumerable icons of vigorous, determined leadership; indomitable virtue; and innocent youth. The message the artist conveyed in using this style was nothing less than a crusade against a vile childhood disease.

Clearly no shortage of resources and goodwill existed for the launching of the NFIP. Thirty-three of the seventy pages of this monthly issue consisted of a broad assortment of commercial advertisements from major corporations— such as airlines, automotive, banks, and steel—that congratulated the president and expressed good wishes for the fledgling organization. O'Connor, working out of his law office, ensured that the foundation maintained even closer Hollywood connections and support than its predecessor. That particular 1938 issue contained nineteen separate pages of celebrity photographs and testimonials. These included radio and stage performers like Jack Benny, Milton Berle, George and Gracie Burns, Al Jolson, Ethel Merman, and Kate Smith. Numerous famous movie stars, such as James Cagney, Joan Crawford, Bette Davis, Rosalind Russell, and the inimitable Marx Brothers, loaned their names and images to the cause. Finally, athletes included Olympic and professional stars like Sonja Henie and Gene Tunney. All of them appealed for donations to save these children and, in doing so, conjured up sorrowful images.[26]

Such "celebrity diseases," as Nancy Tomes labels them, not only raised the public's consciousness but also served as organizational faces and fundraising icons. This phenomenon came to the fore during the interwar years. And the old media, such as the printed page, and new media, represented by movies and radio, fed it. The National Tuberculosis Association, as we have seen, became the "trendsetter" in exploiting these outlets, borrowing "heavily from contemporary advertising and marketing techniques." Endorsements from former presidents Grover Cleveland and Theodore Roosevelt elevated the NTA's profile. Revelations by author and playwright Nina Wilcox Putnam and baseball pitcher Christy Mathewson about their personal battles with tuberculosis expanded the audience and inspired people to contribute to the campaign against this disease. NFIP founders consciously modeled its operations after the NTA. Its use of media and celebrities, however, overshadowed the association's efforts. Tomes labels this the "celebrification" of polio, with movie stars like Jean Harlow, Ginger Rogers, and Robert Taylor willingly lending their names and campaigning to raise funds.[27]

A thirty-two page pamphlet, "'To Unify the Fight:' A New National Foundation for Infantile Paralysis," issued in early 1938, introduced the new organization to the public. It utilized stirring rhetoric, reflecting unyielding determination and irrepressible optimism, and resorted to pithy wartime slogans like "A Call to Arms!" "Organize–Mobilize" and "Forward March!" Such jingoism attempted to mobilize the American public in a "War on Infantile Paralysis." The nation had to marshal its financial and human resources to combat this dreaded disease, the pamphlet said, urging readers to "Enlist under the able direction of the President's committee and go into this fight to *win*." It enumerated a breathtaking agenda consisting of four points, which would drive the foundation's efforts for the next two decades. It would first embark on scientific research to find a means of immunizing everyone. Second, the foundation would provide "epidemic first aid" by supplying "orthopedic supplies and equipment" (e.g., iron lungs), medical personnel, and volunteers during outbreaks. Third, it would assure "proper care" through free braces and surgery. Fourth, and finally, the foundation would sponsor rehabilitation efforts to prevent "human wreckage." This involved aftercare treatments either at therapy centers or, where such facilities did not exist, by sending visiting nurses and other services.[28] "The NFIP, although a *private* foundation, assumed many of the financial and health functions that we associate nowadays with *public health*."[29] A massive publicity campaign blanketed the American public in the weeks leading up to the first March of Dimes campaign. "Walt Disney produced a special Mickey Mouse cartoon. Warner Bros. made two appropriate short subjects . . . A publisher's council enlisted the proprietors of 4100 newspapers; a medical council represented 400 public health officers; an orthopedic council got support from 1000 specialists; there was a motion picture council, and councils of women, hotels, sports writers, fraternities, and educators."[30] It proved to be an unqualified success. Between 1938 and 1945, it raised more than $49 million and treated 77,000 patients.

The March of Dimes became the crown jewel of the NFIP. It sponsored an event during the last two weeks of every January. Five key reasons, according to historian Stephen E. Mawdsley, explain its unqualified success. First, summer polio epidemics remained a constant reminder of this disease. Reported cases increased somewhat steadily from 4,033 in 1942 to 57,628 in 1952. Second, in lieu of health insurance, contributors saw their donations functioning as a kind of an investment; that is, a form of polio insurance. Third, the public witnessed concrete and visible benefits through the payment of medical bills. Between 1938 and 1960, the NFIP spent "$315 million on medical, hospital, nursing, and rehabilitative care for 325,000 polio sufferers." Fourth, the public's faith in science translated into confidence in the foundation's ability to find a solution. It spent $55 million on research and $33 million for fellowships and scholarships to train "medical students, postgraduate physicians, research, experts, physical therapists, medical social workers, and nurses." Fifth, the foundation exploited superb marketing techniques, with heavy use of celebrities and media, to repeatedly and effectively convey its message.[31]

The NFIP created an elaborate organizational structure that claimed 3,100 county chapters nationwide. Such local reliance represented an asset, on the one hand, because residents knew their territories and had personal contacts. Furthermore, the national office ensured that a major share of donations remained in those communities, thus giving an incentive to raise ever more funds. Philadelphia's 1953 financial contributions covered hospital patient expenses, rehabilitation hospital and home costs, treatments at hospital clinics, physical therapy at patients' homes, transportation, brace and shoe purchases, and social worker services. That local chapter also subsidized artificial respirators, including a plastic bubble that encased the child's entire head, eliminating the cumbersome and painful collar. These services totaled $113,892. "By the 1950s, the National foundation had developed the perfect form of philanthropy for the burgeoning consumer culture. The concept of philanthropy as consumerism—with donors promised personal benefits—was to a great degree the contribution of the March of Dimes."[32] On the other hand, this policy "sustained local customs of racial segregation or exclusion." This matter remained unresolved for the next two years, as NFIP officials "understood that recognizing black chapters would not only risk white opposition and add complexity to the Foundation structure, but also serve as a tacit approval of racial segregation."[33]

The NFIP likewise excluded African American volunteers in both the North and the South. Its leaders debated whether or not to use individual African Americans to collect donations. This vacillation evaporated against the backdrop of 1943's severe epidemic; with 12,450 reported cases, local "campaign chairpersons in the North and South became motivated to encourage the limited participation of African Americans in fundraising activities." An uneven pattern of regionally segregated fundraising resulted. Such local variations did not sit well with foundation officials, who preferred a "coordinated national effort to reach African-American communities with the March of Dimes." According to Mawdsley, two pressing demands on the national office forced a solution. First, the sharp rise in polio cases, with 19,029 reported in 1944, drained its coffers. "In fact, one specific epidemic that year in Hickory, North Carolina, required the Foundation to allocate approximately $400,000 to treat 454 patients (a rate of $881 per capita or 1/30 of their 1944 gross income)." The foundation desperately needed more human and financial resources to replenish its coffers. Second, they could no longer postpone the need to desegregate. Returning African American veterans, having fought European fascism, were now ready to challenge American racism. This became apparent in a 1944 confrontation when "African-American volunteers in Pittsburgh, Pennsylvania, refused to relinquish funds they had gathered in their community to the local white Allegheny County chapter."

John W. Chenault, resident head of the Tuskegee Infantile Paralysis Center, suggested a solution: appoint an African American executive to focus on African-American communities during the forthcoming 1945 fundraising campaign. He recommended Charles H. Bynum, then assistant to Tuskegee's president. NFIP officials agreed and hired him on November 1, 1944. "Bynum had become the first African-American executive to be employed by a national health philanthropy."[34]

He maintained a twofold and interdependent agenda during his tenure between 1944 and 1954. In particular, he "addressed the lingering disparities in racialized polio treatment"; in general, he "furthered the African-American medical civil rights struggle." Bynum accomplished this by expanding the foundation's reach, building interracial coalitions, and ensuring that African American children received better health care. In pursuing this plan, Bynum operated in a comprehensive manner. Mawdsley points to six specific elements. First, Bynum improved acute care for African American patients. Second, he extended convalescent care to them. Third, he directed NFIP grants to African-American "hospitals, training centers, and medical schools." Fourth, Bynum "fostered close alliances with the National Association of Colored Graduate Nurses, as well as influential black professionals." Fifth, he customized the foundation's fundraising techniques by targeting African American communities with a "series of special black posters, film trailers, and pamphlets." In 1952, Bynum developed a leaflet, "You Can Help Too," that featured an interracial theme depicting African American, European American, and Latino children and medical professionals. Sixth, and finally, he ensured that the 1954 national field trial included African American physicians and children. Bynum's broad approach transcended Tuskegee, expanding the NFIP's reach to African American "professionals and medical training centers" throughout the South.[35] Bynum became known as "Mr. Polio" in the black press because of these initiatives.[36]

Poster Children

The public's attitude toward those *afflicted* focused on sympathy, which many individuals disabled by infantile paralysis found to be wholly "vicarious."[37] Nothing symbolized this more than the March of Dimes poster child introduced in 1946. Internal debate occurred among the foundation's campaign organizers over how to portray these children: "As cheerful and optimistic or frightened and sad? As moving confidently toward a full recovery or facing a cruelly uncertain future?"[38] They chose the former, "a vibrant model of the ideal polio survivor: well-dressed, well-groomed, full of vitality, needing only the support of the public to be complete. It was exploitive and manipulative, but the cause was worthy, and the campaign worked."[39]

Who served as models represented another difficult decision. "Every parent of every poster child wanted that child to be associated with the March of Dimes," according to Charles Massey, hired in 1948 to organize chapters in Arkansas, Georgia, and Kentucky. "It was," he continues,

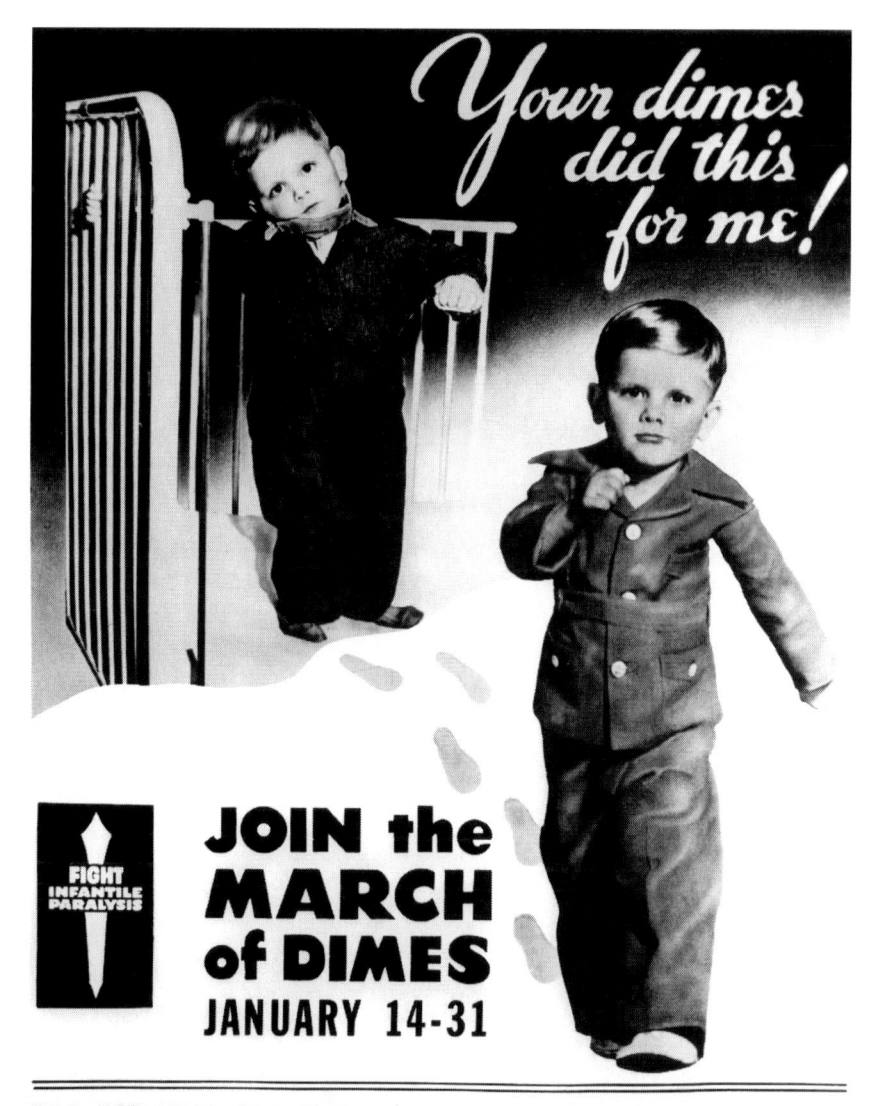

Figure 3.1 Anderson poster. Courtesy: March of Dimes.

almost like a beauty contest in every community. Which child would be selected would depend not just on their appearance, but on the ability to deal with the public, to represent and to be an ambassador for the March of Dimes. We found that the parents were actually promoting their children in this contest, and we were very concerned not to appear like we were exploiting these children. So we would go through all kinds of maneuvers. We would meet with the parents, we'd meet with friends of the family, and so forth, to be sure that this was something they wanted to do.

This occasionally encompassed public appearances. Carol Boyer, a poster child from Washington, DC, found herself displayed for fundraising events as well as for a photo opportunity with Vice President Richard M. Nixon in 1953.[40] This concept "drew on several earlier examples, including the National Tuberculosis Association and U.S. Government War Bond posters, in their use of vivid colors and dramatic depictions" of children, albeit only European Americans until 1947.[41]

Bynum recommended that a set of posters be prepared and distributed that featured an African American child, primarily aimed at African American communities in the South, in order to build trust and support for the foundation's fundraising campaigns. This symbol would demonstrate that the NFIP used its contributions to treat African American children. It also would help erode—he hoped—racial prejudices among European Americans. He could point to a precedent: African American volunteers in "Cook County, Illinois, and Wayne Country, Michigan, had already developed their own posters for an African-American audience." Foundation executives at first balked at Bynum's suggestion. In a seemingly well-meaning way, but one certainly convoluted, they feared that using separate posters, featuring a child from each race, would only reinforce existing "racial divisions." They asserted that the image of a European American child represented a "universal" one, ensuring a unified campaign. But they eventually relented in 1947 and authorized "an order of 3,000 copies of the existing Cook County black poster for national distribution." Nevertheless, these posters were smaller, displayed in predominately African American communities, and eventually featured "light-skinned" children who might "appeal to both black and white viewers." These posters appeared highly effective, since donations increased by 400 percent. Bynum built on this success by using March of Dimes posters to illustrate racial integration: "the Randy Donoho poster (1953) depicted an African-American nurse caring for a white patient and the James Clark Allen poster (1955) showed an African-American physician injecting Salk's vaccine into a white child. In both cases, black professionals were situated in positions of trust providing care to white children."[42]

The poster child, unlike the iron lung, became a positive icon of poliomyelitis. Brenda Serotte, who contracted polio in 1954 at age seven in the Bronx, describes them as "large posters of adorable boys and girls on crutches, wearing metal leg braces. These beautiful, crippled children stood proud and straight as possible or sat in wheelchairs, which heightened their tiny vulnerability." The NFIP used these as rallying points to solicit public donations, as Serotte continues:

> One poignant poster showed a semi-toothless, freckled boy in a cowboy hat, standing with a crutch under each armpit, smiling bravely. "THIS FIGHT IS YOURS!" was the caption under his picture, and in the background stood a huge, scowling GI in combat gear with a rifle. The "FIGHT POLIO!" poster girls, in their delicate, puffed-sleeve dresses and matching hair ribbons,

couldn't have been prettier. One look at these courageous little people, with their luminous wide eyes and their own braces as badges of courage, and your heart caved in.

The NFIP borrowed a long-established tradition of pity and hope, charity and cure, appealing to the non-disabled public through pure sentiment. Widely displayed in storefronts and other public places, they became wildly successful. These children were "highly photogenic; they were picked for that . . . Children who, in another life, would have surely modeled clothes or tap-danced their way to fame and fortune."[43]

However, these posters also have elicited some widely divergent responses, leaving us with a complex legacy. Serotte tends to cast them in an ambivalent light; she simply did not want to be pitied. "Thank goodness for those posters. Although I was carefully guarded from seeing one, eventually I did, and that's how I know what I looked like. Otherwise, I never would have." Serotte's parents denied her disability: "There were not pictures of me taken . . . wearing braces, standing with crutches, or . . . sitting in a wheelchair." She fled these images of disability: "I was the opposite of a polio poster child: They were plastered everywhere with their appliances and sweet, sad faces in order to get sympathy; my mother's goal, and later mine, was to always repel sympathy and concentrating on being 'normal.'"[44]

Other individuals disabled by this disease outright resented these posters because they represented a carefully staged portrayal, conveying a wholly sanitized view. Lorenzo W. Milam, who not only contracted polio as a child but watched his sister die from it, sardonically describes them: "Those adorable little girls, in their pinafores, with their clear little blue eyes, and the sweet rosebud mouths. And their little crutches, and their tiny exquisite little braces on their little limbs! What a pretty disease! No drooling or twitching here! No shitting down the leg, convulsions or other indecent exposures."[45] Lenny Kriegel, who contracted polio at age eleven, expresses the complex world of children disabled by this disease: "Our condition is intense, our isolation massive. Society views us as both pariah and victim. We are pitied, shunned, labeled, classified, analyzed, and categorized."[46] Anne Finger, who became ill in the 1950s, focuses on the degree of manipulation by pointing out that only young children appeared in these posters, not teens or adults disabled by the disease; they would not elicit the high level of pity needed to generate ample contributions. However, an already vulnerable child felled by this virus elicited sympathy, assuring donations. Finally, Margaret Marshall, who contracted polio in 1955 while residing in Shrewsbury, Massachusetts, agrees that the poster child campaign certainly proved to be an unqualified success in generating contributions. But at the same time, they occasionally frightened some children. Whenever she saw them, she felt terror: "I would say my prayers, 'Oh please, God, don't give me polio.'" She contracted it at age five. Her worst fear had become reality.[47]

The poster child project backfired in at least one case, producing serious personal and social repercussions. Cyndi Jones, a 1956 poster child, felt special being photographed, appearing on billboards, and starring on a telethon. However, a few short months later, while sitting in her first-grade class, she confronted the reality of disability. Her teacher distributed a flyer encouraging poliomyelitis vaccinations. It contained two pictures. "One was of a young brother and sister, holding hands and joyfully skipping through a field. Over their picture was stamped: THIS. Next to them was a picture of Jones, leaning grimly on her braces, hair curled, decked out in one of her new party dresses. The caption over Jones's said: NOT THIS." She felt immediate rejection. "It had been a lie; she was not special—she and her polio were feared."[48]

In retrospect, disability scholar Rosemarie Garland Thomson maintains that the poster child is "the quintessential sentimental figure of twentieth-century charity campaigns." But her emphasis is not on the poster children per se; rather, she delves into these images' impact on the public. The viewer, usually an adult, can perform an act of "heroism" by donating a mere dime.

> The poster child of the 1940s and 1950s introduced two new elements into the rhetoric of sentiment that disability photography inherited from the nineteenth century. The first is that cure replaces suffering as the motivation for action in the viewer. Whereas the earlier sentimental literature accentuated suffering to mobilize readers for humanitarian, reform, or religious ends, the poster boy's suffering is only the background to his restoration to normalcy that results from "your dimes." Sentiment here, then, replaces the intensity of sympathy with the optimism of cure, testifying to a growing faith in medical treatment and scientific progress that developed as modernity increasingly medicalized and rationalized the body in the nineteenth and twentieth centuries. The second new element is . . . the self-serving opportunity that charity provides the giver for "conspicuous contribution." What is clearest is that this rhetoric of sentiment diminishes the disabled figure in the interest of empowering, enhancing, and enlarging the viewers' senses of themselves.

The poster child campaign operated as a clarion call to action. "Rhetoric is the art of persuasion. By formulating popular photographic images of disability as visual rhetoric, we cannot only 'read' the content, conventions, and contexts of the photographs but also probe the relationship the pictures seek to establish with the viewer. A rhetorical analysis such as this seeks to illuminate how and what the photographs intended to persuade their audiences to believe or do." The March of Dimes sought to mobilize compassion on a mass scale for these young *victims*, to generate donations, supply care and equipment in the short run, and find a cure and ultimately eradicate this disease in the long run. At the same time, these images detached the viewer from the viewed: "This inherent distancing within the photographic relationship replicates the social untouchability of disabled people, one of the most oppressive attitudes directed at them. The disabled figure in western culture is to-be-looked-at rather than the to-be-embraced." Garland Thomson "proposes a taxonomy of four primary visual rhetorics of disability: the wondrous, the sentimental, the exotic, and the realistic." Polio photographs clearly fit into the sentimental category. As she further asserts, "The sentimental places the disabled figure below the viewer, in the posture of the sympathetic victim or helpless sufferer needing protection or succor." The March of Dimes poster children therefore portrayed a "diminished" image "to evoke pity, inspiration, and frequent contributions." This produced "a spectacle of suffering rather than the reality of the suffering." The viewer was cast as "benevolent rescuer and the disabled figure as grateful recipient." For all of the well-intentioned efforts of the Easter Seal Society and the NFIP, they portrayed children with disabilities as helpless victims on their stamps and through their posters.[49]

The National Foundation for Infantile Paralysis's ability to mobilize the American public on a mass scale to raise funds and disease awareness as well as provide treatment and promote research for a cure has become legend. This alone represents a remarkable legacy. Nevertheless, one element remained missing; that is, disability rights. People with physical disabilities clamored for these basic needs as early as the mid-1930s. Roosevelt and NFIP leaders, from all appearances, remained mum. On the surface, advocacy did not appear as a main agenda item, but the NFIP's commitment to disability issues did exist, albeit piecemeal and nascent. First, Warm Springs served as a clearinghouse for various adaptations, such as automobile levers and house modifications. Second, the foundation tried "to find ways to make streets and sidewalks accessible for the disabled in wheelchairs." A 1954 grant to New York University, for instance, resulted in a curb-climbing wheelchair.[50] Third, the mere existence of a polio network, vis-à-vis newsletters, established the groundwork for a later, vital disability rights movement. Humane reasons certainly drove early aftercare endeavors. Disability, however, transcended the physical realm. It had created an incredibly challenging individual and social problem. The gravity of this is reflected in Philip Lewin's quote of a polio child's prayer in his authoritative 1941 work, *Infantile Paralysis*: "Oh Lord: Restore me to that state of mind and body in which I was, when you created me."[51]

A Social Crisis

"The chief terror of the disease," Flexner publicly stated in 1916, "lies in its appalling power to produce deformities."[52] A 1947 study revealed how his concern had grown at an alarming rate. Of the 163,998 cases reported in the United States between 1926 and 1946, about 140,000 survived the infection; 33 percent of these remained physically disabled to one degree or another. Age seemed to be a significant trait, regardless of the region. This disease continued to strike down young children well into the 1940s. Another study conducted between 1939 and 1944 focused on the "Chicago-Detroit" area and established that 89 percent of those infected were younger than the age of sixteen. And a 1942 analysis of northeastern states found a 70 percent rate for the same age group.[53] Paralysis sparked a traumatic social and emotional metamorphosis, embedded in the framework of disability.

Lenny Kriegel, who had contracted polio at age eleven, a resident of the Bronx, explains his anger about this life change: "The loss of my legs enraged me . . . Its arbitrariness, its naked proclamation of what I could and could not do, of what I could never do . . . [This] rage was testimony to the triumph of the virus."[54] His future had assumed a profoundly different trajectory. Young children, in general, would never experience adolescence in its truest sense, and adulthood had become another reality. Permanent paralysis signaled the end of one self at the same time as it marked the beginning of another self—a death followed by a birth.

Children embarked on an excruciating journey from the illusion of being able-bodied to the reality of being disabled as it hurled thousands of them and their families into this complex world. What does this mean? Disability operates, first, as a "system for interpreting bodily variations; second, it is a relationship between bodies and their environments; third, it is a set of practices that produce both the able-bodied and the disabled; fourth, it is a way of describing the inherent instability of the embodied self." It objectified children; it cost them their humanness. People perceived them differently, avoiding or fearing them if they saw them at all. When they did, their presence proved to be embarrassing or created discomfort. The seer and the seen exist in the public realm of disability. "The dominant mode of looking at disability in this culture is staring. Staring," Garland Thomson contends, "is the social relationship that constitutes disability identity and gives meaning to impairment by marking it as aberrant." The starer is "normal"; the disabled person is not. Starring represents an act of "exclusion from an imagined community of the fully human."[55] This assumed many manifestations. For Charles L. Mee, who became ill at age fourteen in Barrington, Illinois, it began at the hospital. After surgery that transplanted a thigh muscle to his abdomen, purportedly to help him walk, Mee found himself declared a success story and regularly displayed, virtually naked, to visiting physicians. He felt like he was in a freak show. "I was reduced to something even less than an object: I was specimen." That operation proved to be ineffective.[56]

To elaborate, first, disability did not operate as an "isolated, individual medical pathology" but rather functioned (and continues to do so in most cases) as a "social category on a par with race, class, and gender." The "impairment" experience always has been a subjective one, historically a moral, social, and/or political categorization of human beings. It became even more so with the medicalization of society, during the late nineteenth and early twentieth centuries, when it "created a special role both for the disabled person in society, and for disability as a social variable."[57] Disability therefore does not necessarily represent an organic phenomenon, one merely confined to a biological or medical condition, but is socially conceived, "in part by cultural definitions and in part by the demands and limitations of social and physical environments."[58] Society's narrow definition of "normal," the experience of social rejection, and the existence of environmental impediments all converge to create the disabled world. Disability thus transcends medical labels: Physical diversity does not operate as a pathology or represent deviance because it challenges the concept of the "norm." It does not connote aberrance but instead "arises from the interaction of physical differences with an environment." It represents a universal experience, not one relegated to particularism. In fact, everyone is temporarily non-disabled.[59] Able-bodiedness exists on borrowed time. Aging, an accident, or an illness will introduce disability. This forces a fundamental question: What is the norm?

This concept represented a product of mid-nineteenth-century thinking, one that connected to the "western notion of progress." The emerging idea of "evolution" created a sense of the normal; that is, "the average, the usual, and the ordinary." At the same time, it introduced the abnormal (i.e., the "*sub*normal"), which implied the primitive or savage.[60] A social hierarchy thus emerged based on social Darwinism, and disability served as a mark of inferiority.

Garland Thomson writes that both normal and disabled operate as "cultural constructions . . . [T]he 'physically disabled' are produced by way of legal, medical, physical, political, cultural, and literary narratives that comprise an exclusionary discourse . . . *[A]ll* forms of corporeal diversity acquire the cultural meanings undergirding a hierarchy of bodily traits that determines the distribution of privilege, status, and power." Traditional ideas have thus maintained narrow and fixed sets of dualities: attractive and repulsive; beauty and ugliness; independence and dependence. Social stigma accompanies disability; it denies "human agency." It defies the canon: "The disabled figure operates as a code for insufficiency, contingency, and objection—for deviant particularity . . . the disabled body is a spectacle—sympathetic, grotesque, wondrous, or pathological."[61]

Second, physical impediments defined disability. Individuals in wheelchairs not only found themselves blocked by insurmountable obstacles, such as stairs, but also experienced considerable discrimination. Deemed a hazard by apparently blocking the audience's access to exits in case of an emergency, ushers ordered Marilynne Rogers to leave a concert hall. She saw it differently: "It seemed to me that in case of a fire I'd be the one to get trampled. I was the one taking a chance. I left highly insulted." Extremely visible in their wheelchairs, they also suffered either from public displays of pity or social rejection, leading contradictory lives. In the former case, well-intentioned individuals showered them with sympathy, publicly humiliating them. In the latter case, their presence offended many people. "I was asked to leave a restaurant," Rogers recalls, "because it bothered the other customers."[62] Rogers, like others disabled by this disease, discovered her lack of rights, and her existence proved to be a subordinate one. As a result, she led a highly restricted social and cultural life.

Third, public policies legitimated this construct. Legislation and local laws reified disability, which represented nothing more than "a complex of constraints that the able-bodied imposes on the behavior of physically impaired people."[63] The "ugly laws," for instance, attempted to bar any human perceived as repugnant from the streets. Late nineteenth- and twentieth-century state and municipal statutes segregated the unsightly, broadly defined at times to include beggars, immigrants, racial groups, sex workers, and of course individuals with disabilities. Chicago's 1911 ordinance became the most notorious. These various laws did not, in fact, contain the word "ugly," but to historian Susan M. Schweik, it serves as a euphemism used to refer to numerous versions that included the words "deformed persons," "diseased or maimed persons," or "diseased or mutilated limbs," as well as "mendicants." She writes, "The ugly laws are part of the story of segregation and of profiling in the United States, part of the body of laws that specified who could be where, who would be isolated and excluded, who had to be watched, whose comfort mattered. Thinking about these ordinances in the terms of segregation reveals the crucial importance of space and placing in the constitution of American disability"[64] These policies upheld segregation on railroads and issued beggars' licenses to people with disabilities. Americans further reinforced the subordinate role of individuals with disabilities. The Vocational Rehabilitation Act of 1920 etched this in concrete: "This law's assumption that the value of physically impaired people is defined by gainful employment resulted in denying them the same opportunities of citizenship accorded the ablebodied population . . . the understanding that the government did nothing more to achieve their integration into society probably promoted the disabling belief that social marginality is a natural consequence of serious physical impairment." This legislation, along with that passed under President Roosevelt's administration, accentuated the "visibility of this favored class of handicapped citizens." Political scientist Claire H. Liachowitz adds, "Each of these administrative and legislative strategies may have sanctioned the negative attitudes of society toward those incapable of work, making integration of the 'subgroup' even less likely."[65]

Fourth, having become socially objectified, each child with a physical disability also had to cope with a new self-image. Prior to infection, many of these children may have perceived such individuals as deficient and less human; now, though, they had to grapple with this profound identity transformation. For them, the normal had become abnormal; the strong had grown weak; the independent had turned seemingly dependent. Fred Davis, based on his 1954–55 sociological research on the impact of this disease, writes that

> attempts, if any, to be accepted by "normals" are doomed to failure and frustration: not only do most "normals" find it difficult to include the handicapped person fully in their own category of beauty, but [the child disabled by polio] shares the "normal" standards of personal evolution, will in a sense support their rejection of him. For the fact remains that, try as he may to hide or overlook it, he is at a distinct disadvantage with respect to several important values emphasized in our society: e.g., physical attractiveness; wholeness and symmetry of body parts; athletic prowess; and various physiognomic attributes felt to be requisite for a pleased and engaging personality.[66]

This represented a common metamorphosis. Hugh Gregory Gallagher, a polio survivor himself, grew up during the 1930s and 1940s. Before he became paralyzed, he detested people with disabilities: "I would cross the street, rather than pass by a severely handicapped person." For him, disability conjured up a carnival sideshow oddity, one of nature's mistakes. "People with disabilities were seen as pests; they were also the objects of fun. People with physical deformities were exhibited at freak shows . . . [They] were cooed over or laughed at in traveling shows and vaudeville acts."[67] This included children disabled by infantile paralysis: "The polio Frog-Boy performed at circuses in New York in the 1940s."[68] These images extended to mass audiences as well, through the silver screen and television. Jerry Lewis, a leading comic in both mediums in the 1950s, became "a great hit with his gibbering imitation of the retarded and his grotesque burlesque of persons with cerebral palsy."[69] This new self-identity began to take shape as children moved from hospital care to rehabilitation.

INSTITUTIONAL TERRAIN

The institutionalization of children became commonplace by the early twentieth century. "Between 1890 and the early 1920s, the number of children housed in some form of institution grew from sixty thousand to more than two hundred thousand." The preventorium, for example, operated as a residential facility for children with tuberculosis. The first opened in 1908 in Lakewood, New Jersey. "The preventorium blended features of a hospital, sanatorium, and school, while endeavoring to imbue its patients with the values of an idealized middle-class home life." They grew rapidly. Between 1910 and 1940, forty-five existed with 2,783 beds.[70]

Edith Reeves Solenberger's 1918 Bureau of Education survey included "thirty-seven hospitals, convalescent institutions, and asylum homes," representing ten orthopedic hospitals, fourteen convalescent facilities, and thirteen asylums that serviced 2,500 children. Uneven regional distribution hindered treatment, according to this study. Twenty-seven of these care facilities were located on the East Coast, with nine in the Midwest and one in the West; the South had none. And the majority of these were situated in or near the densest population concentrations, with ten in New York City and Philadelphia alone. Most had opened within a 17-year period, from 1891 to 1908, covering the Progressive Era. Solenberger simplified these into three categories to offer clarity, but some functions certainly overlapped. As the twentieth century unfolded, all three of them would play key roles in treating polio patients. Finally, Solenberger overlooked private and public special education institutions, a formative phenomenon at the time of her publication, a more mainstream manifestation to address children with a variety of disabilities. And, of course, outside the scope of her survey and in the near future, the Georgia Warms Springs facility would emerge as a highly specialized philanthropic center to address the rehabilitation of children disabled by infantile paralysis alone.

Hospitals

Most hospitals, Solenberger found, dealt with "comparatively few orthopedic cases," per se. Any inpatient care usually only involved surgery.[71] "By the

1920s surgical admissions outnumbered medical. Ordinary Americans had not only begun to accept the [notion of] hospital [care], they had come to associate it with the surgeon." As a result, few offered physical therapy, with only five having some gymnasium equipment. Fewer still rendered educational services for young patients. Hospital dispensaries, however, provided outpatient care: parents brought their children for checkups by physicians and nurses.[72]

These free dispensaries and hospital outpatient clinics, subsidized by charity, served as the "principal form of institutional care for the [urban] working poor and the indigent" from the late eighteenth through the early twentieth centuries. In 1913, only "13 percent of the sick were admitted to hospitals." Service proved to be poor and superficial, with inconvenient and short hours of operation, causing long waiting times. No privacy whatsoever existed in these settings. Outpatient treatments declined in the 1920s as inpatient admissions increased and hospitals offered more encompassing care. Nevertheless, it remained common in 1940s New York City for patients to be picked up by station wagons and driven to the Joint Disease Hospital in Manhattan three times a week for rehabilitation.[73]

Visiting nurses assigned by hospitals also oversaw aftercare in children's homes, working principally with mothers. For example, in 1912 the New York Orthopedic Dispensary and Hospital employed four nurses who made 8,498 home visits, while surgeons themselves made 7,020. Home visits totaled 15,518, while patients attended its dispensary 27,140 times.[74]

These hospitals, according to Gallagher, were generally grim places, dreary edifices that appeared "indistinguishable from prisons and asylums." Their names reinforced social vilification: Brooklyn's House of St. Giles the Cripple, Philadelphia's Children's House of the Home for Incurables, and the New York Society for the Relief of the Ruptured and Crippled. The latter, founded in 1862 to serve the poor, provided braces, massage, physical training, and surgery. This hospital also maintained a school in addition to inpatient and outpatient care and services. It sent social workers to visit homes to oversee the general welfare of the children, such as giving them clothing. Nevertheless, Gallagher condemns them all as "debilitating" and actually "maiming and torturing" patients. In the most dramatic cases, a few surgeons preferred to amputate affected limbs.[75]

Specialized polio treatment centers only became common by mid-century. Houston, Texas, hosted one of the best-known treatment centers in the United States, the Southwestern Poliomyelitis Respiratory Center, operating as part of a network of care facilities funded by the March of Dimes. Opened in 1950, it was originally housed on the tenth floor of Jefferson Davis Hospital and affiliated with Baylor University's College of Medicine. Because of demand, a new separate, two-story building had to be built. City, county, state, and federal governments covered construction costs, while the March of Dimes supplied equipment, including eight tank iron lung respirators, four Monahan chest respirators, five rocking bed respirators, and a fluoroscope. It also had its own assistive device shop, producing a total of 803 items by 1955. Finally, that institution's social workers mediated patients' return home or transfer to a long-term care institution. It thus represented an example of an all-inclusive facility with critical care, rehabilitation services, occupational therapy, and social services.[76]

Convalescent Homes

These often served as interstitial institutions between hospitals and homes. Generally speaking, they offered the broadest array of services. Their medical staffs consisted of nurses and resident physicians, although they did not conduct any in-house surgical procedures, sending those cases to local hospitals. All such rehabilitation centers had gymnasiums for physical therapy. They also consistently provided schooling opportunities for school-age children. Both public and private examples "maintained organized instruction" such as age grading and individual instruction, usually with city school districts supplying teachers. Vocational education, though, dominated the curriculum. Informal training likewise existed, as children helped with domestic tasks, such as wiping dishes, setting tables, dusting furniture, sweeping floors, making beds, and gardening. This was seen as a "natural fashion"; that is, as Solenberger notes in her study, it "grows out of the life of a large residential institution." It certainly helped to defray operating costs. A number of well-known examples existed, including the New York Orthopedic Hospital in White Plains, the Minnesota State Hospital for Crippled and Deformed Children at Phalen Park, and the Convalescent Home for Crippled Children at West Chicago.[77]

However, the New York Hospital for the Ruptured and Crippled represented the first institutional attempt to confront the "crippled child" as a medical and social problem. Children with physical disabilities had appeared with the onset of the Civil War as beggars on city streets. James Knight, that hospital's first superintendent, set the reform agenda: "He used orthotic devices to correct or brace disabled limbs, a dietary regime and physical exercise, as well as moral instruction, academic education, and vocational training to bring his pupil-patients into conformity with nondisabled norms."[78]

The Gillette State Hospital for Crippled Children, a public facility, opened in 1897 as the Minnesota State Hospital for Crippled and Deformed Children. Although approved and funded by that state legislature, it fell under the auspices of the University of Minnesota's board of regents. They chose to operate the new facility at the existing City and County Hospital in St. Paul, treating children disabled by tuberculosis, cerebral palsy, and clubfoot, among others. Arthur J. Gillette, who had studied with leading orthopedists in New York City and served as an orthopedic surgeon at St. Joseph and St. Luke hospitals in Bethesda, Minnesota, as well as at City and County Hospital in St. Paul, became chief surgeon. The University of Minnesota medical school supplied other physicians. Because of high demand and the need to accommodate the latest medical equipment, the state subsidized construction of a separate and new facility at Phalen Park in 1914, renamed it the State Hospital for Indigent Crippled and Deformed Children, and placed its administration solely under state control. It sat on a large plot of land, with a lake, and had an auditorium, a brace department, a dentist's office, a dining room, a greenhouse, a laundry, a library, an operating room, an outpatient clinic, a swimming pool, wards, and nine acres devoted to growing fresh vegetables. Gillette died in 1921, and four years later the state legislature renamed the hospital the Gillette State Hospital for Crippled Children in his honor. It accommodated 138 patients and, in 1917–18, admitted a total of 426 children, primarily those disabled by tuberculosis. A new wing in 1925 expanded care to 233 child patients. Most of these children had been disabled by tuberculosis, but other diseases, like bone infections, clubfoot, scoliosis, and infantile paralysis, had taken their toll. Polio ultimately dominated patient rolls. Prior to 1917, only 34 children received treatments for this disease; that year alone the figure jumped to 106, and it steadily increased to 321 in 1946. Dr. Gillette had employed a teacher as early as 1898 for the hospital's schoolroom; this teacher followed the standard St. Paul public school curriculum. That district continued to send instructors to conduct classes in the new facility's several classrooms, and it provided textbooks. By 1928, seven teachers taught grades one through twelve. Hospital staff members pushed students, who attended five hours a day, in wheelchairs and entire beds into those classrooms; the latter only received half-day lessons. That institution also provided industrial courses. Here, gender differentiation existed, with girls cooking, learning to keep a household, and sewing, while boys wove baskets, gardened, and learned woodworking.[79]

Gillette Hospital became Jerry McNellis's "[second] family home for many years." Like other convalescent facilities, it maintained a rigid regimen. All of the children in a ward, sometimes consisting of forty to sixty young patients, brushed their teeth at the same time. A nurse also ordered them simultaneously to urinate and defecate into their bedpans; orderlies immediately removed all of those filled containers and loaded them on a tall rack with several shelves. For McNellis, "everything ran like clockwork. Cod Liver Oil. Brush teeth. Urinate. Bedpans. Bed baths. Breakfast. Get dressed. Our daily routine." They then went to occupational and physical therapy sessions, underwent dental and physical examinations, and attended hospital school. Finally, the staff assigned children to complete chores, such as feeding their roommates who could not do so themselves. The "main disciplinarian" ran her ward with "tight control," McNellis recounts. "She was loud and had real command of her ward." Penalties included "restraint in bed" and isolation in a room for two days at a time. If children dropped anything out of their beds, it was confiscated by the staff as punishment. Nurses also used a reward system to control children's behavior. "Good behavior all day got us a back rub or massage before bedtime," McNellis recalls. "Aides, orderlies, and nurses did them. I grew to love massage as a result . . . I think it's psychological: Be good. Don't screw off. Get a massage at night . . . Sort of like Santa Claus—it works until you figure out the scheme"[80]

The D. T. Watson Home for Crippled Children became a renowned treatment center for children disabled by infantile paralysis. David T. Watson, born in 1844 in Washington, Pennsylvania, forty miles south of Pittsburgh, graduated from Harvard Law School in 1865 and began his practice in Pittsburgh. He represented the movers and shakers of the glass, oil, railroad, and steel industries during the Gilded Age: Andrew Carnegie, Henry C. Frick, John Pitcairn, John D. Rockefeller, Sr. and William H. Vanderbilt. Watson willed, in perpetuity, that his estate, Sunny Hill, be used to care for forty white female children with physical disabilities, ages three to sixteen. That country home sat in Leet Township, just west of Pittsburgh along the Ohio River, occupying sixty-eight acres of gardens and woodlands. In addition to the main house, it hosted four additional buildings, two stables, a pumping station, and a water tower. Watson likewise bequeathed funds to pay for patient care and facility maintenance. His will stated, "These children shall be clothed and fed and educated solely at the expense of the charitable organization." They would learn "commonsense" knowledge in basic literacy and "practical" skills in cooking and sewing so they could earn a living, to inculcate them with the "idea of self-support, and encourage them to regular hours of work."[81] Modeled on Swiss tuberculosis hospitals, it underwent renovations encompassing classrooms, gymnasiums, play areas, handrails, and ramps. By the 1920s it hosted one of the first accredited physical therapy schools in the nation. The Watson Home expanded in 1934 with the construction of a 200-room building that contained dormitory rooms, a hospital, and a school. Watson administrators began to admit boys in 1942; four years later the facility boasted 146 beds, with separate wards for boys and girls; polio patients made up 80 to 90 percent of them. "The Watson students attended classes, exercised outside, used canes and tennis balls to play makeshift games of wheelchair hockey in the hallways—and got scolded for the noise they made." Nurses wheeled children on a stretcher onto a ramp that led down into that facility's heated swimming pool for water therapy. At other facilities, a pulley was used to lower patients into the water. Therapists also resorted to marbles and accordions to develop toe and finger dexterity.[82]

Jessie Wright, Watson's medical director, became a leader in the maturing field of physical therapy. She had studied as a physical therapist and then earned her MD at the University of Pittsburgh, where she continued as an orthopedic surgery instructor. She also served as director of Watson's School of Physical Therapy, affiliated with University of Pittsburgh's medical school. Wright was very active at the national level in the American Physiotherapy Association and the American Medical Association. The Mayo Clinic, Northwestern University's medical school, and numerous hospitals hired her as a consultant, seeking her advice about what should constitute the physical therapy curriculum; she readily shared copies of the Watson program of study with them. They also sought her advice about the equipment and facilities needed to run such programs. She became a member of the Special Committee on Poliomyelitis of the Allegheny (County) Medical Society and a charter member of the Society of Physical Therapy Physicians (later the American

Society of Physical Medicine), and she participated on the NFIP's President's Brace Fund Committee and its Committee on Education and Publications. Wright further advised the Veterans Administration on physical therapy, and the U.S. Navy and Air Force sought her help in recruiting physical therapists; she was appointed a consultant on physical and occupational therapy to the surgeon general of the Air Force.

Wright, most importantly, became widely known for her expertise in polio therapeutics; hospitals and physicians both here and abroad sought her advice and copies of her publications. The NFIP's leaders acknowledged Watson as a key institution in 1946 and labeled Wright as a pioneer in the field of poliomyelitis rehabilitation. She spoke at numerous conferences and published extensively as well as traveled all over the country to provide instruction and assistance during epidemics. Wright and her team, for instance, gave treatment demonstrations to local physicians and nurses during outbreaks in North Carolina in 1948 and Los Angeles in 1949. The NFIP covered all of her traveling expenses and honoraria for her services.[83] Wright and the Watson rehabilitation center would continue to play a major role in combating this disease, namely in the development of the Salk vaccine.

Sheltering Arms, a rehabilitation center located in Minneapolis, Minnesota, was formally dedicated on February 21, 1943. The first patients arrived the next day, transferred from St. Barnabas Hospital. But the facility faced initial opposition. Neighborhood residents objected to the licensing of the facility, fearing that they were in danger of infection, and they submitted a petition to city council to block its opening. In spite of neighborhood concerns, the city council approved that hospital's license application. Children of all ages and races came from as far away as Georgia, Ohio, Oklahoma, and South Dakota. Sheltering Arms operated under the auspices of the Episcopal Church and in conjunction with St. Barnabas Hospital, which provided the staff. Wallace H. Cole, professor and director of orthopedic surgery, and Miland E. Knapp, director of physiotherapy, both at the University of Minnesota, oversaw the medical staff. The NFIP officially endorsed Sheltering Arms, and the local March of Dimes chapter subsidized care for some of its patients. O'Connor personally visited that facility in 1947.

It claimed to be the first hospital exclusively dedicated to the Kenny approach, regarding itself as the Elizabeth Kenny Institute, Sheltering Arms Hospital, because only Kenny-trained technicians treated patients there. Children in Ward 1 wrote a sarcastic song, "Polio Packin' Mama," to illustrate their attitude toward this treatment:

> One day we came to Sheltering Arms
>   And boy we started to fuss,
>   Until they laid us down in bed
>   And began a-packin' us.
>   Babe, lay that hot pack down, Babe,
>   Lay that hot pack down!
>   Polio packin' Mama,
>   Lay that hot pack down!

However, Kenny eschewed official affiliation. For her, the Kenny Institute represented the only official location for the study and use of her system. She likewise expressed early objections to this facility's plan to charge five dollars a day for treatment, believing that all treatment should be free. Nevertheless, she made high-profile appearances there. Kenny's visit to ride on the new elevator received a great deal of coverage in local newspapers, as did her attendance at a picnic there in July 1943. More importantly, Sheltering Arms revealed how Kenny's approach could be used for convalescence, not just at the post-acute stage.

Sheltering Arms functioned as a full-service rehabilitation facility. A tree-lined driveway led to a newly remodeled, two-story brick building sitting on twenty-nine wooded acres, equipped with a large ramp to accommodate wheelchairs, a spacious dining room, a sunroom, a library, and a variety of other rooms, ranging from wards to semiprivate rooms. It contained a total of thirty beds during its inauguration, soon expanding to accommodate forty to fifty patients, as well as added an elevator and a dumbwaiter. It provided occupational therapy, consisting of weaving, woodworking, and sewing, as well as orthopedic services. Sheltering Arms also had a schoolroom with a chalkboard and desks located in the basement, where elementary and secondary courses were taught. In 1947, the NFIP's local chapter subsidized its teachers and equipment. It became officially accredited two years later. This classroom accommodated six to twelve students at a time, three days a week. The teacher contacted each patient's school to design lessons and used corresponding textbooks so that a smooth transition would occur for them. This system expanded by 1951 to accommodate more students and additional subjects, like algebra, biology, and history. It grew out of a cooperative effort between the school district's special education office and that facility's superintendent, and it was subsidized by the Minneapolis public education system. In 1952, sixteen-year-old Alice Nelson learned Latin while undergoing treatment there. This was facilitated by a two-way intercom linked to the ninth-grade Latin class at Roosevelt High School, about a mile away. A local group of one hundred mothers raised money to subsidize this service through card parties and other events. Peg Kehret remembers attending school at Sheltering Arms two hours a day in the early 1950s: "Students in wheelchairs got a wooden desktop which attached to the arms of the wheelchair and provided a writing surface. I loved my new desk; for the first time since I got polio, it was comfortable to write. The desktop also made it easier and less tiring to hold a book."[84]

Like other rehabilitation centers, a distinct institutional culture emerged there. Parents could only visit on Sundays. Even then, they had to stand on boxes to talk to their children placed in isolation, speaking through the first-floor windows and balancing precariously on fire escapes to read to them on the second floor. Such loose familial connections eventually caused these young patients to assume a new identity. Closeness between them developed as they shared surgery, therapy, and entertainment experiences. They captured this bond in a tune, sung to the tune of the "Trolley Song:" "Ring! Ring! Ring! Go the ward bells. / Ping! Ping! Ping! Go the tubes. / Bing!

Bing! Bing! Go the wheelchairs / As they crash everything in their way." They competed in Ping-Pong games, played pinball machines, planted seeds in gardens, attended services at the small chapel located next to the hospital (it too had a wooden ramp), and enjoyed visiting animals, like horses. Magicians, circus clowns, singers, and movie stars volunteered to entertain them—all of them together.[85]

Four-year-old Paddy Bird underwent rehabilitation in the 1940s, spending nineteen months at the New York State Reconstruction Home, West Haverstraw, forty miles from New York City in the Hudson Valley. His story typifies this difficult experience for children. The distance inhibited visits by Paddy's parents, who resided in New York City and had to take a train to visit him. This cost money and took time. Loneliness therefore permeates Paddy's story. Sensual deprivation intensified this feeling. With no radios or televisions, his room's window grew in importance, as it served as the only means of entertainment and, more importantly, his sole link to the outside world as he watched squirrels hopping from branch to branch and playing. Sounds took on new meanings for him: hissing steam radiators stand out. Paddy was surprised to find himself in the operating room one morning. A nurse quickly removed his hospital clothing as he protested. The surgeon conducted an arthrodesis procedure, and a short while later he removed part of the cast to gain access to the incisions, letting Paddy watch. Paddy gaped at the "three ugly incisions. One wide and purplish [ran] down the top of his foot. Another, thin and red, [went] from his ankle to big toe. A third incision, also thin and red, [cut] across the big toe. It [had] no toenail. Black shoelace-like stitches [held] the cuts together." Paddy, shocked and embittered, began to whimper; an attending nurse rebuked him for doing so. Since he remained bedridden for so long, he developed bedsores. Finally, Paddy's education proved to be incredibly casual, as a night nurse taught young children, reading to them and teaching them arithmetic and writing.[86]

Davis notes in his 1954–55 sociological study that as an unintended outcome, convalescent homes shepherded children disabled by infantile paralysis through a resocialization process, one that eventually confronted their previous lives and occasionally clashed with their parents' perceptions. Their new lives consisted of a physical environment created for rehabilitation, replete with equipment like dumbbells, horses, inclined walking ramps, parallel bars, and wall pulleys. In this therapeutic atmosphere, very young children, four or five years of age, failed to realize—being exposed to similar children for such a long time—that they were in any way different. Parents, however, interpreted all of this in a more complex way, like one mother who witnessed her daughter wearing braces and standing upright for the first time since the onset of polio: "She really walked awful. She just made it, and it really made me sick because I thought, 'Oh, is that the way she's going to walk?'" Thus, while the child perceived disability as the norm in this environment, her mother, like many other such parents, saw her as a "poor crippled kid."[87]

Rehabilitation proved most difficult for female patients. Many suffered sexual assaults while hospitalized. They never admitted it at that time but did later as adults: "I allowed [the doctor] to abuse me because I would have made my parents angry if I was not doing what I was told. And I was afraid the nurses . . . would have punished me for making trouble. All I could do was stop feeling bad about what he did to me and smile." Confined to institutions because of polio, restricted to their beds because of paralysis, these young girls felt like prisoners. They coped with this debasement by keeping it a secret in the hope of escaping, as another describes it: "Why cry about what orderlies were doing to me at night, to make my parents feel guilty? They were not going to let me come home if I cried and I didn't want to disappoint them. They needed to believe that I was okay so I put on a brave face. I never told anyone about the abuse ever." The complexity of their feelings overwhelmed these children. They had been taught to revere the doctor's authority as well as to respect adults. They could not undermine these lessons. They feared potential retribution from nurses, the only adult females they encountered on a daily basis. Finally, they cherished their parents' love and did not want to intensify their emotional stress. They therefore silenced themselves.[88]

Asylums

These facilities offered permanent residency for their patients. "The asylum was the first of a multitude of institutions opened during the 1800s in the United States that aimed to provide residence, treatment, and education to individuals with formally identified disabilities." In 1817, the Connecticut Asylum for the Education and Instruction of Deaf and Dumb Persons opened in Hartford, Connecticut; it "initiated institution-based special education in the United States." Many others followed, specializing in children with a variety of needs. The Massachusetts Asylum for the Blind (later the Perkins Institution) and the New York State School for the Blind opened in 1832, while the Massachusetts School for Idiotic and Feeble-Minded Youth followed in 1851.[89]

Asylums continued into the twentieth century, fulfilling a largely custodial function. They maintained in-house nursing staffs, relying on local hospitals when the need arose. Moreover, they provided little physical rehabilitation, with only light exercise without equipment. Asylums did provide some in-house education. This sometimes involved personnel arrangements with local school districts. The Chicago public school district, for instance, sent a teacher to provide "bedside instruction" for twenty-five children residing at the Home for Destitute Crippled Children. Otherwise, asylum homes put residents to work, ostensibly to learn cooking, housekeeping, and sewing skills. Some examples of these residential homes included the House of the Annunciation for Crippled and Incurable Children in New York City and the New England Peabody Home for Crippled Children at Hyde Park, Massachusetts. More often than not, these institutions barred African American children with disabilities. The House of Saint Michael and All Angels opened in Philadelphia in 1886; staffed by Episcopalians, it proved to be the exception, hosting African American children from other parts of the country. The first public example was the Minnesota State Hospital, opened in 1897.[90] However, it was the adults and children housed at Polk State School for the Feeble-Minded of Western Pennsylvania who would play a crucial role, like the patients at the Watson Home for Crippled Children, in the development of the first polio vaccine.

Pennsylvania's state Department of Public Welfare officially opened Polk State School in 1897 with great fanfare. Over two thousand people, many of whom were political dignitaries, attended the inauguration. Its official institutional goal read, "To provide suitable training for all children in Western Pennsylvania who, by reason of mental deficiency, are unable to receive instruction in the common schools; to provide manual training and suitable employment for older children who, by reason of mental deficiency, are unable to care for themselves." It represented an impressive, cutting-edge complex for that era. The 2,100-acre facility, located eighty miles northeast of Pittsburgh, consisted of sixteen two-story, red brick cottages flanking the administration building. These contained a chapel, dining rooms, a gymnasium, a kitchen, schools, wards, and wood and metal shops. The grounds included horse and cow barns as well as acreage dedicated to farming.[91]

Polk State School housed 353 children at first; this figure jumped to 1,399 in 1907 and 1,840 (904 boys and 926 girls) in 1916. This exceeded its official capacity of 1,720, yet still there was a waiting list of 152. The students' ages ranged from five to twenty-one. Medical personnel assigned them to classrooms, gymnasiums, and shops based on their perceived abilities. Polk's school included a principal, two music teachers, five kindergarten teachers, four primary teachers, two "advanced" teachers, two manual training instructors, four girls' industrial teachers, and one physical training teacher. The gymnasium provided instruction as well as treatments.[92]

This school, like many similar facilities, emphasized manual and industrial training to prepare inmates for practical contributions. Industrial classes included basket-weaving, crocheting, embroidery, leatherwork, rug making, lacemaking, and woodworking. Most boys toiled on the farm, draining and clearing land, cultivating crops, and caring for livestock. They also built roads and concrete walkways and repaired fences. With 600 acres allocated for dairy herds, 100 for corn, 75 for garden crops, and other acreage dedicated to apples, oats, and potatoes, it helped to sustain that institution's population. Residents also spent time in the broom, carpentry, mattress, shoe, and tailor shops, and they prepared food in the bakery, painted the facility's buildings, and knitted stockings and caps. Typical entertainment and recreational activities included birthday parties, circus day, musical entertainment, picnics, playgrounds, and softball games. The state auditor's report for the 1927–30 period labeled Polk as a "model institution."[93]

Polk would remain relatively unknown outside of that state until Jonas E. Salk utilized it as his second field-trial site in 1952. By that time, it had suffered a serious decline. It grappled with severe overpopulation, at 132 percent of capacity with a waiting list of 1,300 applicants. In 1955, the kitchen could only operate at 50 percent of its capacity because of structural failures in that sixty-year-old building; its floors needed to be reinforced because the steel supports had disintegrated. And at least one of the resident's cottages needed to be replastered because of serious deterioration.[94]

Polio and Disability

Children prior to the onset of poliomyelitis experienced the joy of total physical freedom, riding bikes and scooters, running, skipping rope, swimming, and walking. The world served as their playground. They threw balls in their backyards and on baseball fields, hid under bushes and porches during endless hide-and-seek games, jumped hopscotch squares marked with white chalk on concrete sidewalks, climbed trees to eat fruit, and flew on the swings at local parks. For many, this disease ended all of that: it quickly and profoundly inflicted physical limitations on them. During initial infection, huge steel cylinders swallowed their entire bodies in attempts to keep them alive. Worse than this virus, though, an able-bodied world ensured that physical impediments, which easily could have been rectified, denied them freedom. Forget about pushing a wheelchair across grass or gravel. The lack of ramps isolated these children. What they could do and where they could go was severely restricted.

Children rarely found any solace after they completed rehabilitation. They had become the "other." Nine-year-old Marilynne Rogers's first venture into public, after surviving the initial polio infection, both repelled and angered her. She had not been prepared for how people would visibly react to her appearance as a nurse pushed her down the street in a wheelchair. Hugh Gregory Gallagher recalls how people blessed themselves with the sign of the cross as individuals disabled by poliomyelitis wheeled by on sidewalks. Robert Gurney contracted the virus in small-town Minnesota at age seventeen. As he recalled: "Outside of school . . . sometimes people would look at me like I had some contagious disease." Susan Richards Shreve lived this same life: "The main problem for polios was to persuade others that although the effects of polio remained, the disease had gone. We were not contagious. That's all I knew. I'd said it often, from the time I was little, to anyone who questioned my health or looked askance." In yet another case, an individual recalls a "stranger accused me of 'upsetting people,' saying 'You cripples shouldn't be allowed in public!'"[95] Their mere appearance proved offensive. Mee describes how people frequently talked about him in their presence, referring to him in the third person: "Well, he's one of the lucky ones—at least he can get around in a wheelchair, you know; he's not in an iron lung."[96] Children disabled by infantile paralysis became "socially erased,"[97] evoking Ralph Ellison's eloquent, poignant portrayal, in the *Invisible Man*, of the African American experience. Walking with his braces and crutches one day in the late 1940s, Kriegel fell as he stepped off the curb to cross a Bronx street. Unable to right himself, he remained sitting in the gutter. The only assistance he received came from two African American men who pushed through the crowd of bystanders, picked him up, and escorted him across the street. "When we reached the other side, they asked me whether I was all right, whether I wanted them to walk me home." He politely declined. This incident proved to be profound, symbolizing for him a new and diminished social status.[98] In sum, individuals with physical disabilities either became objects of fixation or repulsion, or they simply did not exist. The amount of therapy, the number of surgical procedures, or being fitted with apparatuses to restore some mobility made no difference—American society never fully accepted children disabled by infantile paralysis.

Chapter 4

Wheelchair Gladiators

The sharp smell of the gas coiled into the back of my throat, the smell becoming a taste. The world began to spin . . .

—Anne Finger

A mother's recollection of visiting her son for the first time at a rehabilitation center paints a brutal picture. She found him bound to a frame: "I don't know exactly what this strapping down is for . . . he's got a strap around his neck and that irritates his neck something awful . . . I guess it's there for some purpose. But I would like to know exactly what good it's doing." Such parental shock proved to be common. In these settings, medical professionals did not routinely inform parents about their children's treatments. Fred Davis noted in his thorough ethnographic study that parents, even well into the 1950s, would too often only learn about these procedures as they entered the ward. There they would see that their child might have had surgery or wore a cast. The contraption described in this case was used to correct scoliosis.[1] Rehabilitation represented just one phase at the post-acute, or convalescent, stage. At the same time, the emotional and social reality of physical disability gradually dawned on these young patients—a profound transformation to be sure.

The Vermont Plan

No systematic method of therapeutic care existed in the immediate aftermath of New York City's massive 1916 polio epidemic. For this, health authorities turned to Robert W. Lovett, who had extensive experience. On the heels of its 1914 epidemic, Vermont's health officials feared that "unless something was done in the way of treatment, the amount of resulting disability and disabling deformity would be very great." That state's board of health assigned Lovett, an orthopedic surgeon at Boston's Children's Hospital and a professor at Harvard University Medical School, to address this challenge. Sizing up the enormity of this task, he immediately recognized that he could not undertake home visits for each patient, a common practice for physicians at that time. He chose a temporary alternative: "The first series of free, public clinics for poliomyelitis in this country were conducted . . . in December 1914 and January 1915, in the state of Vermont." Lovett and his assistant used these clinics to examine patients and advise parents about care and treatment. Lovett revived these clinics the following July when, assisted by his colleague Ernest G. Martin, a physiology professor at Harvard, he devised a systematic method to measure muscle strength before instituting a regimen of massages, electrical shocks, and exercise. They equipped children with braces, corsets, and splints as well. This time Lovett employed nurses to conduct follow-up work. This effort ground to a halt when the United States entered World War I in 1917, as Lovett and his staff served in the armed services. They resumed these clinics in May 1919 after returning to civilian life; follow-up work continued to increase, braces were made and used, and surgery began to be instituted. In the latter case, Lovett noted, "many parents were opposed to having operations performed and a great deal of time had to be spent in educational work before the necessary permission could be secured." Vermont's aftercare medical facilities and services continued to expand through the early 1920s to address the needs of children with disabilities. Parents paid for these services, but if they were unable to, the state covered any expenses through its "Spinal Fund." Finally, Lovett expanded the number of trained nurses available to treat patients.

Lovett's scheme included sending many of Vermont's young patients to Boston's New England Hospital for Women and Children, where forty-eight underwent surgery. Moreover, while there, twenty-two had their tonsils and adenoids removed, six were diagnosed with sight problems and fitted with glasses, and teeth were cleaned, removed, or filled. This represented comprehensive health treatment that revealed the rudimentary health services otherwise available for children at that time. Lovett notes, "Everything was done to keep [the children] contented and happy." This involved "automobile rides or in the electric cars" as well as sightseeing activities. In this way, Lovett stresses, "convalescence instead of being just a number of dreary days to be dragged through became a thrilling adventure from beginning to end." Charles S. Caverly, Vermont's health department director, writing at that time, points out that this "plan of holding free public clinics for the maimed [sic] children, following an outbreak of Infantile Paralysis, has been since adapted in other states, notably New York, after the 1916 epidemic, and has become known as 'The Vermont Plan.'" As epidemics unfolded across the country during the next four decades, several orthopedic rehabilitative approaches gradually emerged that strongly resembled this original large-scale effort. Bodies altered by disease needed to be reconstructed.[2]

Rehabilitation

Hospitals admitted acute cases, stabilized patients, and then released them. The recovery process usually began there too, involving two parts:

immobilization and hot compresses combined with physical therapy. No prescribed time frame had been formulated for such institution-based treatment, "and the release was rarely permanent."[3]

Major recovery, otherwise known as the late subacute or early convalescent stage, began as early as four to six weeks but certainly occurred within six months. At this point, orthopedists performed "test movements . . . without pain in the muscles." Treatment followed a familiar routine. It relied once again on immobilization through the application of splints or plaster casts. Physical therapy involved heat, applied by infrared lamps, heating pads, or shortwave diathermy, to avoid atrophy as well as restore some movement through exercise; underwater therapy could be used as well, possibly involving several immersions a day. Massage also occurred, with "light stroking and kneading."[4] In drastic cases, orthopedists resorted to surgery. This "chronic" period ended, as Northwestern University orthopedist Philip Lewin declared in his 1941 medical text, *Infantile Paralysis: Anterior Poliomyelitis*, "when spontaneous improvement can no longer be observed, i.e., in about one to three years."[5]

Medical and social interpretations of disability created distinct notions of rehabilitation. Medical rehabilitationists focused on mechanical corrections of individuals and "measured the success of rehabilitation by how much function one regained through medical interventions including physical therapy and surgery."[6] Their aim was to fix "physical abnormalities," transforming bodies to fit into a *normal* physical world. In doing so, they "absolved society of any complicity in the exclusion of people with disabilities from such social functions as employment, marriage, and even access to public institutions such as schools or government buildings."[7] Too often, this became a dehumanizing experience for young patients. Eight-year-old Karen (Bruber) Boche from St. Paul, Minnesota, describes how she felt while being treated at Gillette State Hospital for Crippled Children: "I would sit on this table . . . with six or seven doctors around me. They would all examine me . . . They talked about me, but not to me. They had me walk, and they would talk about the way I walked . . . I was extremely embarrassed."[8] Lenny Kriegel also saw this during his two-year stay at the New York State Reconstruction Home: "[The physician] saw in me a body, an object for his probing science. Never did I feel that I was a fellow human being for him."[9]

Training to Breathe

Acute and post-acute stages for respiratory patients required intense medical care; that is, acute care involved a life-and-death struggle for patients entombed in artificial respirators, while post-acute treatment involved stabilization and the beginning of the weaning process. Therapy only began during the convalescent stage while the medical staff continued to ease patients off of these machines.

This proved to be a slow and grueling task that required a medical team, consisting of a nurse, an occupational therapist, an orthopedist, a physical therapist, a psychiatrist, a psychologist, a social worker, a teacher, and a vocational counselor, working in close coordination. They had several options. Attendants could simply shut down the machine, thus compelling patients to assume more responsibility to breathe on their own. Hugh Gregory Gallagher noticed that his therapist "took to dropping in on me in the night hours, unaware. Returning from a dinner party, she would stop by, hoping to catch me asleep . . . [S]he would turn off the respirator and, with a stopwatch, time how long it was before I awoke from suffocation. At this point, laughing, she would turn the respirator back on and proceed upon her way." They sometimes could open a porthole, also while patients slept, to drain pressure, slamming it shut if the occupant suddenly awoke, gasping for air. They could likewise slowly adjust the respirator's pressure to force a patient's diaphragm to compensate. Finally, they could simply remove them from their iron lungs for increasingly longer periods of time, causing them to huff for air in order to reawaken—as believed at that time—their respiratory systems. By the 1950s this all culminated in switching patients to rocking beds if they could tolerate it; this rotation followed the sequence from chest respirator to rocking bed to unassisted breathing, with hopefully the tank respirator only used at night. The ultimate goal was to completely eliminate any dependence on that machine.[10]

Actual therapy followed a highly calculated approach. During the first two to four weeks, physical therapists worked with them in their own rooms, gradually shifting these efforts to the physical therapy department, which involved exercises in a heated pool or some form of hot packs applied to patients' extremities. This progressed to using standing beds to reintroduce patients to a vertical position, a serious weight-bearing challenge. This would hopefully lead to reclining in lounge chairs, which consequently meant a transition to wheelchairs. Once this was accomplished, occupational therapists began to teach functional skills like eating, turning pages in a book, and writing. Throughout this entire process, physical therapists introduced exercises to develop short-term independent respiration. Glossopharyngeal breathing—often referred to as "gulping" and "frog-breathing"—operated as the preferred approach, beginning in the early 1950s. Therapists taught patients to use their mouths and throats in "what appeared to be a swallowing action" that actually involved the "gulping of air trapped by the pharynx and then forced through the larynx." It could take up to several weeks to develop this technique. Younger patients experienced the most difficulty in learning it; adolescents and adults achieved better results. Since patients were unable to manage this while sleeping, they remained dependent on respirators at night.[11] The objective here was to minimize, or perhaps even eliminate, any need for tank respirators.

This was not always the case, though. Lawrence Becker contracted polio at age thirteen in 1952 in Nebraska, where he resided with his family. He became paralyzed, immobile, and unable to breathe, and ultimately he was placed in an iron lung. He recalls the weaning procedure, which simply deprived him of air, as "quite brutal. It was with a stopwatch, literally . . . They would give little prizes for each advance." The supervising physician only restarted the pump when Becker turned blue. His doctors, eventually convinced that he no longer needed it, discharged him. He suffered from tachycardia, however, and they prescribed that he sleep in an artificial respirator every night.[12] And, of course, some weaning cases completely failed. On the third day in the hospital, nurses introduced nine-year-old Marilynne Rogers to an iron lung: "I remember they opened the respirator; it seemed really huge, and they laid me on the tray with a mattress on it, and then they sent me through the hole at the front of the big roller part. Then they closed up the collar and told me to relax. They told me I'd feel much better, and I did. I could breathe more easily." During the next seven months, staff members moved her in and out of it, but her breathing failed repeatedly.[13]

Generally speaking, after nine to twelve months of this rehabilitation regimen, respiratory patients were discharged to their homes. But this too required a methodical approach. Two weeks prior to a patient's release, for example, the Southwestern Poliomyelitis Respiratory Center scheduled orientation sessions for family members, or caregivers, to train them about diet, use of equipment, the dangers of infection, and the urgent need to maintain outpatient physical therapy and monitoring.[14]

Physical Therapy

Two events during the first two decades of the twentieth century laid the groundwork for the growth of modern physical therapy. One was the increasingly heavy demand for polio aftercare. While immobilization and splinting of affected limbs served as the standard treatment, it also produced muscle atrophy, weakened limbs, and reduced joint flexibility. Partial or complete recovery therefore required therapy. New York City's Hospital for Deformities and Joint Disease represented a prime example during that city's 1916 epidemic. This six-story facility gave free treatments and distributed braces. It employed forty trained masseurs to provide mechanical, reflex, thermal, and electrical massages. The latter procedure involved the application of two to twelve minutes of electrical current—which proved quite painful—to relax muscles that caused the paralysis. The hospital's managers estimated that its staff treated between 1,500 and 2,000 cases of infantile paralysis during that epidemic. World War I represented the second influence, involving large numbers of soldiers with disabilities because of severe wounds suffered in that bloody conflict. Together with the demand for polio aftercare, the war stimulated the growth of schools for physical training, often associated with normal schools, in California, Connecticut, Massachusetts, Michigan, and Ohio, to teach professionals how to use massage and hydrotherapy to "reconstruct" people with disabilities. "By 1919, 45 hospitals throughout the country had physical therapy facilities and employed more than 700 reconstruction aides . . . Treatments consisted of exercises, including corrective exercises, passive exercises, sports and games, massage, hydrotherapeutic modalities, and assistive and adaptive equipment."[15]

Limb immobilization remained the preferred approach for treating infantile paralysis through the 1940s, aggressively twisting and fixing limbs in the proper position and locking them into place with splints and casts. In 1939, fourteen-year-old Robert Huse, who had contracted infantile paralysis at age six while residing in Lowell, Massachusetts, underwent a spine suspension procedure, common before 1950, to correct scoliosis; this treatment had been delayed until he reached adolescence. Without any prior notice, one day an orderly pushed a gurney into his hospital room and moved him onto it. They entered the operating room, and the orderly quickly lowered a leather strap that had been suspended from the ceiling, a muzzle-like device that he attached to Robert's head. The doctor at this point informed him, "[We] have to string you up for a while, Bob, and this will put some pressure on your mouth." Shocked and dismayed, Huse immediately heard a pulley turn and strain as he felt himself being raised into a perfectly vertical position that aligned his body, namely his spinal cord, perpendicular to the floor. Completely conscious, Huse recalls, "[My] teeth sank into my lower lip and blood dribbled from the corners of my mouth. They worked quickly now, wrapping my trunk in strips of gauze dipped in plaster of Paris . . . As the wet plaster added more weight to my body my teeth sank deeper into my lower lip, and my head felt as if it were going to explode." After the physician and his assistants completed this application, building a cast, they let him hang for a while, waiting for the plaster to harden, extending his misery. Huse's ordeal was wasted, because that cast cracked the next day. The doctor then resorted to the former approach, strapping him into a rack and encasing all of it in a cast, periodically adjusting the straps to straighten his spine. This approach was just as macabre, as Huse explains: "Through the many long nights that were to follow, screaming with pain, I begged my mother to take off the splints and allow me to bend my legs. With tears streaming down her cheeks she would shake her head and explain to me over and over again why I must keep my body straight."[16]

Following these kinds of orthopedic procedures, "therapists forcefully pulled and pushed joints to move them to their normal position." This proved to be painful and dangerous, as one patient recalls: "The physical therapist pushed up so hard on my foot that she broke the tendon on the back of my leg." Fitted metal braces followed, and therapists worked with patients to help them walk using crutches. But some went too far for one child; "[They] had these rubber truncheons, like short rubber nightsticks . . . Some would hit us if we fell down, even if they pushed us down in order to teach us balance." As Richard L. Bruno, an expert on post-polio syndrome, summarizes, "Physical therapies were often administered as if patients were on an assembly line, without explanation, without parental consent, and certainly without patients' consent. Children, isolated from parents and totally dependent on staff, had no choice but to allow therapists to do what they wanted, in spite of pain and fear."[17]

Polio patients had complex reactions to wheelchairs and braces. Some feared them because they starkly symbolized permanent disability. Early examples neither adjusted nor reclined. This not only produced extreme discomfort in the short run but also resulted in scoliosis in the long run, since the paralyzed occupant would often sag to one side. By the 1930s improvements made them practical and affordable. George S. Salomon, a former patient at Warm Springs, developed a folding, lightweight wheelchair with removable wheels, providing portability. The Colson Company of Elyria, Ohio, manufactured this folding "invalid" chair, and according to a 1933 advertisement, the company also produced one with "fully adjustable leg rests and back, anti-tipping device, and complete rubber bumper equipment." Finally, the Real Courage Association, located in Battle Creek, Michigan, advertised a folding wheelchair for $9.50.[18]

Through mobility, however, wheelchairs gave children a modicum of independence. "The moment my dead buttocks touched the woven-straw seat," Lenny Kriegel relates, "I found . . . freedom . . . I was free now." This had many meanings. He and his mates now wheeled themselves to the convalescent home's school, which met for ninety minutes each morning; this gave the sense of a truly shared experience reminiscent of their previous lives. In general, he no longer had to rely on others for movement; he could go where he wanted, when he wanted. Finally, it symbolized "the way home," the next step in his journey.[19]

Children often personalized their wheelchairs. Peg Kehret, while undergoing rehabilitation at Sheltering Arms in Minnesota, named hers Silver after the famous white steed of the famed radio cowboy, the Lone Ranger. Wheelchair antics seemed to be common as well. Kehret became known as a "daredevil" and popped "wheelies."[20] Jerry McNellis became a "wheelchair gladiator," one of the children who purposefully crashed into one another at the Gillette State Hospital for Crippled Children. "At times kids would get bumped over backwards in those fights and all sorts of damage happened both to kids and their wheelchairs." Too often those trusty warhorses would be sent to that hospital's repair shop. They also used them for racing competitions. New steel wheelchairs, rather than old wooden ones, worked best, McNellis recalls, because they would stay straight instead of veering right or left at breakneck speeds.

> We'd race downhill from school past peeds (pediatric ward) and go as far as we could coast. There were contest rules. Push yourself as fast as you could, then once you went past a certain point you couldn't push anymore, just coast . . . Once we came to a stop, someone would put . . . a mark on the baseboard of the wall to note our distance . . . On one of my runs . . . I ran into a nurse . . . who was carrying a big tray of thermometers. Mercury and glass splattered all over. I can't remember how much I hurt the nurse.

That track accident resulted in a temporary moratorium, imposed by the medical staff. Jerry, meanwhile, spent a great deal of "extra time in bed" as punishment.[21]

Kriegel and his mates played basketball, croquet, football, Ping-Pong, and softball in their wheelchairs. But their most ambitious adventure involved a wheelchair assault, purposefully patterned after a horse cavalry charge. He and his friends had just seen one on the weekly movie at the New York State Reconstruction Home, in West Haverstraw, New York. They conceived a plan to invade nearby Garnerville in order to purchase candy, otherwise forbidden by the medical staff. In a well-executed maneuver, they snuck out of the home in small groups of two or three after dinner, and all thirteen of them rendezvoused on the grounds near the gate. They wheeled out onto the road and descended on the unsuspecting target in two highly organized groups, with one invader imitating a bugle call with his voice. The first wave of six chairs struck first, followed immediately by the second one, consisting of seven attackers. The sudden and totally unexpected appearance of a phalanx of children streaking downhill in their wheelchairs completely stunned that town's residents, who just stood stupefied on the sidewalks. A local police officer quickly arrived to question the boys. He related that the crowd feared that they remained contagious. Kriegel and his comrades assured him that they were not and proceeded to acquire their booty. Nevertheless, the uneasy townspeople avoided them. As Kriegel and his troops departed, he spat on the street before the lingering crowd gawking at them; everyone retreated a step, cowering from imagined infection. The boys returned to the home, where their bedridden mates cheered them as a night nurse watched helplessly. This swashbuckling episode represented three key characteristics growing out of the rehabilitation experience. It served as a revolt, escaping the mind-numbing physical therapy regimen. It also expressed their newly won freedom, thanks to their wheelchairs. Finally, their act of defiance as they exited that town cemented their realization of having become social pariahs because of their disabilities.[22]

Wheelchairs sparked such opprobrium, as many others discovered. Adolescents found this particularly troubling, as Alice R. Thrall, of the Warm Springs "wheel-chair brigade" noted: "Obviously, it is the common lot of us who are bound to our chairs to be stared at. In public we feel as conspicuous as the animals in a circus parade."[23] Even Kriegel's "large, ungainly, magnificently ugly throne on wheels" assumed a profoundly different identity once he returned home. It marked him as abnormal, and thus he no longer wanted to be associated with it. After a year of disuse, he asked his father to donate it to a local hospital. He relied solely on his braces and crutches for mobility. Standing erect partially restored his masculinity.[24]

Fifteen-pound leather and steel braces functioned as the next logical stage of increased mobility, and it was commonly regarded as a more acceptable one, since children could now at least stand upright. The first public campaign to subsidize braces occurred before the 1916 New York City epidemic even ended, as we have seen. Custom-made braces supported weak, paralyzed legs, but children had to relearn how to walk: a slow and tortuous process. As she propped herself up on her new "walking sticks" for the first time, Peg Kehret recalls, "I had to think about the sequence of each step: lift right stick and right foot, move them forward, put them down. Lean on stick for balance. Lift the left stick and the left foot, more them forward, put them down. I felt as if bricks were glued to the soles of my shoes."[25] Fitted with a pair of leg braces for the first time at age twelve, Kriegel stood precariously on them, clinging to his crutches and feeling as though he had been "created in the laboratory of Mary Shelley's Dr. Frankenstein." This provoked a startling dilemma: "I was alive and standing. But, at that moment my mind just whispered the word 'cripple' to me. I had ignored the word until then, ignored the words and all of its implications." He resented braces, angered at what they symbolized. He now began to feel like the "other," a sentiment reinforced by his female coach. Physical therapists typically taught children how to fall and then pull themselves upright. Acquisition of this skill overcame fear of falling while preparing them for a future of such spills. Kriegel provides insight into her motive: "She knew that mine would be a future so different from what confronts the 'normal' that I had to learn to fall into life in order not to be overwhelmed."[26]

Leg braces certainly provoked serious psychological and social conundrums. An eight-month longitudinal study conducted by three psychiatrists at the University of Maryland's School of Medicine, begun during the summer of 1954, focused on a group of children disabled by poliomyelitis. The researchers discovered what seemed to be a counterintuitive emotional toll; that is, many of those children regarded braces as a symbol of failure, because they embodied disability. The longer they remained bedridden or in wheelchairs, the children told the researchers, the better they felt about their chances of recovering the full use of their limbs. Being prescribed braces and released from the rehabilitation center spelled the end of any further progress, in their minds. After returning home, many vented their bitterness, occasionally manifested through violence. A nine-year-old girl attempted to burn her crutch and, having failed that, used it to attack her non-disabled sister.[27] According to historian Daniel J. Wilson's analysis, "Not all polio survivors could shed their braces, but those who could generally did so as soon as possible, even if, from a strictly medical point of view, they might have been better advised to keep wearing them. The temptation to appear more normal by discarding the braces was simply too strong." Some preferred wheelchairs to braces since they offered comfort, mobility, and stability.[28]

Finally, physical pain plagued users of braces. Although seemingly custom fitted, they were never perfect and could prove to be extremely uncomfortable. The bracket on Dee Van Balen's brace pinched her right leg: "That hinge continued to get stuck on my skin, and we never figured out how to stop that from happening." This repeated irritation permanently scarred her right leg.[29]

Surgery

Surgery remained rare until the late nineteenth century, but by the early twentieth century, the "golden age of surgery" had emerged. Due to physiological discoveries, innovative instruments, and new anesthetics, confident doctors plunged ahead in their endeavors to cure patients. Still, such medical procedures remained crude and in development. During the 1918 influenza epidemic, for example, physicians performed thoracic surgery to drain pus from the rib cages of patients. It proved to be ineffective.[30]

Doctors resorted to drastic measures with severe polio cases. Orthopedists Alfred H. Tubbey and Robert Jones, in their 1903 medical text, *Modern Methods in the Surgery of Paralysis, with Special Reference to Muscle-Grafting, Tendon-Transplantation and Arthrodesis*, describe tenotomy procedures (i.e., cutting tendons) on hamstrings:

> In dividing the hamstrings the classical transverse incision must be avoided, and parallel incisions are better made along the tendons of the semitendinosus and biceps. By lifting the skin and using a hernia director, the deep fascia over the popliteal region can be sufficiently divided. The drawback to the transverse incision is that it indefinitely prolongs treatment, as it gapes the movement an attempt is made to extend the joint.[31]

Surgeons followed this with a process called "forcible correction"; that is, placing the "contracted limb" into a "plaster bandage" and eventually replacing this with a mechanical apparatus.[32]

In 1910, by its third year of epidemics, the Massachusetts State Board of Health disseminated a list of possible surgical treatments to "correct deformities" caused by infantile paralysis. Arthrodesis denuded ankle, elbow, foot, hip, knee, shoulder, and wrist joints "completely or in part" of cartilage. Because this fused these bare-boned surfaces, orthopedists hoped to provide some stability for limbs and joints, thus compensating for any loss of muscle control.[33] Fasiotomy involved a skin incision to relieve pressure on a joint, while myotomy allowed a joint or limb to relax by slicing a damaged muscle to release undue stress. Osteotomy realigned leg bones by chiseling or sawing a wedge of bone and then fusing the exposed surfaces together to straighten the leg or make limbs more even.

Lovett also strongly endorsed surgery, for two reasons: "correction of fixed deformity" and "improvement of function." The first had to be performed as soon as possible, as part of the initial hospital stay. Tenotomy could be used to correct an ankle joint by attaching a silk ligament to the Achilles tendon. Hip repair involved "prolonged stretching" through the use of a "plaster jacket with a carefully molded pelvic part and a plaster leg." Or a complex surgical procedure could be used, after which the patient remained hyperextended in a full-body cast. Surgeries "intended to improve existing muscular function," usually relating to the arm, hamstrings, or foot, involved tendon or nerve transplantation. A grafted tendon substituted for a paralyzed muscle. To "secure stability," generally focusing on the shoulder, elbow, hip, knee, or ankle joints, Lovett recommended arthodesis; that is, removing a bone or cartilage to lock the joint.[34]

These operations, as Philip Lewin counseled in 1941, served to "improve muscle function, improve static stability, correct deformities, and make it possible for the patient to discard braces." This only occurred, he directed, after the ages of ten or twelve (with the onset of pubescence) or, for older patients, "within a year after the acute attack." However, children as young as seven underwent this surgery. Some of these procedures continued to require a plaster cast to freeze a limb in place or in a certain position, affording support.[35]

Three concerns justified such medical procedures, according to national nursing organizations as late as 1948: "to correct deformities; to secure stability of joints and; to improve function." These usually involved tendon transplants or nerve crushing, used in an attempt to regenerate the nerve. Following these operations, young patients once again had to be "immobilized in plaster." Nurses had to make sure that the cast remained sterile, to avoid infections, and that it did not create circulatory problems.[36]

Bruno's 1995 survey of former polio patients reported that 20 percent had been "hospitalized . . . for an average of six months for a variety of orthopedic surgeries."[37] Specialists implanted silk ligaments and transplanted muscles. The latter treatment proved to be excruciatingly painful, relocating them from one part of the body to another. Susan Richards Shreve's childhood memories about this particular operation remain crystal clear decades later: "The shin muscle, which controlled my ability to lift my foot, was moved to serve as a calf muscle and held in place for the several months I was in a cast by wires strung through the muscle and a 'rubber button,' with holes for the wires located externally on my heel." For the most part, these medical procedures never completely corrected paralysis; but, it was reasoned, they reduced *deformities* (as they were perceived) and occasionally increased mobility.[38] Surgery therefore proved to be relatively common in an attempt to normalize bodies.

Experiences during surgery and afterward only added to the emotional and physical trauma of these young patients. Although six years old at the time, Anne Finger vividly remembers the morning of her first surgical procedure at a hospital in Utica, New York, during the 1950s. As the nurse pushed the gurney into her room, her senses shifted into high gear:

> I remember the smell and feel of the ancient brown leather covering the thin mattress set upon the wheeled gurney to which I was transferred . . . I saw the leather itself. The leather had become mottled with use, and deep creases veined it . . . Beneath a thin veneer of disinfectant scent was a smell of body odors; the acid smell of someone else's fear, the baser and even more frightening smell of shit and blood . . . Like the sheet on my hospital bed, the sheet across the gurney was stiff.

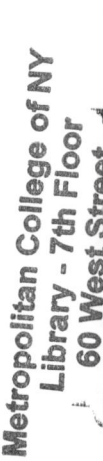

That nurse wheeled her to the elevator, which deposited them in the basement, and they entered the corridor, rolling toward the operating room. Finger recalls the frightening sights as she lay face up on the gurney: "Exposed pipes ran overhead, painted with dark brown paint . . . Here and there were red valves . . . At other places the pipes were fitted with various valves and clamps . . . I closed my eyes, I couldn't look. I clenched my eyes shut as I was wheeled down that long, terrifying corridor." On one level, this scene appears to be taken directly from a horror movie depicting Dr. Frankenstein's laboratory. On a deeper level, the pipes and valves represented metaphors for her anatomy that was about to be invaded and tinkered with. The operating room did nothing to allay her anxiety.

> My eyes opened and I saw row upon row of lidded jars. I was transferred into a cold metal table and saw a light fixture above me. It was on a swinging arm, and the light fixture itself was made up of many hexagonal shapes.
>
> The ether mask, lowered down over my face, made the whole world go black. The sharp smell of the gas coiled into the back of my throat, the smell becoming a taste. The world began to spin . . . As I spiraled down into unconsciousness, I flailed my arms and legs while the nurses restrained me.

Finger's multiple surgical procedures left her with long-lasting bitterness, reaching well into her adulthood: "Surgery seemed an instrument of humiliation, a strange and irrational ritual of degradation."[39]

In the operating room, when anesthesiologists attempted to lower the gauze-covered strainer or mask over children's faces to administer ether, the children often panicked, fighting the feeling of being smothered as they inhaled an irritating and unfamiliar gas. A 1912 editorial in the *Journal of the Indiana State Medical Association* extolled the use of pleasant odors, like oil of orange or wintergreen, in order to reduce their anxieties, concluding that anyone "who has had any experience with anesthesia among children will be delighted to find a method wherein the child lies on the table, breathes with apparent relish that which we have only been accustomed to see it resist and fight against."[40] It did not work, as Moira recounts. She had contracted polio in 1952 and endured dozens of procedures, remembering them as nightmares.

> Almost every summer from the time I was two years old I would have another operation. No one would tell you what they were going to do . . . The night before you got an enema and were shaved . . . In the operating room I would pretend that the ether was working and then try to rip the mask off of my face and get away. I knew the ether would make me throw up later for hours. When I did awake I was in pain and nauseous.

All young patients awoke dizzy, their heads spinning with a terrifying buzzing noise seemingly ringing in their ears, and discovered a kidney-shaped throw-up pan as their bedside companion in the recovering room. While in this stupor, they often noticed blood oozing from their plaster casts.[41]

Gail Bias's memories of the grisly procedures she underwent, beginning at age six, reveal the impersonal, clinical routine manner of the hospital staff. She vividly recalls the smell of the antiseptic scrub the night before each one, the chill of the cold operating rooms, the constricting leather straps that bound her to the operating table, and the sheer terror of knowing her body would be cut open. Bias describes the ultimate frustration: "You couldn't even cry any more because of all the medication they had given you." Her second operation, at age ten, involved the transplantation of a heel cord. For her third surgery, at age eleven, Bias relates, "They broke all the bones in my left foot and reconstructed it to be more like a normal foot." Two weeks later, her fourth operation "involved a 'bone block' to stop that [right] leg from growing. That way there wouldn't be such a big difference between my legs." Bias eventually became addicted to the medication given her to kill the pain.[42]

Kay Brutger's experiences represented one of the most extreme cases. She contracted poliomyelitis at nine months of age in 1950 and underwent four highly intricate and dangerous procedures over a twenty-nine-year period. The first occurred when she was six. She recalls extreme emotional and physical trauma during this initial episode. The former involved being separated from her mother and father for the first time; she reflects, "[It] made me feel very lonely and frightened." That operation caused her extensive pain: it "involved putting a plate in my right leg, an ivory 'screw' in my right knee, and attaching an artificial cord up over the top of my right foot." This required seven incisions and over a hundred stitches, and little Brutger was encased in a plaster cast. Although they lived two hours from Minneapolis, where she was hospitalized, her mother found local lodgings and took a taxi each day to visit her young daughter. These additional living expenses compounded the family's already heavy medical financial burden.

Brutger's second, equally delicate operation came at the age of eleven. Paralysis had caused uneven growth of her limbs, causing her left leg to outgrow her weakened right leg. The surgeons decided to impede the development of her *good* leg by, as she recalls, "putting staples in the [left] knee area. During that same surgery, they also operated on my left foot. That foot sort of turned in when I walked . . . The surgeon tried to turn it back the way it was supposed to be." This highly complex surgical procedure left her with a "trick knee."

Brutger's third procedure occurred when she was seventeen years old, to correct the trick knee. In this case, the doctors sliced her entire thigh open, cutting through previous scar tissue, and inserted "eight screws and two plates" in her knee and thigh. She awoke from the long operation in a body cast. This six-month imprisonment required her parents to install a hospital bed in their living room, and Brutger grew deeply depressed. Her despair grew when the doctors removed the cast. It had been improperly applied and consequently removed skin from her feet. After all of this, she discovered that her left foot had been set at the wrong angle, and it remained that way, even after extensive physical therapy.

At the age of thirty-five and experiencing excruciating pain in her left leg, the legacy of crude earlier procedures, Brutger underwent her fourth and final operation. The surgeons once again had to cut through the previous incision in her thigh. Although this operation was equally complex, Brutger remembers a largely positive outcome: "The doctor ended up taking out all of the old screws and plates. He also realigned the kneecap, which apparently had not been positioned correctly during the previous surgery. While they were in there, they found a lot of scar tissue, which was apparently the source of my pain, so they cut out as much of that as they could. The doctor also used arthroscopic surgery to repair the cartilage and ligaments around the knee."[43]

Clearly, many extreme attempts to overcome the ravages of infantile paralysis in children's bodies proved to be fruitless at best and intensified pain and anxiety at worst. Medical historian Gareth Williams points out that "properly controlled trials of physical therapy were few and far between, making it impossible to measure or even prove the benefits of particular regimens. Nevertheless, intensive physical therapy seemed to sustain, improve, and even restore strength in many cases."[44] Children saw this process not only as physically demanding but also as emotionally draining. Whether successful or not, it often led to "depression and despair."[45] Some felt deep anger, actually resisting therapy. Kriegel strongly resented his braces and learning to walk with them. In his view, this process simply reduced him to a "cripple." These emotions intensified for those who never showed any progress. Finally, the post-rehabilitation period proved to be a shock. The recovery process had operated as a joint effort, one involving the therapist and the patient. In the aftermath, the lone child with a disability now had to come to grips with social reality, a personal struggle to be fought alone. While the former proved to be relatively finite, with an end in view, the latter offered no terminal point.[46] As late as 1948, a physician described the medical attitudes and treatment approaches as "ignorance, impotence, and insecurity."[47] Well-meaning surgeons and desperate parents persisted nonetheless. They believed that some progress could be made. Some even clung to the belief that they had actually witnessed it. However, the body's natural response to nerve damage—that is, the attempt to "sprout" new nerve fibers—only created the perception of improvement by various treatments, including Sister Elizabeth Kenny's method, as we have seen.[48]

Ward Culture

Time assumed a different meaning while "undergoing more surgeries, post-surgical rehabilitation, and outpatient care." With no ready access to clocks, children measured its passage through natural cycles —through the daylight shining through windows, or noting seasonal changes by watching falling leaves and snow.[49] A huge gulf loomed before them, seemingly endless.

Professional articles for nurses stressed that an "especially homesick or distraught" child had an "'abnormal' attachment to his/her mother, or was unstable." They also recommended "wholesome" activities for children, to distract them and fill in the long healing periods: "good books (not comics!), nature films (no cartoons—too stimulating!), and classical music." Many of these attitudes fit into the prevailing childrearing paradigm that continued through the 1940s, involving a "strict adherence to a by-the-clock routine. The regimented and mechanistic care of children in hospitals was encouraged by authorities." No one realized then that "maternal deprivation and separation" caused serious emotional damage. In retrospect, one nurse summarizes professional medical culture at that time: "We weren't as understanding. We weren't as empathetic. We didn't meet their needs with far better understanding and treatment of their psychological needs."[50]

On another level, sociologist Fred Davis says, the convalescent hospital became a surrogate family, albeit a highly regulated one,

> by the assumption on the part of personnel of many parental functions; by the duplication of the ward of many of the familiar activities and diversions of the home (e.g., television, games, picture and comic books, group play, etc.); by a reward and punishment system, both formal and informal, which reinforced good behavior and cooperative attitudes as these are defined by the treatment personnel; and—most important perhaps—by the fact of living in a milieu in which illness is the norm rather than the deviation, a condition that permits the child to assimilate the hospital's universe of special meanings, goals, and evaluative rankings.

As a result, Davis continues, young patients moved from "severed" emotional ties with parents to "loosened" connections. Irregular or rare parental visits to rehabilitation centers contributed to this development. These institutions strictly limited visitation hours, usurping control of these children's lives. Sometimes sheer distances proved too great for casual travel, or work obligations limited the amount of time parents had to devote to such reunions, or they simply wanted to avoid seeing their children with disabilities. Therefore, parental visits once a month or two to three times a year became a common pattern.

A unique ward life thus unfolded. Children did not consciously identify the hospital as a substitute family, Davis found, but it certainly became associated with the only other adult-dominated, large-scale institution they knew: the public school. "In the classroom, what happen[ed] to one child by way of instruction, assignments, and promotion more or less happen[ed] to all. Hence, the oversimplified view of the children on the ward that all 'polios' who were there must . . . be more or less alike, and that what happened to one would very shortly happen to the others as well." Since neither the medical staff nor their parents told them, children gauged the seriousness of their illnesses based on who went home first and who left the hospital last. As each day passed, it grew more apparent how disabled each one was.[51]

In spite of the pain, fear, and loneliness many children felt while being hospitalized, the ward became their world. Here they built their own social and emotional networks. They gave each other and themselves nicknames, such as "Leadfoot." After the staff switched off the lights at night, these bored young patients devised elaborate spitball fights. As Arvid Schwartz recalls, "Eventually, we would make enough noise that the nurses would come down, and we'd catch hell. But really, what could they do to us?" Gail Bias competed in wheelchair races against other girls in her ward. Charles L. Mee recalls how they, like all children, found ways to be playful, if not manipulative: "One boy perfected a technique for getting his wheelchair up to high speed and then flipping it forward just in front of the nurses' station, sending him belly flopping to the floor so that the pretty young nurses would rush over and pick him up and fawn over him." These patients developed other forms of entertainment while confined to the hospital. Len Jordan and his mates chased able-bodied people with their wheelchairs. He also participated in many pillow fights, watched puppet shows, and made arts and crafts. And they ultimately found the intimacy of companionship. Susan Richards Shreve fondly writes, "Nighttime in the ward was cozy. We giggled and whispered. We sang together and told outrageous stories of what we might do when we got out. Often someone would start a story and it would go around the room from bed to bed, each of us adding to it when our turn came. Those nights were as close as I got to a sense of family . . . as close as I felt to belonging to a group."[52]

Robert Huse discovered a "flourishing caste system" of an "elite group of older boys" who ran everything, operating as a small, tightly knit society. In addition to the predictable hospital routine, three leaders oversaw their peers' activities. Such was the case at seven o'clock in the evening, when all of the young patients tuned their radios to the same station. "By having all the radios playing one program, those without [radio] receivers were able to listen together with the rest of us. It gave us all something to look forward to and made us feel less lonely . . . I was to learn," he continues, "a great deal more of this unique oligarchy in the coming months and its influence on the lives of patients of the East Ward at the Shriners Hospital" in Lowell, Massachusetts. For example, when a patient returned from surgery, he would receive a sudden and touching surprise; his ward compatriots loaned him all of their precious comic books to let him know that he was not alone.[53]

While individually struggling with their own lives, they looked after one another, more often than not. Twelve-year-old Kehret found herself assigned to a bed next to a boy in a respirator. As she slowly regained limited mobility, she would help him each day: "I began reading aloud to Tommy. I quit only when my voice got hoarse, but even then he always begged me to read just one more page . . . I felt sorry for Tommy who was still stuck in the iron lung." As she progressed with her physical therapy, she used her free time to explore the facility and socialize: "I spent a lot of time visiting patients who didn't get any outside company . . . I began reading aloud to the little kids every day."[54] Surgery proved to be terrifying to all of them. The veterans, as one young patient recounts, served as surrogate parents: "When someone was going to surgery the next morning, especially if it was their first surgery, those of us who had been 'upstairs' would explain what it was like, what to expect before and after. When they came back down from the recovery room we would sit by the bed and hold their hands."[55]

The world of the ward had yet another side. Jean Johnson and others undergoing physical therapy at the D. T. Watson Home for Crippled Children, near Pittsburgh, retaliated against cruel nurses and hospital staff members by creating more work. They maintained an innocuous appearance while playing surreptitious pranks: "We'd go in and leave the showers on and put the plugs in the tubs. We'd spill our food on our beds and then say, 'Oh, it was a mistake,' you know." They cooperated to plot and execute their revenge in unique and clever ways: "When we pulled one of these capers, you'd get somebody with hands to help somebody that could use their feet. I mean, we had to take a combination of bodies to be able to pull these things off, so that you knew people by what they could help you with, or what they were able to do, not by what they *couldn't* do. Which, of course, is essentially opposite to the view of the outside world."[56] These children, in short, fashioned a world of their own, one that thrived on emotional support and mutual aid and grew out of their own personal and collective context.

External forces also contributed to this unfolding social world, as volunteers and medical personnel provided entertainment. For instance, the staff at Houston's Southwestern Poliomyelitis Respiratory Center organized trips to the circus, ice shows, movie theaters, picnics, restaurants, and rodeos for patients. "Because some patients on these trips had to be accompanied by their breathing devices, many of these outings required a great deal of advanced preparation." Nevertheless, traveling together on such adventures, sharing laughs, and discovering new experiences added to their camaraderie.[57]

And of course the ward routine blurred the lines between hospital and school. This began quite early in the string of polio epidemics. In September 1920, Bird S. Coler, New York City's commissioner of public welfare, ended outpatient rehabilitation clinics, moving those children into hospitals as resident patients. His office also assigned a public school teacher to each building. Because of their disabilities, they had been unable to attend school. "Under the new plan," *The New York Times* announced, "their minds will be developed as their treatment progresses." A tutor visited Marilynne Rogers once a week to give her lessons at Minnesota's Kenny Institute during the 1950s. Some convalescent homes even provided classrooms. Teachers and students used public library books as well as regular textbooks, loaned by local school principals. Little or no formal teaching occurred; self-directed learning dominated, with children studying on their own under the guidance of instructors. "There were three or four of us in our class," Schwartz says, "and we were all about the same age. I was in my wheelchair; there was a boy who was in a respirator, and a girl was wheeled down there in her bed . . . I went there about three months. They sent a report card to my principal in Wood Lake. He looked at it and said I passed! So that's how I did my seventh grade." A different standard existed for African American students. The Houston public schools were a case in point. While administrators sent homebound teachers to the Southwestern Poliomyelitis Respiratory Center to keep children academically abreast with their classmates, they did not provide that service for African Americans until 1951.[58]

The hospital environment in general and ward life in particular represented more than a clinical setting, a place merely for medical diagnosis and treatment; it hosted more than passive and dependent patients. There, school-age patients nurtured peer relationships, created mischief, assisted one another, and continued their education. They had to, because medical treatments for them required long stays in some cases. There, children grew close. And it proved to be extremely difficult emotionally for those with severe paralysis to watch their roommates arrive, improve, and then leave. Yet they remained; they knew the score. More importantly, this offers us a brief glimpse of the power of human agency. As Kehret boasts, "We had the kind of camaraderie that I imagine exists between soldiers who have fought together during a long and difficult war. In our case, the enemy was polio. Our battle medals were wheelchairs, back and leg braces, and walking sticks, and we wore them proudly. We were survivors."[59] And young patients did not always celebrate being discharged from these institutions. Fidel Gonzales left his Texas hospital at age sixteen filled with anxiety: "I felt something had been taken away from me . . . My friends, my hospital, my bed, my nurses, my doctors—I wasn't going to see them again. It just felt like the world was coming to an end." As historian Heather Green Wooten concludes, "Life in the polio wards had, for many patients, become a safe cocoon from the outside world—one of support, acceptance, and camaraderie."[60] Disability had crafted a new norm among the children in these wards; they knew this would not be the case in the outside world.

Within a span of several days, children moved from the world of the able-bodied to that of the disabled. What meaning did this have for them? People now perceived them either as helpless, incapable of being historical actors, or as heroic, overcoming incredible obstacles to assume celebrity status. In either case, disability has often been portrayed as a lonely experience requiring rehabilitation and acceptance of a new life—in sum, individually adapting to it. Those who supposedly overcame it demonstrated personal courage and determination, a more acceptable cliché for the able-bodied majority. Regardless, they were stigmatized, losing dignity as well as rights.[61]

Portrayals of people with disabilities shaped these perceptions. The first, the "Tiny Tim" character, has long projected helplessness; that is, a "sad, unlucky, disabled person, in need of pity and charity."[62] Charles Dickens introduced the public to him in his 1843 classic, *A Christmas Carol*. Bob Cratchit, Ebenezer Scrooge's poor, overworked clerk, enters his humble abode with Tiny Tim perched on his shoulder, returning from church services. Dickens vividly describes him: "Alas for Tiny Tim, he bore a little crutch, and had his limbs supported by an iron frame!" Dickens portrays him not only as physically fragile but also as having a feeble voice. He builds this imagery as he describes how Tiny Tim's "little crutch" thumps on the wooden floor, slowly moving toward the table with the Christmas goose, to sit by his father's side. Even the mere sight of him softens Scrooge's sternness.[63] This representation of a child with a physical disability would resonate a hundred years later.

Televised fundraising events portrayed the "worst American cultural notions about people with impairments," presenting them as helpless victims, thus emphasizing the "worst stereotypes." Individuals with disabilities have criticized these shows as being "the most despised aspect of disability history."[64] Disability scholar Rosemarie Garland Thomson takes this analysis a step further:

> Jerry Lewis's Telethons testify not only to the cultural demand for body normalization, but to our intolerance of the disabled figure's reminder that perfection is a chimera. As a cultural emblem for the restricted self, the disabled body stubbornly resists the willed improvement so fundamental to the American notion of self. Indeed, lurking behind the able-bodied figure is the denied, and perhaps intolerable, knowledge that life will eventually transform us into "disabled" selves. In the end, the body and history dominate the will, imposing limits on the myth of a physically stable self progressing unfettered towards some higher material state.[65]

The second case, known as the "supercrip," performs at a "superhuman" level to overcome incredible obstacles, ones that even a person without disabilities would find difficult. Olympic track star Wilma Rudolph and President Franklin D. Roosevelt exemplified this.[66] But it was more complex than this.

Disability wore the mantle of medical authority and scientific objectivity but produced a subjective reality. It connoted prejudice. Society manufactured stereotypes and constructed obstacles to fundamental social interaction. The mere act of meaningful work became problematic: "The new clinically disabled category defined the person with a disability as a figure excluded from economic opportunities and therefore without free agency, self-determinism, and self-progressing—the ennobling attributes of the liberal American individual." Yet another, but rarely acknowledged, cultural stereotype arose: a disabled woman as "asexual and unfeminine."[67] Work and sexuality have operated as fundamental social experiences, ones that define the human condition. This process of classifying people, a social construct, became embedded in everyday life and in basic social contexts.

Modern media in general and the movie industry in particular, during the twentieth century, became "so intertwined with other institutions" that they played key roles in fashioning the dominant culture,[68] maturing as poliomyelitis epidemics raged throughout the country. The cinema, a manifestation of popular culture, entertained mass audiences and became the most pervasive visual medium during the pre-television era. And unspoken, exaggerated representations endured, with filmmakers freely exploiting the spectrum of emotions. The public's gaze became profitable through such "visual consumption."[69] This medium did much to reify public perceptions of disability. "In the early twentieth century, the predominant social identity enjoined on people with *physical* disabilities was 'the cripple.'"[70] Movie characters with "orthopedic impairments" received special attention as early as the second decade of the twentieth century. Cast as antagonists, their repressed anger over their condition, and their frustration as rejected lovers because of their hideous appearance, ultimately led to their downfall. This became instantly symbolized in the visual image of the "hunchback" or any other characters with "distorted spines."[71] Mass culture, simply put, reduced "cripples" to social pariahs.[72]

The sideshow's greatest popularity occurred between 1840 and 1940. A physical anomaly usually marked such "curiosities"; appearance thus defined the display, and the sale of photographs and pamphlets exaggerated it. Nineteenth- and twentieth-century audience responses differed, though. During the former, freak shows projected them as "inferior, subhuman, and dangerous." These displays remained "an accepted part of American popular culture" well into the twentieth century. However, due to the "growth of organized charities, the rise of professional fund-raising, and the invention of the poster child," they now elicited pity from viewers.[73]

Early cinema embraced this freak-show image of disability, exemplified in the extreme with Metro-Goldwyn-Mayer's 1932 release of *Freaks*. Early in the film, the sideshow barker promotes "monstrosities" that consumers pay to view. While they find the sight of children with disabilities playing or appearing in public places abhorrent, as we have seen, they willingly spend money to gaze at them in a carnival setting for entertainment. But this does not represent the only subtle message. Tensions exist among circus performers themselves. Most of the able-bodied abuse, demean, exploit, and patronize characters with disabilities. The latter feel animosity toward the former who hold them in such contempt. The main plot centers on Hans, a small person, and Cleopatra, a big person. He is smitten with her, and she leads him on for her own amusement and that of Hercules, her able-bodied boyfriend, who works as the strongman. Another small person sees what he does not. Hans continues to woe Cleopatra, but the film also consists of a variety of vignettes portraying each person's disability. Hans, who had inherited a fortune, gives Cleopatra expensive jewelry, which she then gives to Hercules to sell. She hatches a plan with him to marry Hans, kill him, and split his estate. She gradually begins to poison him as early as their wedding feast. Everyone attends, and they all grow intoxicated. When Hans's peers attempt to initiate her as "one of them," she cruelly rejects them, furiously screaming "freaks" at all of them. Offended and suspicious, Hans's friends combine their disabilities to spy on her, realize her murderous intentions, and unite to protect one of their own. They inform Hans about her plan. He thereafter secretly spits out the poison, disguised as medicine, that Cleopatra gives him for his so-called illness. Hans's friends unnerve her by continuously and visibly watching her, ultimately confronting Cleopatra and Hercules. The climax comes with them slaying Hercules while Cleopatra mysteriously turns into part duck and part human, a freak. She has become one of them. This movie was re-released in 1948 under various titles, one of them being *Nature's Mistakes*.[74]

Other productions, benignly labeled "horror films," projected people with disabilities in a variety of sinister roles: things—not people—who sparked anxiety or abuse. These movies clearly exploited "able-bodied fears," and audiences loved them, much to the glee of cinema moguls. The director of *Freaks*, Tod Browning, had already established his cinematic reputation with *Dracula*. Pity surfaced as well, with the symbol of the "Sweet Innocent" exemplified in the person of Tiny Tim, portrayed in *Scrooge* in 1935 and *The Christmas Carol* in 1938.[75] Whether as monsters or victims, "they were represented as incapacitated for real participation in the community and the economy, incapable of usefully directing their lives, disruptive and disorderly, antithetical to those defined as *healthy* and *normal*. They were socially devalued."[76]

This became institutionalized for children disabled by poliomyelitis, who "were segregated in the 'special' classes and schools that had been expanding since their advent around the turn of the century. The vast majority of handicapped youngsters were completely excluded from public schools. Rehabilitation professionals favored educating them in more 'appropriate' settings such as hospitals. Moreover, public resistance to educating them at all, whether in special or general classes, seems to have intensified during the 1930s. Those allowed entry were often stigmatized."[77] As Edmund J. Sass, disabled by polio, retrospectively points out, this disease struck at "a time when there was no concern for handicapped rights or accessibility, a time before political correctness, when a person with a physical disability was just a 'cripple.'"[78] And many of these children internalized these attitudes. Michael Davis's left leg remained one inch shorter than his right, and only after years of therapy did he partially recover the use of his left arm. In the process, even two years later, he felt like a "freak and didn't want to look and act like one."[79]

Families too often contributed to disability's stigma. Fred Davis's sociological study found that households with children disabled by infantile paralysis pursued some form of adaptive behavior or coping strategy to one degree or another, manifested through either normalization or dissociation. The former proved to be the most common, while the latter was less so. "Normalization was found in families in which the polio child was relatively young, only moderately handicapped, and closely related in age to one or more siblings, and whose family functioned in a more or less equalitarian fashion." This process, always forced, attempted to restore social relationships and routines, to assimilate the child back into society; it appeared to be fraught with rationalization and denial by the child and the parents. Dissociation occurred "when the polio child was older, severely handicapped, and either an only child or far removed in age from his nearest sibling, and whose family functioned in a more traditional fashion." Deeply embarrassed, the family members attempted to separate themselves from the social world because "they themselves regarded the crippled child as somehow 'different.'"[80]

"Emotional Maladjustment"

Psychological considerations were noticeably missing from many rehabilitation programs. Between 1932 and 1940, the modest amount of literature that existed casually categorized individuals disabled by infantile paralysis as manifesting pathological behaviors, such as being demanding, embarrassed, emotionally maladjusted, lazy, prone to temper tantrums, resentful, and selfish. Both the medical and psychological communities knew that physical disabilities exacted a heavy emotional toll on children, but they remained unclear about the actual impact.

A clinical study, compiled by a medical social worker, followed the lives of one hundred patients, between the ages of eighteen months and fifteen years, who had been discharged from the Orthopedic Clinic of New Haven Hospital during the 1943 polio epidemic. The study ran from September 1, 1943, to April 15, 1944, a major period of physical recovery and social readjustment for them. Fifteen had been released to the Children's Community Center for convalescence, sixteen went to the Newington Home for Crippled Children, and the remaining sixty-nine returned home directly after discharge. This report concluded that these children experienced more "difficulties" than children recovering from other diseases. Thirty-eight percent of them displayed serious "behavior problems," generally manifested as markers for clinical depression: antisocial behavior, eating problems, frequent crying spells, insomnia, intransigence, irritability, and general withdrawal. Three theories emerged from this analysis to explain this phenomenon. First, the poliovirus itself inflicted serious, and sometimes permanent, physical and emotional damage. Second, this disease struck already vulnerable children the hardest—those already susceptible to a multitude of problems, those with a "constitutional inferiority." Third, polio irreparably traumatized them, beginning with the shock of parental separation during hospital admissions. Then the realization of contracting a highly feared health menace further devastated them. Finally, these children recognized that physical disability often meant social ostracism.[81]

The National Foundation for Infantile Paralysis (NFIP) seemingly made a commitment to this area when Morton A. Seidenfeld became director of psychological services in February 1946. That organization's total knowledge, accumulated between 1932 and 1951, could be distilled to four key points, as Seidenfeld clinically pointed out to nurses, parents, and physical therapists: first, be a good listener, to give the child a chance to "get it off his chest"; second, maintain a tight schedule that distracted children from "vegetating," or wallowing in self-pity; third, communicate with patients about their treatments, because providing information relieves apprehension; and fourth, do not coddle them. For Seidenfeld, helping the disabled child learn how to lead a normal life was "fundamental," because no emotional differences existed between children with and without physical handicaps. In sum, the individual disabled by this virus held the sole power to overcome social attitudes and physical obstacles. It merely represented one's outlook, a matter of "good mental hygiene."

After two years, Seidenfeld expressed disappointment in the lack of enthusiasm or financial support by the NFIP for psychological research. He saw that the NFIP's leadership's "evasion" and "resistance" to this initiative had "completely emasculated" the program, that "phase of poliomyelitis research that most everyone wants to 'duck.'" This lack of empirical data hindered any meaningful psychological assistance. The foundation not only minimized the need for psychological research but also failed to even implement training programs to address the emotional needs of children disabled by polio.[82]

This was desperately needed. The emotional transformation from being able-bodied to being disabled did not usually unfold in a clear-cut, linear fashion. As Mary Grimley Mason expresses it in her memoir, "I think some part of my mind always remained able-bodied and functioned as an observer, creating a double consciousness. At times this second self took over and I acted without awareness of my disability. I felt like a 'normal' person. At other times, this other self withdrew in sadness and I felt different and alienated."[83]

Left to their own devices, people with disabilities acted in many different, and sometimes nuanced, ways.[84] Individual action involved the "overcomer."[85] Collective responses represented another expression of agency. The New York League of the Physically Handicapped initiated sit-ins, strikes, pickets, etc., to protest the discriminatory policies of the Works Progress Administration (WPA) and the Emergency Recovery Act. The Great Depression intensified the problems of the people with physical disabilities. The much-heralded WPA, while attempting to relieve serious unemployment, blatantly discriminated against them. Disability historians Paul K. Longmore and David Goldberger note how anger against the federal government's biased policies spawned an organizational response. Founding members rejected the stereotypes of villains, victims, and overachievers; instead, they sought self-dependence and dignity. The league, an all-inclusive association, included many polio members. Hyman Abramovitz, who wore leg braces and used a crutch due to childhood polio, served as an early leader. "Forming not as the League of Polio Survivors, but as the League of the Physically Handicapped and rarely even mentioning impairment, they concentrated on discrimination rather than diagnosis. Their activism sought to alter public understanding of disabilities, shifting the focus from coping with impairment to managing identity, from experiencing polio to engaging in politics." Abramovitz led a sit-in at the New York City Emergency Relief Board (ERB) on May 29, 1935. The protesters focused on meaningful and well-paying work as their fundamental goal. They made two demands on behalf of the disabled: jobs and integration. In a show of worker solidarity, the Writers Union, the Young Communists of America, and the City Committee of the Unemployment Council joined the dissenters as picketers the next two days. On May 31, ERB administrators vacillated: they at first cut off food and then decided to feed the squatters, but they isolated them from any contact with the press. Finally, on June 6, the police arrested eleven protesters, "eight of them handicapped." The sit-in ended that day. League members staged an additional protest outside of the WPA's New York City headquarters on November 9. Better organized, identifying with the unemployed in general, and using radical labor tactics, they picketed for three weeks and again in January 1936. WPA officialdom, after stalling for months, relented and created the Bureau for the Physically Handicapped, providing jobs for some 1,500 workers.

Nevertheless, League leaders recognized that the New York branch of the WPA did not represent the source of their problems; rather, the federal government did. Thirty-five members traveled to Washington, DC, and staged a sit-in until WPA director Harry Hopkins agreed to see them. While he conceded to the protesters' request for a meeting, Hopkins remained steadfast in denying any WPA discrimination and angrily bolted from the gathering. League members appealed to President Roosevelt for a hearing, but he rebuffed them. In August 1936, the League submitted a formal list of grievances to Hopkins and Roosevelt. The president never responded. As Longmore and Goldberger point out, Roosevelt, by all accounts, saw disability as a personal struggle, but League members recognized it as a social issue. They staged another protest in Washington, DC, in June 1937, but to no avail. In sum, they had achieved a pyrrhic victory: the League won short-term, local gains in New York City yet failed to reshape federal policy toward the disabled.

People disabled by polio struggled to create a positive self-identity and sometimes resorted to activist methods to achieve it. They wanted "not just jobs but valid social identities." League members saw themselves as "handicapped," not "cripples," "paralytics," "invalids," "paralytic victims," or "helpless crippled people," labels that proved demeaning at worst and patronizing at best.[86] Many perceived themselves neither as less than human nor helpless.

"Useful Citizens"

Manual training, as we have seen, appeared to dominate the educational agenda for children with infantile paralysis. This concept grew out of the broader progressive education movement that unfolded between 1880 and 1920. As each state passed mandatory attendance laws, enrollment increased dramatically. In order to accommodate such large numbers while at the same time recognizing that most school-age students did not move on to higher education, they had to be prepared for work. Business leaders, operating from a human-capital perspective, likewise supported industrial training, because they needed more productive workers in order to compete with other industrial powers like Germany and Great Britain. All of this converged with federal legislation: the Smith-Hughes Act of 1917. It formalized and institutionalized vocational education as an integral part of the public education system. "Schooling would serve as a bridge to a job and perhaps meaningful work." However, this notion undermined using public schooling as a mode of social mobility; in short, it limited equal opportunity.[87] "During the first half of the twentieth century . . . the disabled body was constructed primarily in terms of the industrial body, or the productive body, or the ergonomic body."[88]

Society saw people with disabilities as potentially less productive and concomitantly dependent. This situation was morally wrong and had to be rectified. These children needed "reclamation," as the editor of the *Hospital School Journal* opined in 1919.[89] A clear institutional response to this disease unfolded, albeit somewhat unevenly. One of these, Vermont's first rehabilitation facility subsidized through philanthropic support, opened in January

1921. This "school and home for crippled children" located in Proctor was, according to Lovett writing in 1924, "built especially for these children. In addition to a staircase, an incline to the second floor is provided so that children with long braces and crutches may ascend easily." It provided a "real home atmosphere" with a garden, a gymnasium, a playroom, a sun parlor, "an open fireplace, a piano, a victrola, couches, well-filled book shelves, and toys to delight the heart of any child." Schooling continued as well: "Lessons are given to them in shorter periods than in the schools for *normal* children and in addition to the regular schoolwork, cooking, sewing, and handicraft are taught, as well as music for those of special ability." Teaching these children such vocational skills appeared to be part of the natural order of things.

That same year, Vermont's state health department conducted a study of individuals disabled by polio and found that "because of their . . . isolation from suitable work [they] were unable to contribute materially to their own support." It inaugurated a vocational training program that, in largely rural Vermont, involved a visiting teacher "who shows them the various possibilities in the way of making articles and instructs them in the one that they select." This included creating toys, making baskets, producing needlework, and weaving rugs. Follow-up visits ensued to monitor progress, providing raw materials, collecting their finished goods to sell, and paying them for their work. "Aside from the economic value of enabling these remade individuals to discharge their debt to the community," Lovett concludes, "the moral effect of this work on the patients themselves can be scarcely be overestimated, for through it they have acquired independence and self respect and have become useful citizens."[90] Paternalism and morality, values embedded in this educational venture, would prove uplifting to the non-disabled observer.

Human-capital notions certainly contributed to philanthropic support. At the same time, and reflecting Progressive reformers' attitude toward disability, philanthropists simply deemed individuals with disabilities unproductive. Rockefeller Foundation officials early on reasoned that since the "eventual ability of a paralyzed child to earn its living is largely dependent on the extent to which its muscular functions are destroyed, the per capita expenditure would seem to be amply justified as an investment."[91] Brooklyn's Seaside Hospital is an institutional example of this outlook. It opened in the autumn of 1916, devoted strictly to the aftercare of children with physical disabilities. Seaside's primary goal consisted of avoiding muscle atrophy in order to prevent "deformity." Treatment involved casts, consisting of metal and plaster of Paris, supplemented with a "long time in bed, with proper support to back, to arms and to legs and feet, and with gradual assumption of reclining positions and continuance of the specially indicated support." It operated with the strict motive of avoiding disability. Such care therefore solved a "large economic community problem. By far-reaching preventive measures, it transforms a *cripple* into a *worker*. It frees the community from expense and obligation."[92]

Social rehabilitationists focused on aligning disability with these public attitudes. They perceived disabled people as "shiftless." This "victim-blaming practice" saw dependency as pathological.[93] By 1935, Henry H. Kessler, a recovery specialist, noted that polio caused 27 percent of disability in New York City, 41 percent in Cleveland, and 51 percent in Chicago. The major problem, as he saw it, was that "child cripples are adult disability problems." This existed because general hospitals discharged orthopedic patients "too early." Thus they had little or no institutional therapeutic support.[94]

Progressive reformers saw education, vis-à-vis vocational training, moving individuals with disabilities from a perceived state of parasitic dependency to that of a potential economic and social asset. A good American male citizen worked, after all. "Through work, men contributed to the economic well-being of the nation, set an example for younger generations, and symbolized the most prized aspect of the American character—independence." Women with disabilities became social outcasts for two reasons. First, they appeared repulsive, absent any sexuality. Second, they were unmarriageable because of the additional responsibilities they would load on the shoulders of their husbands and the burden that the stress of being wives would place on their frail bodies. These rehabilitationists, focusing their efforts on both male and female children, built some twenty hospital-schools between 1890 and 1924, ranging in size "from modest facilities of less than thirty 'pupil patients' to large institutions with hundreds of beds." They provided both medical treatment and education, with the latter stressing "moral, vocational, and academic" guidance and skills.[95]

That moral component became encapsulated in psychological terms, as John F. Landon and Lawrence W. Smith articulate it in their 1931 textbook, *Poliomyelitis: A Handbook for Physicians and Medical Students*. The "mental attitude of the 'cripple'" remains paramount throughout the convalescent and residual paralysis stages. The "cripple" psychology, they elaborate, becomes a label for those "handicapped individual[s] who [are] satisfied to sit back and let others wait on [them]." To avoid this mindset, Landon and Smith emphasized that "definite plans for economic self support should be considered," principally through schooling.[96] In sum, normalization dictated the rehabilitation regimen for children disabled by polio.

Disability represented a fundamental economic problem. Not only did society lose productivity, Kessler argued, but the "disabled have, up to the present time, always been considered as a permanently dependent class." Only through the inculcation of certain work skills and attitudes, as he saw it, would they cease being a drain on society, becoming productive citizens once again. Therefore, the "disabled person is an individual problem of vocational adjustment." Education presented a conundrum, however. It operated as an apparent solution, but it remained largely inaccessible. In Cleveland, 32 percent of children with disabilities were not in school in 1915; in New York City, that figure was 21 percent. They were instead supposedly educated at home.[97] Special classes and schools developed through the public education system attempted to address this perceived problem. Nevertheless, society's expectations (i.e., normalization) and the realities of disability remained unreconciled until World War II.

Howard A. Rusk, an internist in St. Louis, profoundly influenced modern rehabilitation policies and practices. After enlisting in the military in 1942 and working in a Missouri Army Air Corps military hospital, he began to conceptualize a comprehensive convalescent program for military personnel recovering from combat injuries. It began as a transition program from being a patient to returning as a soldier. This required physical conditioning, to be sure, but it included academic and military studies (i.e., occupational therapy); that is, to expedite the recovery of wounded troops, they rebuilt engines, studied radio codes, and planted victory gardens. His goal involved bringing "severely injured men back to mental as well as physical health," encompassing their educational, emotional, and occupational needs. Moreover, early ambulating following surgery, Rusk discovered, hastened healing: "We were fighting a desperate war, and … we needed all the manpower we could find . . . Our initial aim had to be to send them back to duty in the best possible condition and in the shortest time. If they could no longer do their previous jobs, we should help them choose jobs they could do, and then retrain them." Pragmatic as well as humanitarian reasons drove Rusk. This innovation resulted in shorter and improved recovery, bringing it to the attention of military brass. They replicated it at 253 Army Air Corps bases, officially becoming the Army Air Force Convalescent Training Program. As Rusk recalls, "There was no precedent for rehabilitation programs on a large scale in the military . . . [and] no extensive civilian programs, either."[98] Before leaving the military, Rusk also ensured that the reorganized Veterans Administration adopted this same model.

With the end of the war and as "growing numbers of polio epidemics made child patients rather than wounded soldiers the defining focus of physical therapy work, the site of practice shifted from veterans' hospitals to children's hospitals and children's rehabilitative centers."[99] Rusk embarked on "rehabilitation in civilian life, where the concept of rehabilitation for the disabled was virtually unknown or unaccepted, even by the medical profession." He wanted to restore the "whole person . . . not just the part of him that had been damaged. They had no concept of the emotional problems which followed disability, or the problems of job placement." In December 1945, he accepted the chair position of the new department of Rehabilitation and Physical Medicine at New York University's medical school. The formal dedication of the permanent home of the Institute of Rehabilitation Medicine occurred on January 25, 1951, and nine-year-old Margaret Ann Flick, confined to a wheelchair because of polio, cut the ceremonial ribbon. That facility included administrative offices, a cafeteria, a gymnasium, a library, an occupational therapy department, and patients' rooms. And it catered to patients with physical disabilities from all over the world, not just those paralyzed by poliomyelitis.[100]

Brenda Serotte, who contracted this virus at age seven in 1954, while living in the Bronx, went there as an inpatient for follow-up care with the goal of eliminating the need for her "Milwaukee brace," a body brace made of leather and steel running from the neck to the pelvis. She underwent occupational and physical therapy, and she attended "Hospital School" at the institute. Because of its predictable routine, it grew familiar and secure, ultimately becoming a "new home" for Serotte. "We had school until lunch; afterwards everyone went to the physical therapy room for individual help." There, therapists relentlessly drove their patients, demonizing disability. "Unless you wanted to be a 'helpless cripple,' synonymous with 'hateful devil,' you fought, you fell, you climbed, you stretched, you kept working." They especially pushed those disabled by infantile paralysis: "It was believed that we could accomplish more than others, accident victims or those born with birth defects, could. I was indoctrinated with the idea that I could do *anything*, miraculous things . . . And if I did not reach my goal, it meant that I didn't work hard enough, trying my best . . . No doubt, it left some of us, who failed to scale Mount Everest, furious with ourselves and depressed."[101]

Rusk succinctly summarized his approach as "mind could overcome matter."[102] His combination of physical and occupational therapy represented a "ground-breaking emphasis on looking at the whole person." But it still worked within the medical paradigm, not seeing disability as a social issue.[103] This certainly represented an incremental improvement over what had preceded it, moving it to a highly technical, if not mechanical, routine of physical and emotional recovery. Yet disability remained a largely individual challenge, though the NFIP subsidized the Self-Help Device Research Project undertaken at Rusk's institute. This study collected information about "devices and gadgets that might aid disabled persons in the performance of daily activities of life and work." The institute's staff tested these appliances as well as designed and developed others.[104] Nevertheless, Rusk's compelling assertion that motivation, "exploiting to the fullest, the patient's remaining abilities," drove his technique; at the same time, it minimized the "physical and emotional consequences of poliomyelitis."[105] Therefore, by the 1950s, recovery involved "hard work, determination, and pluck." It became, in short, the "Horatio Alger cripple story."[106] This required no cultural realignment in able-bodied perceptions or environmental adaptations. For those disabled by polio, no fundamental change occurred, as they remained the "other."

"A Polio's Paradise"[107]

Another therapeutic option existed, where individuals paralyzed by this disease did not have to worry about being perceived through their disabilities or fear mistreatment. Many likened Warm Springs to heaven. Often, after many years of entering one hospital after another—depressing institutional settings for children—the mere glimpse of Warm Springs gave them instant respite. To Shreve in the 1950s, it appeared to be a resort, "more like a hotel than a hospital, like a spa it had once been at the turn of the century. White-painted brick buildings surrounding a wide expanse of lawn with trees and flowers, winding cement walkways, the southern calm of a balmy afternoon." Rather than a forbidding multistory brick edifice, like typical hospitals and rehabilitation centers, it exuded warmth, sitting amidst tall oak and pine trees; rather than the drab paint and stark architecture common to medical settings at that time, it provided young children with disabilities with an almost enchanted physical world. They attended school during the morning hours and therapy in the afternoons.[108]

Roosevelt's annual Thanksgiving visits became major events. Mary Grimley Mason, who contracted polio at age four in 1932, went there for therapy. She won the privilege, through a lottery drawing, to sit next to the president and his wife, Eleanor, at dinner. Mary felt incredibly self-conscious. In an interview published in *The Philadelphia Inquirer*, Eleanor revealed that Roosevelt had cut Mason's turkey for her in an attempt to help her relax. Children also performed musicals for the president during those visits.

They did not feel like outsiders in this social context. Small cottages operated as patient dormitories, rather than large wards, and had a "housemother" who wrote a weekly letter home to each child's family.[109] Moreover, all felt wedded together through the common bond of disability. This commonality spawned strong emotional relationships at key points in their lives. This was the case with Lorenzo W. Milam. As a teenager during the summer of 1953, he experienced a spiritual and social resurrection while at Warm Springs. A combination of effective rehabilitation and unfettered social interaction—watching movies, playing cards, frolicking in wheelchairs with peers, dating, drinking, and engaging in sexual exploration—helped them to recover some parts of their lives. As he expressed it, "For being crippled in the environment of three hundred other upwardly mobile cripples has its own special distinctive rapture. We speak the same language. Our bodies know the same limitation. Our restricted world is restricted commonly among the three hundred of us, and especially the dozen or so who make up our age group."[110]

Shreve, who arrived at Warm Springs in 1950, recalls a similar feeling; in her words, those who inhabited Warm Springs became a "substitute family." Nothing symbolized this tight-knit group more than Thanksgiving Day, when a long line of patients in wheelchairs and stretchers excitedly proceeded across the grounds to Georgia Hall. Shreve describes "a sense of family . . . a colony of outsiders whose lives were dignified by kinship to a man like us who had been president of the United States." As they crowded into the large room, they found "candlelit tables with white tablecloths set in a U. On one side of the U were the patients on stretchers, pushed up to the table on their stomachs so they could eat. And on the other side of the U were the wheelchairs. There were no regular chairs at all, no need for a chair except at the far end of the table, the half-circle of the U, an empty chair where Roosevelt would have sat had he been there." At Warm Springs, they were all the same. As Shreve expresses it, "At Warm Springs I would be one among equals."[111]

Warm Springs operated on levels other than just treatment. It served as a source for innovation for people with disabilities, collecting, archiving, and distributing sketches and plans for many adaptations to facilitate mobility and overcome architectural impediments. Patients published many of these in the *Polio Chronicle*. "Do You Drive, Polio?" featured photographs of mechanical modifications to automobiles to permit "parals" (i.e., the paralyzed) to drive—levers operating foot pedals represented one example. "The Electric Eye" explained how photocells, or "light-sensitive devices" or "electric eyes," offered assistance in crossing streets, controlling lights at home, and opening doors. In "Going Up," the Architectural and Mechanical Hints Group of the National Patients' Committee noted that it had on file "complete information provided by manufacturers of different types of home elevators"[112]

Warm Springs thus operated as a clearinghouse for information and the heart of a network linking individuals disabled by polio throughout the country. Patients themselves began to publish and distribute various newsletters, from the *Polio Chronicle*, to *The Crutch*, and finally the *Wheelchair Review*, in the 1930s. They sent them to donors as well as to those disabled by this disease. This outreach process gradually built a national community, one whose awareness of the need for disability rights grew each year; this was a place where individuals with disabilities led real lives.[113] But it was not totally inclusive. Since it resided in Georgia, a Southern state committed to *de jure* segregation, it did not treat African American patients.

Tuskegee

African American children who contracted polio faced the most intense social rejection, because they battled two prejudices: race and disability. A severe epidemic struck the previously unscathed South in 1936. Until that point, most medical experts claimed that African Americans remained immune to this virus. That year's epidemic destroyed that myth and revealed a serious medical void: "Those institutions capable of treating poliomyelitis effectively were either too far away to permit travel for poor rural blacks or were open to whites only." The Children's Bureau reported in 1939 that African Americans had access to a mere thirty beds in the entire Southern region; otherwise, they had to sit in segregated waiting rooms or in hospital basements, awaiting their treatments.[114]

The Warm Springs facility, located in the deep South, conformed to dominant white prejudices, as its 1929 pamphlet declared: "The spirit of Warm Springs of the Old South is carefully nurtured and preserved. Here the lightheartedness of the darky help abounds."[115] It hired African Americans to work as cooks, custodians, waiters, and wheelchair pushers but did not admit African Americans for treatments. As a result, many during the 1930s perceived Warm Springs as an "elite" refuge.[116] Because of exclusion, others objected to fundraising activities like the President's Birthday Balls. In Texas, the "Harris County Afro-American Medical Association refused to purchase tickets to the Houston Negro Ball." Dr. Mary F. Waring, president of the National Association for Colored Women, expressed her discontent in a letter addressed to the Warm Springs Foundation: "Children are deserving of a fair start in life and all children should be given the chance to develop normally, if possible."[117] Only reluctantly and after considerable prodding from Eleanor Roosevelt did Warm Springs begin to accommodate young African American patients. This proved limited, though: "While [President Roosevelt] was happy to dedicate the building of the new Warm Springs Negro School in 1937, after it had been constructed with the support of the Julius Rosenwald Fund, blacks were never admitted to Warm Springs for treatment, except as outpatients, during his lifetime." Whether it was the context of Georgia's long and dubious segregationist tradition, or Roosevelt's "unthinking racism of his class," the concept of "separate but equal" permeated Warm Springs.[118]

The emergence of the National Foundation for Infantile Paralysis in 1938 marked an institutional shift. Criticized by African American journalists and pressured by African American doctors through their organization, the National Medical Association (NMA), Basil O'Connor began to explore "solutions to resolve the disparity in convalescent treatment," addressing a serious social and public relations challenge for the fledgling foundation. In doing so, he sought the advice of Midian O. Bousfield. Having graduated from Northwestern University Medical School in 1909, Bousfield became a leading African American physician, serving as NMA president in 1933–34 and appointed as director of the Negro Health Division of the Julius Rosenwald Fund in 1939. He suggested the development of a "Negro Warm Springs" facility. O'Connor asked Paul de Kruif, secretary of the foundation's General Advisory Committee, to investigate its feasibility. Finally, on May 22, 1939, O'Connor publicly announced a new NFIP project: the Infantile Paralysis Center for Negroes. The foundation granted the Tuskegee Institute $192,253, over the next four years, to construct, equip, and maintain a 36-bed facility. It would provide care and after-treatment for African American patients, establish a brace shop and train "Negro orthopedic brace makers," and train doctors, nurses, and physical therapists.[119] "At the time," historian Stephen E. Mawdsley writes, "this was the largest grant ever made by the NFIP to a single institution, the first grant awarded to a black institution, and the only grant made for a construction project." Tuskegee's Infantile Paralysis Center was formally dedicated on January 15, 1941, with O'Connor delivering one of the inauguration addresses. It operated as a special unit of the John A. Andrew Memorial Hospital on that campus, which had opened in 1913 to provide health care to African Americans in the South, as well as extension programs, health clinics, midwife courses, and nurse training.[120]

The NFIP's sponsorship of Tuskegee's polio facility fit into the broader context of white philanthropies and African American social institutions. Julius Rosenwald, president of Sears, Roebuck, and Company, ran his fund from Chicago. From 1917 to 1927, it subsidized the construction of schools in the South for African Americans as well as Meharry Medical College. After 1928, it "broadened its mission to include medical care." However, historian Vanessa Northington Gamble asserts, in a more fundamental way, "the Rosenwald Fund worked to establish and maintain racially separate institutions, viewing its support of such facilities not as encouraging Jim Crow, but . . . as a pragmatic response to the racial realities of American life." The General Education Board represented another example. It maintained a broad education agenda that encompassed basic and higher education, teacher training, and medical education, providing an "annual appropriation to Meharry College" beginning in 1916 and to Howard University in 1920; this involved upgrading preparation for African American medical students as well as subsidizing internships. The resolution of racial problems did not represent part of its mandate either. All of these white philanthropies, Gamble adds, designed their programs "to operate within the framework of a segregated society."[121]

John W. Chenault, head of orthopedic surgery at Andrew Hospital since 1937, served as director of the new polio care facility. He had graduated from the University of Minnesota's medical school in 1931 and served as a Rockefeller Scholar in orthopedic surgery at the universities of Chicago and Iowa. His initial contribution to the fight against this disease involved research that showed the "rising number of poliomyelitis cases among children being seen at the hospital. In the absence of studies correlating poliomyelitis with racial incidence, Dr. Chenault . . . showed that 15.3 percent of all crippled Negro children seen at Tuskegee Institute were victims of infantile paralysis, a significant percentage considering that blacks were thought to be immune." He had also worked with George Washington Carver and his peanut oil massage therapy, finding some promise in this approach for children disabled by this virus.[122]

The Infantile Paralysis Center occupied a three-story building, containing a brace-fitting room, a gymnasium, a heated swimming pool with a hydraulic lift, a kitchen, a schoolroom, patients' rooms, stainless-steel Hubbard tanks, a sundeck, treatment rooms (e.g., plaster casting), and whirlpools, while surgery took place at the Andrew Memorial Hospital. Chenault oversaw a physician, five nurses, two physical therapists, one occupational therapist, and various assistants. The Alabama State Crippled Children's Service supplied two special education teachers. This center primarily accommodated African American children from the South but welcomed patients from as far away as Illinois, Ohio, New York, and Texas, admitting a total of two hundred patients between 1941 and 1948; their stays ranged from ten to eighteen months. The staff ensured that they celebrated all holidays and every patient's birthday. Six-year-old Clara Yelder, who resided in rural Alabama, received treatment there. For fun, she and other young patients listened to the radio and raced their wheelchairs. That center not only treated polio patients but also disseminated information and trained African American nurses, physicians, and physiotherapists. Bousfield appealed to O'Connor in 1941 to promote the new facility, and the foundation responded by producing fifty thousand booklets that were circulated among African American newspapers, physicians, religious leaders, and teacher associations, among others. The foundation ultimately invested a total of $414,356 in this clinic over a period of six years.[123]

Nevertheless, Warm Springs remained a bone of contention, "a symbol of persistent inequality" for African Americans. With a far more sophisticated medical staff and elaborate facility than Tuskegee, it employed African American domestics and custodians yet accepted no patients of color.[124] Moreover, Tuskegee's polio center, later termed a "Negro medical ghetto" by a critic, proved inadequate to serve all of the needs of the African American community.[125]

One other lone exception, the Gonzales Warm Springs Rehabilitation Hospital for Crippled Children, in Texas, opened in September 1941 with two eight-bed wards and two large therapeutic pools. On the surface this facility appeared to replicate its Georgia counterpart; two differences stood out, though. First, while Georgia's Warm Springs center received national support, the Texas version relied on individual donations as well as local and state subsidies. Second, and more important, the Georgia center succumbed to segregation pressures, but the Gonzales hospital admitted all children: African Americans, Latinos, and European Americans shared the same wards. Due to circumstances unique to Texas—likewise mired in the Jim Crow South—it became "the only racially integrated rehabilitation hospital of its kind in the nation."[126]

THE END OF THE ROAD?

Many children worried about returning to their families. Quite a few feared leaving their convalescent facilities, where rigid routines ensured predictability. Home life would be different, but they did not yet know how; the unknown proved unsettling. Kriegel felt "terrified." He had lived in the ward for two years. He mourned the death of his life there. His comrades were there—his equals. There, everyone was the same. He was mobile. No one pitied him. As he departed, his friends gathered on the porch to bid him a sad farewell. He would never see them again. "How I loved them, all of them."[127] Others viewed their departures in almost euphoric terms, as George Durr describes. He had become infected at eighteen months of age in 1931 while living in Peekskill, New York, and because of the toll that virus took on his little body, he did not leave institutional care until age five. The insular nature of hospital life coupled with physical rehabilitation dominated his life during those years, making the outside world totally alien to him. He vividly recalls his impressions of assuming, for him, a new way of being. "I remember leaving the hospital, and I could not walk. I was completely paralyzed from the neck down. They had to strap me into the car. This was my first experience being outside—seeing trees and corn . . . It was just amazing to see houses and roads and cars . . . an unbelievable sight to a five-year-old kid who had been literally strapped or locked into a bed his whole life."[128] He was going home.

Chapter 5

Home Sweet Home

. . . save my children

—Dr. Robert Edward Wilson

Franz Kafka's surreal 1915 novella, *The Metamorphosis*, narrates how the central character, Gregor Samsa, awakes one morning to discover that he has suddenly and mysteriously been transformed into a "monstrous vermin." Lying on his back in bed, with his "pitifully thin" legs waving helplessly in the air, he cannot seem to move his insect-like body. He is revolted by his appearance. That is not all that has changed. Samsa's otherwise normal physical surroundings have become major obstacles; he is unable to extricate himself from his own bed or manipulate the door handle. The transformation of Gregor Samsa, a brother and son, is not isolated. It sparks a series of profound and extreme emotional, economic, and social changes within his family. His parents and their two domestic employees cannot see Gregor beyond his new physical manifestation. His father remains detached at best and outright hostile at worst. His mother and sister confine him to his bedroom to keep him out of sight, only unlocking the door to nervously shove some food on the floor and quickly retreat. Samsa's sister retains some compassion, but she is nevertheless disgusted by his new appearance and disposes of everything he touches. One of the maids is terrified even to be in the house and begs to be dismissed. After several months, his family's collective attitude shifts from treating him with antipathy to bare tolerance. As Kafka describes it, "In spite of his present pathetic and repulsive shape, [Gregor] could not be treated as an enemy; that, on the contrary, it was the commandment of family duty to swallow their disgust and endure him, endure him and nothing more."

Absent Gregor's income, the family slowly slips into poverty. Individual family members find jobs and exhaust themselves in a vain attempt to maintain the household. Pressing debts force them to fire their last housekeeper, sell their jewelry, and rent their spare rooms to boarders. All of this adds more stress as his weary sister continues to provide care for the helpless Gregor, cleaning his room and feeding him. The members of the once-placid family begin to frequently and intensely bicker among themselves; rejecting the once-loved brother and son, the family disintegrates over Samsa's new existence. Every one of his family members finds relief in his death; only then is the family resurrected.[1]

Although a seemingly simple tale, *The Metamorphosis* is suffused with multiple and complex meanings. In its literal sense, it portrays alienation. Samsa has mysteriously become a being who defies the norm, a "creature without a place in God's order."[2] He is unsightly, and his mere presence frightens even his own parents and sister. He feels like a burden to them and grows ever more isolated. *The Metamorphosis*, albeit dramatic and wholly dark, in many ways serves as an apt metaphor for how poliomyelitis unleashed a profound and multifaceted transformation for many American families. Historian Hugh Gregory Gallagher, disabled by infantile paralysis, expresses it best in retrospect: Polio was "not an individual" experience. Like a whirlpool it sucks all family members into a downward spiral.[3]

The institution of the family ground to a halt to await the life-and-death struggle of a child and at times more than one, though multiple cases of infantile paralysis appear to have been somewhat rare. During the 1916 New York City epidemic, 4.2 percent of recorded infections occurred among brothers and sisters, but the 1943 Los Angeles outbreak saw it rise to 9.3 percent. This virus, unbeknownst to families, usually lurked in their own bathrooms. "Inside the family, it spread through the bathtub, the viral particles shed by one bather clinging to the porcelain or towels used by the next."[4] Family members also shared the same toilet. Multiple infections proved to be especially tragic for parents. Such an episode unfolded during the 1910 Iowa epidemic. Seven siblings suffered infection to one degree or another within a ten-day span. On April 22, a four-year-old girl became ill and then suddenly was paralyzed; five days later her nine-year-old sister showed symptoms and shortly thereafter suffered paralysis; a twelve-year-old sister fell ill on May 1 and developed neck stiffness and general weakness but fully recovered; four additional siblings during this period only displayed a "malaise" and some limb weakness. Two years later, in September 1912, the seven-year-old daughter of a St. Louis doctor, Dr. Robert Edward Wilson, succumbed to poliomyelitis. The front page of *The New York Times* reported that the father, worried about the fate of his other three, similarly infected children, said, "I will give $10,000 to the man who can save my children." The article goes on to say, "The pathetic scene in the little girl's room . . . caused Dr. Wilson to go frantic, while two other physicians who had been in attendance were so affected that they had to leave the room."[5] Children's deaths took a heavy emotional toll on parents. The New York City health department released the contents of a contributor's letter to *The New York Times*, which the paper published on August 17, 1916: "Please add this modest contribution to the fund for braces for the crippled children who were perhaps more fortunate than mine . . . *An Easter Flower*—for that is what I have lost."[6] Forty years later four children of a Milwaukee family died of bulbar polio within eight days of one another. The oldest, age seventeen, played high-school football and had seemingly strained his right shoulder during practice. He and his family treated it as a typical minor injury and ignored it. Four days later, on September 14, he awoke with little use of that arm, a severe headache, an earache, difficulty speaking, and observable head tremors. His parents rushed him to the hospital, where his condition rapidly deteriorated; he died late the next day as his youngest sister, age four, was being admitted. She succumbed within thirty hours. Her eight-year-old sister followed on September 19 after complaining of a headache and stiff neck for two days. In spite of artificial respiration, she expired within a thirty-hour period. Finally, the hospital admitted her thirteen-year-old sister on September 21; she passed away within sixty hours. As late as 1956, the entire Rosenwald family fell ill—daughter, mother, and father. They all lay side by side in their respective iron lungs in the hospital.[7]

If the child—or children—survived, then a stressful regimen of recovery began. Returning home immediately introduced serious challenges at the human level. Moving from hospital life (where they had interacted with other children with disabilities for months) to home and eventually school, to be suddenly surrounded by people without disabilities, sparked emotional trauma. For young Charles L. Mee, an unbridgeable "gulf" now existed.[8] Following months of surgery and rehabilitation, the entire household had to adapt to new relationships and alter the physical arrangement of the home itself to accommodate a disabled member of the family. This intense care and new equipment came at a dear price, both emotional and financial. In sum, the entire family unit underwent enormous upheavals because of this disease.

The American family initially proved ill equipped to respond to the shock of childhood disability. Relying on the nuclear model for centuries in Western culture, its size shrunk, coinciding with a steady decline in birth rates from 1800 until World War II. Fewer household members meant more individual responsibilities during medical crises. This institution also struggled in another way. Between 1900 and 1950, its financial state proved precarious. By 1929, 60 percent of American families "earned $2,000 or less a year and were unable to save anything to help them weather spells of unemployment or illness." The Great Depression exacerbated this situation. The traditional idealized image during this dire period paints a picture of remarkable cooperation and interdependence among all members in order to survive. Nothing could be further from the truth. As unemployment and poverty steadily increased, so did domestic violence and child abuse. A catastrophic illness, like infantile paralysis, only added to this stress.[9]

Reactions to this stress assumed a variety of forms. It was not uncommon for some parents, at the beginning of the twentieth century, to abandon children disabled by polio because they saw them as "grotesque."[10] Even by the 1920s, many families typically hid them away in their homes.

Parents in particular and society in general simply denied their existence, as Gallagher says:

> In the 1920s, to be handicapped in some visible way carried with it social opprobrium . . . The well-to-do were able to afford custodial nursing care for their handicapped family members, and the loving family was able to care at home for its crippled loved ones. Many of the handicapped, however, were simply ignored by their families and society. A New York State study of handicapped children found them to be "neglected at home, rejected by the public schools, incapacitated by physical disability and unable to care for themselves." There was very little help for such persons.[11]

In many ways, then, family members often compounded the medical impact of this virus by conforming to social constraints against people with disabilities.

Public responses during epidemics manifested themselves in two distinct ways. Illness either caused local acquaintances to ostracize the affected family or resulted in unifying the community to assist the family. In the former case, people crossed streets to avoid passing directly in front of houses with polio patients, often advertised with quarantine signs. Many next-door neighbors closed and locked their windows facing homes where infections had occurred. One New Haven, Connecticut, family with an infected child could not use their front porch because of a verbal confrontation.

In the latter case, different groups coalesced in a single-minded effort. During North Carolina's 1944–45 epidemic, Hickory's citizens converted an open-air camp situated on the shore of a local lake to a temporary triage center. They undertook the onerous task of quickly converting the existing stone building and expanding it for patients. Volunteers began work on June 22, 1944, and within forty-eight hours completed construction of the first new wooden building. They continued to toil twenty-four hours a day to finish additional ward facilities, with carpenters, electricians, office workers, and parents carrying on through rain and at night, using floodlights. Local businesses and churches donated bed sheets, blankets, electric fans, refrigerators, stoves, and other furniture to equip the wards. A local Army barracks supplied beds, bedpans, and mattresses. The Red Cross and Army Air Corps flew in nurses, while other hospitals sent student nurses. The National Foundation for Infantile Paralysis (NFIP) paid the hotel bills to house all of them. It also sent Don W. Gudakunst, its first medical director (1938–45), to oversee matters, and it provided medical personnel, hot-pack machines, and respirators.[12] The family simply could not fathom how neighbors, in particular, or communities, in general, would respond to this crisis.

Beginning in the 1930s, after over a decade of relentless epidemics, the onset of infantile paralysis marked a profound transformation process for the American family. Marc Shell, disabled by infantile paralysis, dubs the family affected by this disability the "handicapped family."[13] In addition to paralyzing children and inflicting excruciating pain, infantile paralysis robbed them of their privacy, destroyed any sense of intimacy, and ate away at their dignity. Disability also profoundly disrupted family routines and interfered with personal relationships. This disease also proved to be highly conspicuous. In sum, the household experienced tensions, role realignments, spatial transformations, and financial hardships.

The Pathos of Disease and Disability

Polio unleashed a raft of emotions. Quarantine, as we have seen, represented a reflexive response by public health officials. This had a profound impact on household members. Because of placards, everyone now knew that the virus lurked nearby, and friends and neighbors sometimes abandoned them out of fear. During New York City's 1916 epidemic, people sometimes vacated entire tenement houses if two or more cases occurred there. Thirty-eight years later, seven-year-old Brenda Serotte witnessed a similar phenomenon at her Bronx apartment building after she had been diagnosed with infantile paralysis. Perceiving her parents and their apartment as contaminated, their closest neighbors "bought industrial-strength disinfectant and scrubbed down their doors, as if that would bar the microbes from seeping in." Others simply moved out. For months, neighbors snubbed her mother or crossed the street when they saw her.[14]

Extreme stress generated by epidemics, harsh public health policies, and compulsory separation of infected children pushed some parents to the breaking point. In 1916, a week after New York City health authorities forcibly removed Hilda Woltje's three-year-old daughter from her home and sent her to an "isolation hospital," she abandoned her husband in the middle of the night, fleeing with her five-year-old son to hide. She did not want to lose custody of her second child. On August 29, a *New York Times* front-page headline exclaimed, "Oyster Bay Revolts Over Poliomyelitis." It described how 160 residents in that Long Island village, incensed about the "health regulation permitting the forcible removal of children to the hospital" by the sheriff's department, began a "reign of terror" and took over the town meeting, forcing its board members to flee. A "citizens' committee" formed its own sanitary committee, which drafted new rules. Fearful of similar repercussions, other Long Island communities quickly modified their health measures. These actions went beyond New York City and its surrounding communities. In Orange, New Jersey, parents refused permission for their two-year-old son, recently diagnosed with infantile paralysis,

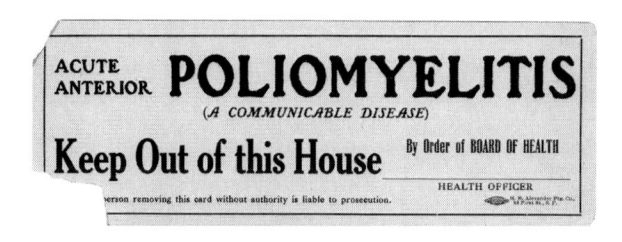

Figure 5.1 Acute Anterior Poliomyelitis (A Communicable Disease). Keep Out of this House.

to be sent to an isolation hospital. Three police officers overpowered the father while a health officer restrained the mother, in order to remove the child from the house. Within that same week, another article, titled "Mob Riots Over Paralysis," reported that on the evening of September 2, near Chambersburg, Pennsylvania, parents battled a health officer, a sheriff, and nine deputies when the officials attempted to prevent young children from attending an ox roast. This "mob" severely beat two of the deputy sheriffs in a melee that lasted well into that night.[15] Parents certainly feared the invisible bugs that threatened their children but could do nothing concrete about them. They did, however, find occasional convenient outlets with those civil servants who compounded these anxieties by separating them from their children. Many simply would not tolerate this violation of their parental rights; it was not enough, however. Health authorities, more often than not, prevailed.

Fred Davis's sociological analysis conducted in the mid-1950s found that immediately following a positive diagnosis, parents began a three-part emotional "inventory" process. First, they evaluated the child's condition, remaining ever optimistic. This glimmer of hope emerged with the near escape from death, reinforced by an implicit trust in medical science and health professionals. Second, and in spite of this sanguine attitude, parents felt guilt because their efforts to protect their child had proven inadequate. *They* had somehow failed! Many had attempted to protect them by purchasing wallpaper for their bedrooms soaked with DDT (dichlorodiphenyltrichloroethane), which was widely manufactured and sold. Although religious beliefs offered temporary solace, families found lasting comfort from the support and aid of others: "After some initial hesitation due to fear of contagion, neighbors and relatives rallied around the family; they inquired after the sick child, expressed condolences, helped with baby-sitting and other household-management problems, sent the child cards and presents, and in some instances even made offers of financial assistance to the family." Third, parents eventually recognized the long-term meaning of this health crisis. Functional households suddenly discovered that they had become dysfunctional. The "crippling" effect of paralytic polio meant "social abnormality, isolation, and, in the eyes of some, visible manifestation of inherent malevolence."[16]

Disability set a new course for families, who embarked on lives they had never anticipated. Anne, who contracted polio in 1951, remembers it as follows:

> My parents were told that I might not make it through the night. Doctors kept an iron lung right outside the door to my room. Since I kept breathing and didn't need the iron lung, my parents were told I would live, but I was likely never to walk again. I was in the Pest House for a month and then moved up the hill to the rehabilitation hospital. I stayed there for over a year. I left the hospital on my own two feet, a brace on my right leg. So I did live and I did walk again in spite of what the doctors said . . . [M]y parents say my recovery was "a miracle."[17]

Escaping death, in Anne's case, appeared to be her parents' only solace. Their daughter now faced a future dominated by orthopedic disability. Poliovirus shattered plans for a son's future, according to one father: "My life is formed around watching him grow up . . . Everything is good . . . Polio kills that. It stops that dream. It cuts it short." A mother experienced a complete breakdown when her four-year-old son entered the hospital. She abandoned her husband and other son for several days, seeking emotional refuge with her mother.[18] Edward O'Connor, who contracted this virus at age ten in 1955, while living in the Bronx, witnessed a tragic manifestation of this stress. With seven children in the family, the economic weight already proved to be overwhelming. The expenses of caring for a child with a disability only exacerbated his family's fragile financial well-being. Facing seemingly insurmountable bills, his father suffered a heart attack as O'Connor was being discharged from the hospital.[19]

For much of the twentieth century, poverty or alcoholism strained American families, sometimes leading to some form of neglect or violence; nevertheless, illness specifically accounted for 20 percent of the causes for attacks on children. Primary and secondary literature rarely hints at severe mistreatment of children disabled by polio. However, Richard L. Bruno, a post-polio syndrome expert, conducted a survey in 1995 and estimated that 40 percent of them reported abuse. The overwhelming emotional and economic pressures that parents felt during the critical period of infection and after-treatment expressed themselves in many and varied ways. Resentment over the loss of freedom, routines, and expectations led to outright violence in some cases. One person reported such an incident in Bruno's study: "When polio struck I was totally paralyzed and my mother screamed into my face, 'Why are you doing this to me?' Mother blamed me for family problems even when they really had nothing to do with my polio." Alice Cote contracted it at twenty-two months of age in 1935 in Attleboro, Massachusetts. Her return home elicited a chilling response: her stepmother beat her with a belt buckle out of bitterness over having to assist her with her rehabilitation exercises. Alice fled to live with an aunt and uncle to escape this maltreatment, but after being frightened by her uncle's sexual advances and isolated because of her aunt's jealousy over them, she moved in with another aunt and uncle. However, because they were in their seventies, they could not assist her with her physical therapy. She changed residences once again to join her sister, whom she found to be inhospitable. Cote's nuclear and extended family saw her disability as a burden—she was not welcomed anywhere. Her unfortunate odyssey resulted in a fragmented life, as she observes: "My first year of high school, I'd been to four high schools. Nobody wanted the responsibility of helping." Nor did Norma Meehan's parents cope well with her disability. They retreated to denial at first. Ill-treatment followed. One morning at age six, during the mid-1950s, she lay naked on her stomach, completely vulnerable. As her mother grew increasingly frustrated with trying to fit her back brace, impatient with the difficulties of dressing her and angry with her younger sister's irritating and distracting behavior, she completely lost her composure and beat Meehan with a belt buckle: "I was struck over a hundred times. It left some scars . . . My mother put Vaseline on it." Her father did not intervene, causing Meehan to feel betrayed.[20]

This disease unleashed a crosscurrent of emotions. Children disabled by infantile paralysis often allude to subtle but clear nonverbal signals in their parents' demeanor or changes in their personality with the onset of polio and its aftermath, reflecting incredible empathy. Parents stood on the precipice. The only occasion when they could visit their children in isolation was when they were on the verge of death. Twelve-year-old Peg Kehret found herself in this situation when she awoke one day to see her parents wearing gowns, gloves, and masks. This was the first time she had seen them since being admitted to the hospital. "As they stood beside my bed, I saw fear in their eyes. I realized they were allowed into the isolation ward now, when they had not been earlier, because I was so sick that the doctors weren't sure I would live." But it was not the disease alone that caused these emotions; disability intensified them. Michael W. R. Davis perceived it very quickly. "Although it was never discussed, I do know my parents were crushed psychologically by my illness." Susan Richards Shreve similarly comprehended the impact on her parents: "I knew that my life stood in the way of theirs. I felt accountable, as if my illness were premeditated . . . Children who are ill *know* this about themselves. They aren't blind to the pain and trouble their illness causes other people who love them. And I can imagine even in my mother a silent exhaustion, a growing irritation, at what had befallen her young life." Shreve saw her parents and brother, but especially her mother, as sacrificing their lives for her. "Caught up in the dilemma of the sick child, the center of attention, I was an inadvertent troublemaker, an albatross around the family's neck."[21] Much went unsaid, but even more was known. Parents' body language, quiet whispers, lost stares, and their seemingly endless fatigue all conveyed clear signals to these children.

Many of these children attempted to shield their parents and siblings from their disabilities. Shreve consciously projected a happy-go-lucky, *normal* childhood for both of her parents, particularly for her mother: "To her mind, I had the generic good fortune of a sunny disposition. Things didn't bother me, she'd tell her friends; my illnesses caused me little of the psychological or physical pain that they might have done in another, more sensitive child, one less able to *roll with the punches*, as my father said of me." Some of these children thus intentionally insulated their loved ones. Shreve cast an image that she thought gave her parents some solace. But it was all an invention.[22]

Conversely, many parents protected their children, producing a complex scaffolding of emotions that provided a fragile deception—which, in truth, protected no one. Shreve reflects on how her parents rushed to build a façade of averageness through their annual Christmas card. "It was so unlike my parents to send out photographs of their children to relatives . . . to the friends . . . as if we were a normal American family. It was as though they were somehow ashamed and wanted to prove to others that we *were* normal now, finally, at Christmas 1950, and that we were all well with our dog in the backyard." They hoped to project the image of an "ordinary" family.[23]

Finally, parents often emotionally insulated themselves as well as their children by discarding toys and belongings that might have rekindled the realities of this disease, of what had been before. Shell draws on his personal experiences to make this point:

> Sometimes . . . polios' beloved teddy bears were discarded simply because they were manufactured by the very popular Steiff Company. Margarete Steiff, who had founded this company many decades earlier, was a wheelchair-bound polio—a fact much discussed in the magazines during the 1950s—and many caretakers believed that Steiff teddies would too morbidly remind polios of their difficult situations. So, I lost my teddy bear, Mr. Doogie.[24]

In the process, his parents colluded to erase that family's collective memory.

Children and parents tried to anticipate the emotional impact of this disease on each other and attempted to respond with what they believed would be appropriate actions, albeit tenuous and inadequate. Both struggled with the trauma, masking their own pain, whether physical or emotional, in order to ease the torment of the other. But these illusions seemed to provide a false sense of security and an elusive glimmer of hope.

SHIFTING ROLES

This disease profoundly reshaped families. Its onset often resulted in isolation, disrupting daily routines and causing fear and dread. Parents forfeited control of their children to medical professionals, literally separated from them for weeks at a time. They patiently and hopefully awaited the outcome of therapy. Failing this, individual family members had to adjust to the homecoming and, concomitantly, to the many and unique needs of a child with physical disabilities.

This deeply affected parents. Ellen Whelen Coughlin, a social worker, published a 1941 article, "Parental Attitudes Toward Handicapped Children," based on her clinical experiences at the Detroit Orthopedic Clinic. She found that disability transformed the family's social dynamic by intensifying interpersonal relations. Parents in particular displayed one of two behaviors, either "constructive" or "destructive." Each of these consisted of various degrees of responses. The most constructive parents emotionally adapted and usually took the initiative to introduce any necessary compensations. Others either accepted their child's disability but failed to initiate sufficient accommodations, or felt disappointment and refused to make any adjustments. Still others totally abrogated all of their responsibilities, surrendering them to public or philanthropic agencies. In any case, children with disabilities received some level of care. Destructiveness, as Coughlin terms it, appeared to be dominated by a partial or complete breakdown by parents, who exhibited a range of feelings such as denial, discouragement, guilt, overanxiety, and overprotectiveness. They felt unsure about how to fulfill their child's enormous emotional and physical needs. Fear proved to be the prevalent trait displayed: "fear of surgery, fear that the child might grow worse, fear that he could never be economically independent, fear of what others in the social groups might think." The inability to cope at all, in the most extreme cases, caused them to shift their attention to their other, able-bodied children, emotionally abandoning their child with a disability. A few even tried to hide paralysis from the public eye. Whether constructive or destructive, Coughlin adds, fathers tended to act detached, while mothers seemed to remain engaged with their child.[25]

Family members significantly adjusted and realigned their roles. Parents assumed additional chores, attempted to cope with intense feelings, and struggled with mounting financial responsibilities. Older and younger brothers and sisters also trod on new ground. Their relationships with their parents began to morph even before the homecoming of a disabled sister or brother. Gripped with fear, parents spent a great deal of time at the hospital and seemed to be perpetually distracted. Once that child arrived home, siblings may have had to compete for adult affection. Or they reveled in their newfound role as the center of attention because of their parents' disdain for disability. Their roles as brothers and sisters likewise experienced dramatic changes. Because of this virus and its disabling effects, the *other* was now ever present. How did this reshape the specific roles and relationships of family members?

Parents

On March 7, 1912, Carolyn McDaniel, a mother in Annapolis, Maryland, wrote to Dr. Simon Flexner at the Rockefeller Institute for Medical Research (RIMR), five months after the death of her three-year-old daughter, who had succumbed to infantile paralysis. She remained "haunted" by the fear that she had somehow inadvertently caused her child's death. The young girl had fallen, hit her head on the floor, and temporarily lost consciousness. In a frantic attempt to revive her, the mother shook her awake. Shortly thereafter, her daughter became ill. McDaniel sought information that linked her reflexive action to her daughter's condition and eventual death. Flexner assured her that no such medical connection existed.[26] Mothers most deeply felt guilt when their children fell ill. In addition to the initial trauma, this virus continued to exact an enormous toll on the maternal parent. Her responsibilities expanded in three distinct ways. Some of this represented a redefinition or expansion of domesticity as bedside attendant and physical therapist. Still another introduced an unintended outcome; that is, a sense of agency, albeit a limited one.

The Vigil

Disease saddled the maternal parent with more work and stress than any other household member, because she usually took command of medical treatments, a traditional role. By the mid-nineteenth century, middle-class wives and mothers certainly oversaw the general welfare of the family, providing a clean, neat, and smoothly operating domicile, ensuring an insulated, emotionally secure retreat for all family members, and supplying the gentle, feminine emotional environment to counterbalance the aggressive, masculine values of the husband and father. And tending to sick children enhanced the woman's utilitarian value, at least in historian Barbara Welter's universe of responsibilities embedded in the "cult of true womanhood."[27] Health care thus operated as a gendered family chore.

Moreover, the American public in general and parents in particular feared hospitals well into the twentieth century. They did not view them as places to be healed but rather as death houses. "Writing a ten-year retrospective on the Babies Hospital of New York City, superintendent Luther Emmett Holt (1897) anguished over the difficulties facing children who required a prolonged stay because of the likelihood of their developing an acute disease while in the hospital." Families, as a result, preferred to treat their children at home. This attitude would only gradually shift at the turn of the century among those of the middle class.[28]

"Home hospital" practices continued well into the twentieth century but now anointed by medical science. While wives and mothers still served as home nurses, the fear of potential infection made their tasks more intense and prescriptive. Hygiene ruled the day: reduce contagion through disinfectants; sanitize the patient's laundry; carefully dispose of the ill family member's bodily discharges; replicate spare hospital rooms by minimizing the pieces of furniture, thereby reducing potential hosts for microbes. It is not surprising, then, that the New York City Department of Health in 1916 promoted cleanliness as the first line of defense against infantile paralysis. Similar recommendations included well-functioning bowels, a nutritious diet, ample fresh air (preferably in open spaces), and an adequate amount of sleep. Finally, it encouraged the use of a mouthwash consisting of boric acid and ingestion of castor oil as a general medication.[29]

With the onset of infection, mothers assumed even more demanding and exhausting nursing tasks, as well as having to adopt a new role by providing physical therapy. Children who contracted the virus during the 1920s and 1930s often remained at home and received folk medicine and parental care. Mothers sometimes even had to diagnose their children, at least according to Anthony DiBona, who contracted polio at about a month old in 1916 while living in New York City. Public health authorities "used to tell the mothers to tickle the babies underneath their feet. If they would retract them, they were all right." His left foot never responded to his mother's touch.[30]

Overwhelmed with fatigue, mothers provided round-the-clock care for their little patients, as evidenced by a pamphlet, *Circular of Information Regarding Acute Poliomyelitis (Infantile Paralysis): Information for the Public*, issued by the New York City Department of Health in 1913. It prescribed a strict hygiene regimen for the patient's room. The department mandated that only one attendant, usually the child's mother, provide care; no other family members could enter the room. The room itself had to be stripped of all unnecessary furniture, rugs and carpets, and wall hangings. All toys had to be disinfected or destroyed. The mother had to wet mop the floor to remove any contagious dust (a suspected vector) and air the room daily. She also had to sterilize all bed linens, clothing, drinking glasses, plates, and utensils with a carbolic acid solution.[31]

By mid-century, home care had become more informed and routine. A 1944 NFIP publication, *A Guide for Parents in the Nursing Care of Patients with Infantile Paralysis in the Home*, maintained a threefold agenda. The first item in this twenty-two-page, second-edition booklet concentrated on "general nursing care" procedures for the attending adult, presumably the maternal parent. This manual expressed, in vague terms, the hope that she was working under the guidance of a certified nurse from the local health department. Nevertheless, the pamphlet directed the mother to dress the little patient in a loincloth, because inflamed nerves created ultrasensitive skin, and included an easy-to-follow pattern for her to make it. This booklet also gave detailed instructions for delicately positioning the patient and concluded this section with careful directions for cleaning the home hospital room as well as disposing of contaminated clothing and other materials. The second part enumerated the equipment needed to properly address the patient's needs. The bed had to be raised to make it easier to lift the dead weight of the patient and, in the case of older children, to "prevent back strain" for the caregiver. This could be simply and cheaply accomplished, the guide continued, by using wooden blocks, preferably with casters to allow for bed mobility. A thick board could be inserted under the entire length and width of the mattress to stiffen it, ensuring that the patient had steady and solid support. Other materials included a rubber sheet or an impenetrable substitute (to prevent bodily fluids from seeping into the mattress), a large boiling pot (to sterilize the loincloths and bedding), and safety pins (to hold the diaper-like apparel in place). While the first two parts of this booklet dealt with initial critical care, the last one emphasized recovery through therapy, as we shall see.[32] This kind of information proved invaluable to most American families, because public health nurses, even by mid-century, were not readily available, especially in many rural communities. For those households that did receive this guide, it was analogous to the Sears catalog of polio treatment.

Nursing for the Poliomyelitis Patient, an authoritative care guide published jointly in 1948 by the National Organization for Public Health Nursing and the National League of Nursing Education, described the needs of families living in such isolated areas. There, it noted, the burden of medical care during the initial period of infection usually fell on the parents' shoulders; again, more often than not, this became the sole responsibility of the mother. She would often relocate her wringer washer to the child's bedroom in order to eliminate excess scalding-hot water from the moist heat packs. It even explained how to use a vacuum cleaner to suction excess throat mucus to prevent strangulation in emergency cases. But home care required more than attending to the physical needs of the patient. The guide cautioned that the "emotional convalescence from the disease is much longer than has been usually appreciated." Feverish young patients cried, acted irritable, and experienced nightmares. Mothers also had to be dieticians, monitoring their child's nutritional needs. Finally, they had to give enemas and laxatives to relieve the patient's constipation due to their sedentary life in bed.[33] Otherwise, any kinds of adaptations both at home and school proved to be minimal at best. Arvid Schwartz, who lived in Minnesota's northern farmland and contracted polio at age twelve in October 1952, recalls absolutely none. "There weren't any aids, you just had to figure out how you were going to make this work and again it wasn't that my family wasn't interested in it. It just that at that time in history of our country, when you were a cripple . . . you either made it or you didn't make it . . . There was [sic] no support groups, no programs, no classes you could go to."[34]

Where public health nurses were available, usually in urban areas, they guided families in cobbling together special orthopedic equipment. A Bradford frame—an elevated hard mattress, reinforced with wood—used straps to immobilize the patient and facilitated the easy use of a bedpan. If families lacked adequate financial resources to purchase one, then nurses provided oversight as the parents, and possibly other family members, improvised the construction of a homemade hospital bed. An ordinary bed could be adapted by inserting a wooden board under the mattress, elevating it by using sawhorses or by threading steel water or gas pipes together and attaching them to an existing metal bed frame. Nurses also directed them on how to convert a corset into a jacket, a vest-like apparatus with straps. This proved to be an especially useful piece of equipment to prevent young children from "twisting from side to side" as well as to give them abdominal and back support to prevent scoliosis. Other homemade hospital equipment, like gurneys, "reading racks," and splints, could likewise be engineered from common household products and furniture. Finally, public health nurses taught the sequence of heat, massage, and exercise to mothers to relieve tissue soreness and restore muscle ability.[35] Charles A. Stone contracted infantile paralysis at the age of six in 1930. His parents never admitted him to a hospital, instead treating him at home. Although they knew he was ill, no one realized that he had infantile paralysis until later: "No one was sure what I had until after I got over the acute stage of the illness. It was only after I was well enough to get out of bed, and I was dragging my left leg, that it was determined I'd had polio." His mother spent weeks massaging his sore body, but his leg never fully recovered.[36]

Sister Elizabeth Kenny traveled extensively to give public lectures about her treatment. "For many disabled Americans and their families Kenny became a hero." In 1943, a New Orleans mother traveled to Minneapolis to learn Kenny's method while her son was being treated at the Kenny Institute. Parents with paralyzed children also "besieged'" her with telephone calls and letters at her home. Kenny's method "demanded a major role for her patients' family caregivers, which in most cases meant the mother."[37] This was especially the case when overcrowded hospitals—a not uncommon phenomenon—delayed the admission of patients because they had no spare beds, as in the case of the 1944 Kentucky epidemic. In the interim, maternal parents assumed the responsibility for emergency care. Michael Davis's mother, who was a practicing nurse, immediately began the Kenny treatment at home after being given directions over the phone. "She went to a secondhand store," he writes in his memoir, "where she bought surplus army blankets, a rubber sheet, and large wash boilers to heat on the gas burners of the kitchen range."[38] This round-the-clock regimen continued until a hospital bed finally became available for him. Parents also extended Kenny's approach beyond acute and post-acute care. "By the mid-1940s Kenny talked more often about teaching mothers to continue the exercises and hot packs she recommended *after* the child had left the hospital."[39]

The last gasp of traditional home care occurred during the early twentieth century, just as infantile paralysis epidemics began to ramp up. "By 1900, the home seemed no longer the ideal site for diagnosis and treatment of severe illness—as it had still been a quarter century before." The hospital, with full-time staff, the latest technology, and medical expertise, replaced it. Still, this transition unfolded at a gradual pace. Once a place for the indigent, who could not afford private care, in mid-nineteenth-century cities, it increasingly evolved into a middle-class institution during the early decades of the twentieth century.

> The American hospital in the period of World War I had become a vastly different institution from its postbellum predecessor. Just as medical theory and practice had shifted gradually . . . so [did] the hospital . . . Medical care was seen increasingly in technical terms, and the hospital population was defined increasingly by physician-diagnosed pathology and not social position. The hospital itself was entering a world of impersonal cash transactions and bureaucratic relationships. It was only to have been expected that human relationships within the hospital would evolve in ways reflecting these new realities.[40]

The expansion of institutional care by the late 1920s thus eroded personal involvement. Instead of sitting at a child's bedside, providing comfort and concomitantly consoling herself, a mother now had to watch detached medical professionals (i.e., strangers) tend to a *patient with a disease* through the glass partition of the isolation ward.

Not all parents kowtowed to physicians, nurses, and hospital rules. Jack Dominik, who fell victim to polio at age three in 1925, remembers that his mother remained with him while he was hospitalized for some four weeks: "She slept on a cot in my room with me, but they couldn't give her any meals there. She only ate whatever I didn't eat from my meals, which wasn't very much."[41] A 1943 survey of parents by a medical social worker in New Haven, Connecticut, found that 92 percent expressed "concern because they could not see the doctor." Many stood outside of that city's hospital and "called to [their] children one, two or three floors above them, in an effort to ascertain, with their own eyes [through the open windows], how the children were."[42] A few parents firmly asserted their authority. In 1949, Peg Kehret had a high body temperature for over a week and began to deteriorate rapidly because of a lack of fluids and nutrition. Her parents' gentle but persistent efforts to coax her to drink culminated in her asking for a chocolate milkshake. But hospital rules banned milk products for polio patients, because they generated phlegm and mucus that could clog breathing passages, further inhibiting the ability to breathe. Kehret describes the tense scene that ensued:

> "You rest a bit," Mother told me. "We'll be back soon." She and Dad went out.
> They returned in less than an hour, carrying a white paper bag. The nurse followed them into the room.
> "I won't be responsible for this," she said.
> "We know you have to follow the rules," Dad said, "but we don't. This is our daughter, and she has had nothing to eat for over a week. If a chocolate milkshake is what she wants . . . then a chocolate milkshake is what she is going to have."
> "What if she chokes to death?" The nurse demanded.
> "If something doesn't change soon," Dad replied, "we're going to lose her anyway."

It worked. Kehret slowly sipped the entire milkshake. Her temperature finally broke—a key turning point. Her life had hung in the balance; her parents acted, though producing a confrontation with a member of the medical staff. A strained standoff existed at first, but her parents prevailed. Ken Handel, who contracted infantile paralysis in Brooklyn at 18 months of age in 1951, describes his parents' response to his initial isolation and hospitalization. Growing desperate because of a lack of information, they crept up the hospital's fire escape to see him through a window; they too grew uneasy with his care, as Handel recalls: "They thought I was not being well treated, but they couldn't get me out." It remains unclear what Handel was referring to, but his parents felt concerned enough to bribe a nurse with $500 to smuggle him out of the hospital. Then, Handel continues, "They put me in a car, under a blanket in the back seat, so that people wouldn't see me. They took me out to Sister Kenny [at the Jersey City Medical Center] in New Jersey."[43] Implicit in this recollection is that his parents felt that orthodox medical approaches proved inadequate for their son, and they acted to correct it, subverting the hospital's care system, if not committing a felony.

Parents circumvented hospital rules in other ways. Rehabilitation represents a case in point. Although candy was banned, they smuggled it in for their children, as Avrid Schwartz reconstructs the Stalag-like sabotage of that rule: "We'd hide the candy because periodically there'd be 'raids,' and our candy would be confiscated. We'd, of course, catch holy hell from the nurses, but we thought it was worth the risk. They even sent a letter home to our parents telling them not to bring us candy, and that worked for a couple of weeks, but then someone's parents would work up the courage to bring some, and the cycle would start over again until there'd be another raid."[44]

Parents did not escape the shock of this illness. Some proved less resilient than others. Some hospital staff members witnessed how mothers, isolated from their sick children, typically grew depressed with each passing day. And some never fully recovered. Susan Richards Shreve's mother experienced a debilitating bout of depression, retiring to her bedroom for an entire year. In 1952, Joe Jamelka, a Texas farmer, saw four of his six children hospitalized for poliomyelitis. His wife became emotionally traumatized and became bedridden. Hospitalization also uprooted parents' lives. Lawrence Becker contracted bulbar polio at age thirteen in 1952 while residing in Nebraska. His father, a congregational minister, and his mother completely adapted their lives to his illness. He spent the better part of a year in the hospital before he was transferred to a respiratory center in Omaha, 160 miles from his home. His parents sold their house and followed him there, with his father becoming a pastor in another church. In yet another case, a desperate mother futilely pleaded with doctors to surgically transplant her healthy muscles to her sick son. Finally, Ray K. Gullickson, who had contracted this virus while growing up on a Wisconsin farm, was transferred to the Minneapolis General Hospital. Shortly after he arrived, the local newspaper and radio, because of a bureaucratic error, mistakenly reported him among that disease's fatalities. His mother, who had just departed the hospital, raced back after hearing this report, only to find him alive.[45]

Home Therapy

On December 11, 1919, H. L. Amoss, of the Rockefeller Institute, responded to a distraught father in Houston, Texas, requesting information about the treatment of "anterio-polio-myelitis" for his two-year-old son. He sent him a copy of Robert W. Lovett's book *The Treatment of Infantile Paralysis* and prescribed rest for several weeks and then a regimen of "gradual muscle retraining." Amoss adds, "In young children the mother, if very patient, is usually the best adapted for this under the direction of an orthopedic surgeon, who from time to time tests the muscles to determine whether too much or too little exercise has been given."[46] In spite of the father's concern and the male doctor's expertise, the child's mother assumed responsibility for and rehabilitation, of course under the supervision of a male physician or, at least, a visiting nurse.

    A mother's death vigil, watching closely to see whether or not her child would survive the initial viral infection, simply drained her. After-treatment proved to be just as exhausting. During the early part of the twentieth century, some 46 percent of polio patients, the largest portion, remained in or returned to their homes following acute and subacute care; the remainder appeared to be scattered throughout a variety of institutions, with no more than 10 percent of them admitted to any one type of institution. Thus, the home operated as the single most critical post-hospital care unit. In Chicago, the Visiting Nurse Association assumed oversight of all children discharged from hospitals and sent home. The association divided the city into ten districts and assigned one nurse, who had been trained by Lovett, to each of them. They treated children and transported them to orthopedists, using a donated automobile, and they taught their parents about care and therapy. Association nurses engaged 746 patients and visited homes 18,478 times between November 26, 1916, and October 1, 1918. The family in general, and the maternal parent in particular, served as the linchpin in overall polio care.[47]

It is no wonder, then, that the 1940 guide for public health nurses, *The Nursing Care of Patients with Infantile Paralysis*, cautioned how they had to give the maternal parent almost as much attention as the young patient. The wife and mother naturally oversaw her usual domestic chores in addition to assuming the role of full-time nurse. According to this pamphlet, she experienced incredible "physical and emotional strain" and required "rest and recreation," yet the guide failed to provide any practical suggestions. The booklet urged, "Sometimes the patient may be placed in a convalescent home for a short time in order that the mother may have a rest." Some parents, like their children, never fully recuperated.[48]

In contrast, those children who fell ill in the 1940s and 1950s generally went to hospitals for their initial treatments. Aftercare then occurred at rehabilitation centers—that is, if they existed or were not overcrowded. Home therapy represented the only other alternative, and that responsibility continued to fall on the maternal parent's shoulders. Aftercare is the subject of the third (and main) part of the National Foundation's 1944 booklet, *A Guide for Parents in the Nursing Care of Patients with Infantile Paralysis in the Home*, described in the previous section. It outlined the purpose of aftercare, listed the materials and equipment (e.g., a wringer washer) estimated the cost, and described the procedure for making heated wool packs. But the actual application of these hot wraps dominated this section. It included not only patterns and measurements for them but also diagrams showing where specifically to apply them on the patient's body (abdomen, back, foot, thigh, etc.).[49] Following his hospitalization, ten-year-old Bill Van Cleve returned home, where his mother laboriously exercised his limbs, imitating Sister Kenny's method. These workouts proved to be highly painful, causing him to cry. He remained bedridden for an entire year, with his mother addressing all of his needs. Susan Richards Shreve, who fell ill at age one in 1940 while living in Toledo, Ohio, writes in her memoir that her mother created and maintained an intense program to rehabilitate her muscles: "My mother figured she could do something about my condition . . . [S]he devised a military regimen of exercises to coax those muscles back to life . . . My mother and I spent days together, all through my childhood, on the floor, on the bed, standing against the wall . . . She made a game of this routine, so it felt pretty much like play for me."[50] Margo Vickery's mother had attended one of Kenny's lectures at Jersey City Medical Center before Vickery contracted polio at age five in 1946. Her parents saw no point in admitting her to a hospital, since the doctor who had diagnosed her said there was little more that medical personnel could do. Vickery's mother proceeded to treat her at home: "She would carry me into the bathtub, take me back to bed, and physically make my limbs move. It hurt her and hurt me." Vickery credited her mother with saving her life.[51]

To assist psychological recovery and pass the time, public health nurses assisted with children's readjustment to home life and coping with disability. This usually involved occupational therapy, such as creating needlework and working on other crafts, and the introduction of new hobbies, like collecting stamps and playing board games. It of course included "bedside teaching" to avoid falling too far behind in their schoolwork.[52]

Finally, some women witnessed the disintegration of their families. Such was the case with Josephine Howard. Not only had she seen five of her six children fall to infantile paralysis, not only had one died from this disease, but her husband had contracted it as well. Public fear proved to be pervasive; it usually manifested itself in quarantine of one kind or another, but it also assumed other forms, as we have seen. Howard's neighbors shunned her: "We were pretty isolated because people didn't want to come around, you know." When he learned that infantile paralysis had struck the family, even the gas meter reader fled from her house in panic, fearing exposure to this contagion. A health official visited her home and essentially blamed her for the infection; Howard recalls that she said "it was because I didn't clean the vegetables. Which, of course, was not true at all." The belief that dietary toxins (contained in fruits, milk, seafood and shellfish, sugar, and vegetables) caused polio persisted until the 1950s.[53] This virus contaminated the entire family, no matter how many members had become ill. And too often, mothers served as scapegoats.

Motherhood has remained a fluid experience over time. The role of a mother shifted due to economic demands, political changes, moral influences, regional expectations, and social-class backgrounds. Mothers shaped history in many ways, many of which remain hidden. Assuming the task as the family's health guardian added yet another chore. Prevention, through a clean household and close care of the children, represented the first line of defense. A long tradition of women serving as home nurses continued well into the twentieth century, and poliomyelitis intensified this duty. Moreover, an unprecedented role for maternal parents grew out of these epidemics. For the first time, they could rally against a disease on a mass scale; instead of just individually fearing and treating it, they could act rather than react.

Foot Soldiers

Gender is rarely highlighted as an integral part of polio's story. Yet home hospitals required mothers to assume the role of a domestic nurse, often saving the lives of their children. The sexuality of young women disabled by this virus became a major impediment to peer acceptance, as we will see. The NFIP's Mothers' Marches added yet another dimension. These campaigns not only raised income for the foundation, but they also reinforced the sympathy evoked by poster children by combining it with domesticity (i.e., maternal emotions). In this process, women not only extended their traditional social roles but also became significant agents for change.

Such activism appeared to be an anomaly immediately following World War II, a time of apparent quiescence. But that simply was not the case. Linda Eisenmann's research on women in higher education during that same time offers an interpretive framework to explain the NFIP's Mothers' Marches. Her concept of "quiet activism . . . marks a particular postwar approach to advocacy that may be different from other eras but that suited the contextually complicated postwar period." It occurred, as Eisenmann argues, with "a quiet voice and a less radical face than found in prior or subsequent periods." And this advocacy usually expressed itself through an organizational base[54]— in this case, the National Foundation for Infantile Paralysis.

The Maricopa County, Arizona, NFIP chapter inaugurated the first Mothers' March, a wholly organic movement, on January 16, 1950. It relied on billboard, newspaper, and radio advertising augmented by trucks with loudspeakers driving through neighborhoods announcing its slogan: "Turn on Your Porch Light, Help Fight Polio Tonight." Homeowners turned on their exterior lights during the evening hours to send a welcome signal to 2,300 volunteers to collect a donation. They raised $45,000 in donations within the first hour and $100,000 the following year.[55]

Elaine Whitelaw immediately applied this highly successful approach on the national level. She joined the NFIP in 1943 as national director of women's activities and played an instrumental role in developing and directing volunteer services. To accomplish this, she created an elaborate and sophisticated national infrastructure, beginning at the local level, to generate donations—a conscious populist approach. During World War II, the NFIP had already begun to collect dimes in movie theaters. Whitelaw introduced several new fundraising measures during the postwar era, launching the annual March of Dimes Fashion Show in January 1945, at about the same time as the late President Roosevelt's birthday on January 30. Fashion designers, like Christian Dior, contributed their services. With actress Helen Hayes serving as host, models included movie stars Joan Fontaine, Grace Kelly, and Marilyn Monroe, who wore jewelry loaned by Harry Winston. Singers Eartha Kitt, Gypsy Rose Lee, and Ezio Pinza provided entertainment. It proved to be an immediate success. This spawned similar, local variations in Baltimore, Buffalo, Chicago, and Dallas, among other cities. The foundation sponsored volunteer-led bowling tournaments, carnivals, dances, polio parades, rummage sales, and wheelchair basketball games, among other events, as well as sewing bees in which mothers created "outsized 'polio blankets' (the forerunner of the AIDS quilt)." And it introduced the "phonathon," which would become a fundraising mainstay for decades. Under Whitelaw's direction, the Polio Emergency Volunteers grew from 3,000 in 1945 to 60,000 ten years later. As director of volunteer services, Whitelaw also oversaw community organization, coordinating educators, health professionals, and volunteers for the national vaccine trial in 1954.[56]

Her supervision of the annual Mothers' Marches, which became month-long crusades held every January, involved locally sponsored troops of women. Parents of what would later become known as the baby boom generation, with police and community support, canvassed neighborhoods to collect donations. These highly organized and well-coordinated porch-light campaigns involved mothers as well as their children going door to door to collect nickels and dimes. They deposited the donations at local firehouses, for example, which served as collection centers. With so much cash at stake, heavily armed police officers guarded these sites and escorted armored cars that carried the donated money. Women embraced and sustained this grass-roots fundraising effort. Charles Massey, who organized local chapters in Arkansas, Georgia, and Kentucky during the late 1940s and early 1950s, describes the response by contributors: "This was a case in which people who lived there invited the solicitors to come in and many times they would invite them in the house to have coffee."[57]

Charles H. Bynum, working within the NFIP on African American outreach between 1944 and 1954, successfully recruited African American women as well. As he visited communities, he purposefully sought out women's organizations, such as the Federation of Women's Clubs, Kansas State Meeting of Colored Women, National Association of Negro Business and Professional Women's Clubs, and National Council of Negro Women. He likewise worked diligently to integrate African American women into the foundation's fundraising activities by directly working with Whitelaw. They collaborated, for instance, to produce a 1951 film, *Mother's March on Polio*, that depicted interracial cooperation in fundraising. "Due to Bynum and Whitelaw's attention to mobilizing the resources of women's groups, the support of such organizations in the March of Dimes grew significantly."[58]

Mothers acted in distinct ways toward this disease and its disabilities. Some of this behavior reflected an extension of traditional domestic roles, while some represented philanthropic activism. They maintained a death watch, assisted in the recovery of their children's health following hospitalization, and eventually provided the resources to assist their disabled children and ultimately eradicate the disease in the United States. This latter action culminated in the March of Dimes, maintaining a populist approach with so-called pocket change. This endeavor relied heavily on public relations to disseminate news of any breakthroughs, which in turn hopefully generated more donations. "Researchers became accustomed to using Madison Avenue methods, and an unprecedented rapport was forged between doctors, researchers, and the people." The results proved to be stunning. "Between 1938 and 1962 the National Foundation's annual income averaged $25 million; its total receipts were $630 million: 59 percent went to medical care, 8 percent to education, 11 percent to research and 13 percent to administration and fund-raising."[59] The Mothers' Marches contributed a major portion of this revenue stream. Mrs. Read, a mother who lived in DeWitt, New York, participated in her community; she summarizes what mobilized these women: "When it comes to protecting children, mothers make the best warriors!"[60]

Sibling Rivalry?

Little has been systematically reconstructed about the direct and indirect impact of polio on siblings. With parents consumed by a life-and-death struggle, distracted by the possibility of full recovery or the lack thereof, and overjoyed by that child's homecoming, their other children generally received less attention, if not becoming completely marginalized. The entire realm of child-parent independence and dependence became transformed. New definitions emerged. Parents tended to be overprotective, at the cost of their able-bodied brothers and sisters. Children disabled by polio who wanted to recapture their former freedom, if not expand it, not only felt constrained by physical limitations but also smothered by overly protective parents. This "independent-dependent" relationship continued to evolve.[61] In sum, this disease and its concomitant disability often had a "corrosive effect on the family."[62]

Infantile paralysis immediately disrupted siblings' routines. Quarantine, a long-held policy of municipal and state health departments, mandated isolation at home, interrupting schooling. Multiple outbreaks within a family frightened officials and the public alike. As early as 1911, Samuel C. Dixon, Pennsylvania's commissioner of health, based on his findings of that state's 1910 epidemic, declared that "members of the patients' families should be excluded from schools during the period of isolation and possible incubation of new cases."[63]

The long-absent patient's reappearance redefined relationships in so many ways. Able-bodied brothers and sisters often found themselves living with a stranger following hospitalization and rehabilitation. Intimate connections to siblings had to be carefully recovered or totally constructed from scratch. George Durr, who entered the hospital at eighteen months of age, finally returned to his family at age five: "When I got home I met my brother and sister for the first time. They weren't allowed in the hospital. I didn't know who they were. The only people I knew were at the hospital."[64] In most cases, though, prior relationships underwent profound change. Infected at age nine in 1949, Marilynne Rogers spent two and a half years away from home. Because of her long absence, she and her brother had to reacquaint themselves when she returned home. At the most basic level, simply playing with brothers and sisters underwent a profound and permanent change. Mary Grimley Mason discovered that she could no longer participate in pillow fights or hide-and-seek games.[65]

Children with disabilities clearly received special treatment of one kind or another. After they returned home, parents tended to indulge them, only gradually implementing a slightly stricter behavior routine. This too often caused friction among siblings, according to sociologist Fred Davis. While parents recognized that their children appeared to be "more mature," they also acknowledged that they acted "more spoiled." As one father recalled, "I'd say I give in to her a lot more . . . [S]he wanted to go see this here Walt Disney movie . . . [I]f Laura hadn't been sick, I might not have jumped right up like that." Many children affected by polio "expected preferential treatment," and parents willingly complied.[66] As the center of attention, Bill Van Cleve's family "spoiled" him; he consequently became highly "self-centered" and selfish, refusing to share anything with his sisters.[67] Ted Kellogg's parents fussed over him, straining already tense sibling relations. As a result, he remained estranged from his older sister well into his adulthood: "Her childhood was filled with Teddy this and Teddy that, because Teddy had polio."[68] Steven Diamond contracted infantile paralysis at age thirteen in 1953 while living in the Bronx. Disability indirectly destroyed his younger brother: "My parents did the best they could do for him, but there was a lot of resentment about me getting so much attention. I went on to be a rather good student, and he didn't."[69] In all cases, siblings, with parental oversight, reshaped their roles in order to cope with the new set of circumstances. Like their parents, many pandered to their disabled brothers and sisters. Robert Huse became ill at the age of six in 1931. When he returned home, he recalls, his sisters "would perform any outrageous task I assigned to them. One evening my supper [served on a tray in my bedroom] was not to my liking, so I had my sister Priscilla throw it out my [second-floor] bedroom window."[70]

The cumulative consequences for siblings could be profound. They sometimes felt guilt. George Rugh, of Belle Vernon, Pennsylvania, became infected at eighteen months of age in 1937. He explains how his sister carried a lifetime of remorse for causing his infection: "My older sister told me that for years she worried that she was the one who made me get polio because she dropped me on the sidewalk. She picked me up and I was okay, but within days I started to get sick. She always felt that if she hadn't dropped me that I might have not had polio."[71] Separation from one or both parents during their sibling's hospitalization (and possible later surgery) caused undue emotional stress on those left behind. Excessive attention to a sister or brother with disabilities could cause a feeling of neglect or anger, much of it becoming internalized. Some of this manifested in learning difficulties or behavior problems at school, or in physical reactions like stuttering, vomiting, or general depression.[72]

Parents divided brothers and sisters in other ways. Anne Finger's strict father directed his worst punishments at her more than at her siblings: "His anger toward me was physical, rage at that body of mine [that] persisted . . . in remaining crippled. His daughter's body—and for him, the operative word in that phrase was 'his'—which walked . . . leaning on crutches, drawing stares, some curious, some sympathetic. Out there for all the world to see, the physical manifestation of the inner state of our family—broken, bent, crippled, wrong." This reached an emotional crescendo one evening when he beat her head against a sofa arm, followed by almost choking her to death.[73]

Twins suffered the most. A 1951 North Carolina study of forty-five families with twins found that 36 percent of identical twins contracted paralytic polio, while 6 percent of fraternal twins had both experienced some paralysis. Six-year-old Janice Flood Nichols cried herself to sleep every night after her fraternal twin, Frankie, suddenly died. He had become ill during the week of Halloween 1953, beginning with a runny nose and a temperature. After he developed breathing problems, his parents rushed him to the City Hospital in Syracuse, New York. Doctors conducted a spinal tap, confirming the presence of poliovirus, and placed him in an iron lung. His condition worsened shortly thereafter, and physicians requested that his parents approve a tracheotomy. They consented, but it was too late; he died on the way to the operating room. Only forty-eight hours passed from the time he entered the hospital until when he died. Nichols had nightmares for months afterward. She also fretted about her dead brother's fate in heaven: "Although I missed him terribly, my early heartache was much more based in worry for *his* well-being." She also felt guilt about surviving. For twins, death sparks distinctly unsettling feelings, as Nichols describes: "Many twinless twins . . . endure an unbearable sense of loss . . . as being disconnected."[74] She never fully recovered emotionally.

In general, then, a brother or sister with disabilities could prove to be an imposition or even repulsive. While they received the lion's share of attention, for better or worse, some also felt a profound sense of helplessness. They sometimes had to depend unduly on their siblings for assistance, as Durr describes: "My brother would get a wagon, and I was brought to school with my brother and sister." Ruth Esau contracted polio at age two in 1919 while residing in Cass City, Michigan. Unable to walk to school, she explains how her nuclear and extended family adapted to her disability: "My mom bought a little wicker stroller and pushed me in that to kindergarten. My brother took me in a little Express wagon or on a sled or on his bicycle. I had cousins that were in high school who would stop with a little pickup [truck] and give me a ride." Some brothers and sisters happily complied; others did not. Finally, many able-bodied siblings did not want to be touched by their brothers or sisters who had a disability; they found the paralyzed limb especially grotesque and avoided it at all costs.[75]

Sibling bonds changed profoundly because of this disease. Parental attention shifted, usually for the worse. Role reversals occurred. Now big brothers and sisters with disabilities had to rely heavily on their younger siblings to perform formerly easy, everyday tasks for them. Brothers and sisters, shouldering these new responsibilities, sometimes perceived their siblings as nothing more than a burden. And still others suffered irreparable emotional damage.[76]

SPATIAL REALITY

Home proved to be a distant dream for many hospitalized children. Because of homesickness, they tended to over-romanticize their memories, saturated with Norman Rockwell images of security, stability, and warmth. Nothing more symbolized their pre-polio lives; simple things dominated, like being able to walk and eat, and the intimacy of their own bedrooms and private lives. Kehret, who contracted infantile paralysis at age twelve in Austin, Minnesota, in 1949, desperately clung to her fantasy: "Home. What a powerful word. It caused pictures to flash through my mind like slides fast-forwarding on a screen." However, standard architectural features created obstacle courses. Carpets prevented them from pushing their wheelchairs, and dining room tabletops blocked their wheelchairs' handles. Bathtubs, fixed faucets, narrow doorways and hallways, sharp turns, and toilet height posed other barriers. Kehret's first-floor bathroom brutally introduced her to her new world called home: "My wheelchair did not fit in it. To get the chair close enough to the toilet, I had to leave the door open [and] I needed help to get off the toilet. The lack of privacy embarrassed me." Because of her paralyzed legs, she could neither play the piano nor frolic with her beloved dog. Disability had alienated her from her own home. "I felt like a stranger in those familiar rooms." She ruefully concluded that trying "to get along in the normal world was too hard." Her dream of returning home, to recapture her former security and life, had turned into a dark nightmare. She came to a brutal realization: At the rehabilitation center, she was like everyone else; at home, she had become an outsider in every sense of the word.[77]

Illness thus wrenched children from one apparently stable reality (the convalescent hospital) to another that seemed to be unsettled and perpetually redefining itself. They quickly discovered that their houses' physical spaces defined their disabilities. Two- and three-story dwellings presented major impediments. Charles Mee attempted to plunge into the *normal* routine of home life: "There was no special equipment for getting in and out of the bath, nothing special to hold on to except the ordinary banister for going up and down stairs, nothing altered in my bedroom. I learned to accept the world as it was and to adjust to it." Lenny Kriegel could only navigate the stairs in his house by sitting and boosting himself up and down on them. A New York couple carried their two daughters, both disabled by polio, from room to room. Robert Lovering's parents took the most dramatic and expensive action, selling their two-story home and purchasing another without stairs.[78] In most cases, though, these obstructions forced families to reconfigure their multistory abodes to accommodate the needs of their recently hospitalized children. They converted rooms to assume new functions. Since children could no longer climb the stairs to their bedrooms, first-floor living rooms or dining rooms hosted hospital beds, wheelchairs, and occasionally iron lungs, while braces stood ominously in the corners of those rooms. Michael Davis, who became infected as he completed seventh grade during the 1944 Kentucky polio epidemic, had lost 25 percent of his body weight by the time he was discharged and returned home. His mother and father moved him into their bedroom on the first floor, closer to the kitchen where wool compresses could be boiled, facilitating hot-pack treatments. Marilynne Rogers's parents converted their dining room into her new bedroom. And Ruth Esau slept with her mother in her mother's bed, which had been relocated to the living room. Unable to reach her bedroom on the second floor, Kehret slept on a cot in the living room. The dining room table became Janice Nichols's physical therapy center.[79]

In the process, the entire household too often surrendered its intimacy, adapting to a new reality. Nuclear families could no longer assemble in their living rooms to host guests, play board games, listen to the radio, or (during the early 1950s) watch television. Extended family members, friends, and neighbors could no longer gather in the dining room to celebrate holidays or birthdays. Privacy disappeared. During the 1916 New York City epidemic, *The New York Times* posted daily the names and addresses of reported new cases and recent deaths. This was not an isolated practice: thirty-six years later *The Houston Chronicle* published the names, ages, addresses, and conditions of reported cases. In 1944, after Michael Davis was diagnosed with poliomyelitis, the Louisville health department affixed a large yellow and black quarantine sign to the front door of his home. A personal illness became a public spectacle. In other cases, visitors knew almost immediately this virus had randomly struck a household; disability advertised itself with a wheelchair ramp leading up to the front porch. And if neighbors and guests did not already know what had happened, they did immediately upon entering homes that had a bed inhabiting one of the first-floor rooms, or even a bulky iron lung dwarfing everything.[80] For children with disabilities, their former solitude had disappeared; children's bedrooms now sat in the middle of the hustle and bustle of daily household traffic. All members of the family, friends and neighbors, or even door-to-door salespersons and other strangers witnessed their every activity.[81] For Regina Woods, who became infected at age thirteen in 1952, disability signaled a loss of her personal space, if not loss of dignity itself. She could no longer bathe by herself at home. Moreover, while she was in the iron lung for most of the day, one of her parents or siblings opened and read her mail to her. Finally, her phone calls became part of the family's discourse, whether she liked it or not.[82] The family's role as a sanctuary from the outside world, as well as the ability of individual members to retreat within the household, disappeared.

EDUCATION

School attendance constituted a major portion of *normal* children's lives. Infantile paralysis abruptly interrupted this routine. But this formal educational process resumed as soon as possible and took many different forms, as we saw with classrooms at rehabilitation centers. In addition to operating as a hospital, the home often became a classroom. Ten-year-old Bill Van Cleve's symptoms occurred suddenly and, he recalls, seemed to be generic: "I was nauseous, hot, achy, and feverish. I was put in the hospital." He had to drop out of the fifth grade because he had been confined to bed care for so long. His local school provided instruction in his home after the hospital released him. Public schools, regardless of their location, followed a similar pattern. The Chicago, New York City, and Pittsburgh school districts operated hospital schools or bedside education programs as a temporary approach for sick children. Such a visiting teacher gave daily lessons to David Kangas while he was hospitalized and also served as a homebound teacher to help him complete tenth grade. While recuperating at home, Charles Mee, who contracted polio in 1953 at age 14, relied on a novel approach to home education, using a speakerphone connected to the school in order to participate in his ninth-grade classes in Barrington, Illinois. In the long term, however, children had three options. They could either resume classes at their school, be assigned to a special school, or learn at home through a "home teaching service," also known as homebound instruction.[83]

As we have seen, disability has been traditionally viewed as a "pathology." Medical professionals, as well as the general public, saw people with disabilities only as patients, the subjects of treatment, or as victims afflicted with disease. People with disabilities therefore appeared one-dimensional, with no personal or work lives. Many historians have unwittingly contributed to this dehumanization. But this historiography has recently been changing, as "historians have increasingly addressed the sociocultural experience of illness and public discourse about disease, health, and health care." Within this new narrative, people with disabilities have functioned as "historical actors."[84] And the lives of children disabled by polio, in particular, become humanized when viewed within the context of their families. This disease fundamentally transformed family members' roles, internal relationships, and public image. Emotions became strained among family members, sometimes beyond the breaking point. The household now operated as a miniature hospital and school, with most, if not all, activities overshadowed by this virus. With these added responsibilities, the already precarious household budget teetered on the precipice of impoverishment.

Financial Crisis

Families, with little or no assistance, grappled with the enormous financial pressures that poliomyelitis imposed on them, because few had medical insurance. Hospitalization during the 1916 epidemic threatened the family's economic well-being. A series of state commissions, between 1915 and 1919, gathered statistics about health-care coverage and found that from 25 to 35 percent of employees had it but that it seldom extended to family members. Coverage proved limited in other ways. In Ohio, it only amounted to paid sick leave, excluding any cash benefits to pay medical bills. Illinois, Massachusetts, and Pennsylvania discovered similar situations. California's study observed that extended illnesses contributed to half of the destitution rates. A New York commission concluded that the lack of insurance caused many to neglect their illnesses, ultimately creating the "development of a mass of chronic ailments."[85]

In 1927, the Committee on the Cost of Medical Care, a philanthropically subsidized initiative, began a five-year national study of the delivery of medical services to Americans. Haven Emerson, the former director of New York City's health department during the 1916 polio epidemic, served as a member. Its final report, according to medical historian Alan Derickson, stresses that "99 percent of American families could not set aside enough money to be assured that they could meet any medical emergency." Poor and working-class families, more often than not, skipped any medical care because they could not afford it. Paying for even the simplest of procedures exhausted the family's income and savings, forcing them to secure loans to compensate for the shortfall of funds. "By the end of the 1920s, medical bills could bankrupt all but the wealthiest citizens." This report concluded, without any reservations, that "health-care bills were the leading cause of indebtedness among Americans." Hospital costs for the treatment of children ill with infantile paralysis proved to be extremely expensive because of all of the specialized equipment and the need for intensive staff care.[86] A potential financial cataclysm loomed over every household.

The economic calamity of the Great Depression, Derickson continues, further eroded access to physicians and hospitals. A California investigation found that 20 percent of "relief recipients" in that state "received no medical care when ill, whereas only 9 percent of sick high-income residents . . . went untreated." Poor and working-class families delayed necessary but prohibitively expensive surgical procedures, exacerbating their original medical conditions. Sixty-seven percent of Californians could not afford a simple appendectomy.[87] And the March of Dimes had not yet organized sufficiently to subsidize hospital and home care expenses. "In 1939," according to polio historian Daniel J. Wilson, "only 6 percent of the population was covered by private health insurance." With a median annual wage in 1940 of $877, American families could ill afford such enormous expenses. But this would change during the 1940s.[88]

Postwar America experienced an explosion of commercial health insurance, driven both by labor union demands and by an affluent public. "Whereas only about one American in eleven had hospital insurance in 1940, ten years later one in two had it."[89] For those who did, the paternal parent's employer provided it. Yet this too often proved inadequate. The first year of hospital care for polio ranged from $2,000 to $3,000. Even after being discharged, families with children disabled by poliomyelitis incurred $75–$150 a month for continuing treatments, equipment, and supplies. They remained ill prepared for this medical crisis, since "in the early 1950s it cost approximately $15,000 annually to care for a patient in an iron lung." With average annual wages at $2,992 in 1950, "paying for a severe case of polio remained difficult for many families."[90] Finally, for many parents, the dream of subsidizing professional rehabilitative services remained out of reach.

These expenses forced drastic actions in some cases. After suffering with poliomyelitis and coping with disability for five years, Marilynne Rogers needed to qualify for additional income. This meant that she had to legally disconnect herself from her family, an action she recalls as purely pragmatic: "When I was 14, I heard about Social Security disability. In order to apply for that I had to go to court to claim my independence and be adopted as a child of the court so that I could get benefits. From then on, I got a small income and used that to pay for things."[91] Although certainly a statutory formality in this case, the family as an institution became yet another casualty of this virus.

Most household members, however, relied on less extreme measures to compensate for this seemingly endless financial drain. They typically employed any or all of four strategies; these involved internal responses as well external aid. First, following a long tradition, the maternal parent largely compensated for the lack of health insurance, fulfilling whatever medical responsibilities she could. This transcended the traditional hygiene regimen as well as the usual temperature-taking and tucking-into-bed routines. Providing round-the-clock care proved to be a demanding job and required an entirely new skill set, as we have seen. Through her *free* labor as a home nurse, she subsidized critical medical and therapeutic care to secure the household's financial survival. Second, as the family underwent a series of role adjustments throughout this experience, hard financial decisions had to be made as well. At that time, families adhered to a conventional patriarchal structure, with a working paternal parent and a stay-at-home maternal parent. And those wrestling with the emotional and financial demands of an ill child and subsequently adapting to disability usually maintained this intrafamilial structure. Fathers faced with these added expenses, in many cases, sought better-paying jobs.[92] This could uproot the entire family, since they might have to relocate. Third, some of these young people themselves attempted to contribute to the household's income. David Kangas, feeling the pinch of the household's budget shortfall, sought a job in his city painting parking curbs from his wheelchair: "I made a little money, and it really gave me a boost in terms of my self-esteem."[93]

External assistance provided a fourth option; that is, charities and government aid. Local fraternal organizations included the American Legion, Elks, Kiwanis, Lions, Rotarians, and Shriners. These generally operated in a highly diffuse manner until the 1930s. During the Great Depression, county and state governments assumed some treatment costs. This shift from the private sphere to government support expanded as epidemics exacted a steady toll. The state thus began to play a larger role in rehabilitation. "The Social Security Act's grant-in-aid program for Crippled Children's Services was a significant force in shifting the balance from community to state."[94]

But philanthropic groups continued to play key roles, only now coordinating their activities with the public sector. The NFIP by the 1940s appealed directly to state health officials to report cases directly to its local chapters. It made the same request of physicians. The NFIP instructed local chapters that if "the high cost of polio care would result in undue hardship, force the family to sell a car, mortgage its home or otherwise drastically lower its standard of living, the chapter should offer to pay for all or that portion of the cost that cannot be reasonably met."[95] The foundation spent some $315 million on "medical, hospital, nursing, and rehabilitative care for 325,000 polio sufferers."[96] Arvid Schwartz's rural Minnesota family lacked health insurance, but the March of Dimes paid 90 percent of all of his hospital and care bills. Fred Davis's sociological analysis points out how the NFIP's community representatives sensitively contacted parents of children admitted to hospitals. "Repayment not being expected, nothing was said about it, although many parents voluntarily promised to make repayment, in part at least. Interestingly, a few of the parents . . . held the view that the financial aid extended them by the Foundation was a form of insurance payment, a return on their contributions over the years to the March of Dimes and other Foundation fund-raising drives." Such charity, however, vitiated physicians' attitudes toward patients and families. Davis speculates that when parents received NFIP subsidies and doctors knew it, they felt "less compulsion" to be completely forthcoming about a child's diagnosis and treatment than for the "same patients under the more usual fee-for-service arrangement." While Kangas's family absorbed enormous hospital bills for his ten months of care, the local March of Dimes helped by paying some of them. Finally, the NFIP purchased iron lungs in order to loan them to families so that their children had the opportunity to go home, and even paid parents $40 to $50 a month to subsidize home care.[97]

The financial burden imposed by this disease and its concomitant disability proved to be especially hard on single-parent families, as Julie Silver and Daniel J. Wilson found while collecting their oral histories. With the death of her father, Ruth Esau's mother had to earn all of the family's income and pay for her special equipment in cash. Her short leg required a custom-made leather shoe that attached to an iron brace that extended to her hip. The shoes alone cost 13 dollars, Esau asserts, "which was a lot of money because she only made a dollar a day." Other single-parent families did not fare so well. Samuel McKnight contracted infantile paralysis from his mother, who had fallen ill while pregnant. She died shortly after he was born in 1949 in Connecticut. His father, distraught over her death and overwhelmed by the responsibilities of caring for a son disabled by polio, abandoned him to be raised by his maternal grandparents.[98] For an African American sharecropping family in the South, already eking out a subsistence existence in a very modest two- or three-room home without electricity or indoor plumbing, this disease proved to be catastrophic. "A mother might receive a check from the State of Alabama, Department of Pensions and Security, Aid to Dependent Children for some of her children, while others might not be eligible." The NFIP ultimately subsidized much of this treatment.[99]

Children disabled by poliomyelitis required intense care and special equipment. All of this cost households dearly. Parents could not possibly foresee this crisis, and so their budgets usually did not account for such a dire medical catastrophe. Prior to the 1935 Social Security Act, state relief agencies, and the NFIP, no reliable financial safety net existed. Individuals paralyzed by polio pointed out very early on, through their newsletters, that disability caused poverty. Some family units at that time made rational choices to meet this contingency. In other cases, individual members made difficult decisions that threatened that institution's very coherence: disability shattered many households. Exorbitant costs of and lack of access to allopathic medical treatments caused many to turn to unconventional palliatives or outright charlatans in the vain hope of fiscal relief and potential remedies.[100]

Medical Alternatives

The emotional strain of seeing their children suffering from the virus or being disabled caused many parents, out of desperation, to turn to extreme means to find a cure. It was also a cheaper alternative. As early as July 2, 1916, New York's health commissioner, Haven Emerson, had to caution city residents about "quack and advertised remedies and preventives of the disease." Later that month, officials at the U.S. Department of Agriculture warned the public about unscrupulous individuals exploiting epidemic fears to sell "worthless concoctions," useless treatments, or ineffective remedies.[101] Dominik vividly describes his home therapies in 1925:

> I recall my mom giving me rubdowns with goose grease. When I was given a bath, they were supposed to put salt in the water and make waves . . . I also remember a medicine that came in a square can. It was kind of a yellowish color, and my mom would rub it on my legs. I think it was called Viavi . . . There were also some capsules that I took with meals, and I got a shot glass full of some liquid that I had to take with lunch every day. That was particularly vile tasting stuff . . . I think the stuff that I drank was bought from a door-to-door salesman. I suppose there were all sorts of medicines being sold back then that didn't really do a darn thing.[102]

This experience was not unique; people resorted to alternative palliatives as preventives and cures well into the twentieth century. During the apocalyptic 1918 influenza epidemic, terrified individuals spurned emerging modern medicine, which appeared impotent against this particular disease. To prevent infection, they kept an ace of diamonds in one of their shoes, inhaled the acrid smoke of burning corncobs, tied cucumber slices to their ankles, wore necklaces of chicken feathers, carried a potato in each pants pocket, ingested strychnine, applied vinegar-soaked flannel strips to their chests overnight, chanted voodoo spells, and drank ample doses of gin, among other measures. An Oklahoma physician confidently recommended that teeth and tonsils be surgically removed. "Science, in the early decades of [that] century, was a strange amalgam of wisdom and silliness, triumph, experimentation, cruelty, progress, and naiveté." It was simply the "temper of the times."[103]

Parental treatments often incorporated traditional folk remedies or new miracle cures to supplement the grueling therapy they employed. Parents also occasionally chafed at the hospital's impersonal atmosphere and the medical staff's clinical detachment. And many different "healing movements" operated on the "principled rejection of orthodox medicine in favor of alternative healing philosophies."[104] Folk and homeopathic medical approaches had deep cultural and gendered roots, and they endured even in the face of modern medical developments.[105] Thus, the child's return home from the hospital freed the family from the orthodox mindset, allowing some parents to pursue other means of treatment. Many proved to be novel and seemed effective. Other options grew out of sheer despair or financial exigency.

Other Choices

Alternative medical practices occupy the "ground between domestic and professional medicine," operating often as "an extension of domestic care." And parents, searching for elusive cures, turned to this "organized and self-conscious alternative to the dominant profession."[106] Their reasons are essentially irrelevant. What is important is that their actions were rooted in a long tradition, one dating back centuries and part of a larger historical context. Seeking other treatments, in fact, represents a distinct genre of illness pathographies. Literary scholar Anne Hunsaker Hawkins sees these choices as characterized by a series of dichotomies: agency versus passivity, a focus on the patient rather than the disease, and relying on "natural agents and processes" instead of technology. Medical science had truly wrought remarkable breakthroughs. Yet it produced an unintended outcome, as Hawkins posits: "While the alliance between science and medicine was strengthened, the link between the medical and the humanities became ever tenuous. Medicine's primary concern shifted away from the welfare of the individual patient and toward the diagnosis and treatment of disease."[107]

Women appeared to be the most prominent practitioners. "Plant medicines, whether in the form of food, teas, or poultices, formed the core of rural American household health care" since the colonial period.[108] Women healers functioned as "specialists in infant care" and nursed sick relatives, but they mainly served as midwives.[109] The German-born homeopathic movement progressed steadily throughout the nineteenth century in the United States, resulting in a flurry of asylums, hospitals, medical schools, and publications. "Women figured prominently in the rapid growth of the new school of medicine. Children's dislike of nauseating and disagreeable doses of drugs prescribed by regular physicians contrasted with their positive reactions to the small pleasant tasting doses of homeopathic remedies, which provided an 'entering wedge' for the system." Women also maintained high visibility as chiropractors and naturopaths among Christian Scientists as they disappeared from revamped medical schools after 1900. Reformed medical education required devout and intense graduate work, sacrificing personal lives and costing exorbitant tuition fees, all of which virtually drove most women from the profession.[110] Homeopaths believed that the Indian grass pea (*Lathyrus satirus*) represented the "most perfect antidote for prevention and cure of polio."[111]

Chiropractors advertised during outbreaks that they could prevent infantile paralysis by aligning patients' spinal cords. Others claimed to be able to cure it by resetting misaligned bones in children's spines. This process of luxating (i.e., the realignment of dislocated vertebrae to alleviate pain and illnesses) was not new, having emerged in the 1890s. Lenny Kriegel's parents secured the services of a neighborhood chiropractor, who treated him at home. He experienced no improvement whatsoever; however, as he reflects, this futile effort seemed to be meant more for his parents, their feeble grasp of hope. They simply could not confront the fact that one of their sons was now permanently disabled, and they jumped at every opportunity to escape this reality.[112]

Finally, some individuals disabled by this disease grew so despondent that they sought religious miracles. David Kangas, who caught the disease at age fifteen in 1952, recalls one such incident:

> A group of faith healers came to town, and some of the people at the hospital said, "We're going to the healing tent; do you want to come along?" . . . The guys who went were all in their 20's. I remember them coming back from the healing tent and telling us what happened. They said that the preacher had put his hands on them and told them to rise and walk. But, of course, they couldn't. They were still in the wheelchairs when they got back.

Fred Suite, Jr., went as far as to bathe in the waters at Lourdes in an attempt to be healed.[113]

There Is No Place Like Home?

Disease and disability inflicted incredible emotional, physical, and financial stresses and strains on the family. As Fred Davis's sociological research found, parents experienced a clear sequence of responses. At first, they gushed with optimism. This "honeymoon period" lasted only a few weeks, though, with parents desperately embracing an "unrealistic" expectation for recovery. They refused to accept the permanent transformation of their unimpaired child to one with even minor disabilities, and they adopted a wide range of coping strategies. Some parents still hoped for total recovery, denying obvious atrophy. In other cases, parents postponed corrective surgery, perceiving what they thought was steady progress. In still other cases, they desperately clung to a mind-over-matter belief that sheer will and determination on their child's part would ultimately overcome polio's physical limitations. As one mother expressed her early hope for her son, "Well, I think that Marvin will be all right. I mean, I think he'll help himself a lot to walk again." Some doubt typically surfaced after about ten weeks. With the fading of the optimistic "glow," parents entered a "moratorium" period. Marvin's mother reflected this emotional recalibration: "I have no idea. I mean, I just don't know. I know that my husband and I'll do everything we can . . . and I think Marvin will walk some day without his brace." During this time, some parents still grasped at the goal of full recovery but just saw the need for additional time, while others substituted a more guarded hope of piecemeal recovery. After several more weeks, Marvin's mother continued to express hope, but with less conviction: "I guess I don't expect anything for the two-year period. I mean . . . the leg'll get a little stronger, then he could walk without the brace." Daily contact with their children caused parents to continuously reevaluate the situation. At the end of eight months, Marvin's mother expressed even more uncertainty; although wavering, she still refused to submit to reality: "I don't know. I thought—I had more hopes. Now I don't know, I mean I thought if it would improve a little bit more, it would have improved by now."

Only very reluctantly did parents accept the fact that their perceptions of once healthy, active, and energetic—that is, *normal*—children would never return. Finally, for those who showed no marked recovery, parents sometimes experienced an emotional collapse; their quixotic hope for positive change clashed with the reality of a static state with no possibility for full, or even partial, recovery. Marvin's mother expressed this despair: "Well, you know, the two years are almost up. So I guess we can't expect any improvement any more." Davis asserts that the "moratorium mentality gave way to a more resigned sense of disappointment regarding the child's ultimate outcome."[114]

Returning home proved evocative for young patients. The sheer happiness of escaping a feverish illness, pain, death, and ultimately the hospital, coupled with the sight of familiar landmarks and happy memories of their pre-polio lives, overwhelmed many of them. However, home now presented frustrating obstacles: where previously they strolled across the lawn, it now presented a new challenge to mobility; where once they unthinkingly skipped up the front steps, they now meant a major physical effort, both time-consuming and painful; and relaxing in the once-comfortable sofa swallowed unsuspecting victims, trapping them in its deep clutches. Mia Farrow returned home to find that everything had changed. Her parents literally took her doctor's advice and disposed of everything, burning all of her toys and bedroom furniture and bedding and giving her pet dog away. The carpets had been replaced, walls repainted, lawn reseeded, swimming pool drained and refilled with fresh water, and furniture newly covered. Even her brothers and sisters had been sent away. She "wasn't allowed to see them or any other children for months." Loneliness represented another problem. These children underwent a desocialization process when they entered the hospital and resocialization while they remained in post-acute therapy. As Huse discovered, without the constant companionship provided by ward patients, many returning children who had spent extended time in rehabilitation felt instantly isolated, if not outright homesick—they missed their friends there. They had to endure yet another acclimation. A sense of vulnerability suddenly loomed large. Hospitals and convalescent centers maintained rigid routines, to be sure, but they also conveyed a feeling of security. Everyone knew what to do; predictability prevailed; no surprises existed. All of that disappeared as they resettled at their homes. For iron lung patients, hospitals often had generators to compensate for power outages, but not their families' homes. Fire also elicited great fear. Medical facilities had fire extinguishers readily available, but homes usually did not have them. Care centers also had wide hallways and ramps. Children with disabilities did not always find these physical accommodations at their homes, and often they felt trapped. Finally, medical staffs, with their combined expertise, maintained a 24-hour presence, but if a crisis occurred at home, who would intervene?[115] As Lenny Kriegel, who contracted the virus in 1944 at the age of eleven, writes, "There are moments when one forgets that no one lives by choice in Kafka's house."[116]

The American family proved to be a resilient social institution, as we have seen. Nevertheless, during the early years of polio outbreaks, many parents hid their children with disabilities, embarrassed by their stigma. Only after over a decade of relentless epidemics did the household begin to implement wholesale adaptations. Still, even by the late 1940s, not only did some families refuse to provide care for their infected children, but a few even discarded the children outright. Such was the case with Alice. She had resided at a convalescent hospital for ten years, since the age of three. As she described it, "[My] parents refused to take me. They didn't want a big old crippled-up blob on their hands for the rest of their lives." In some cases, parents expanded their responsibilities to include these castoffs by informally adopting them, at least while they remained hospitalized. Kehret's parents, seeing this situation at the Sheltering Arms center in Minneapolis, Minnesota, became a surrogate family to many deserted girls. As they visited every Sunday, like clockwork, they observed that her four roommates had been alone for months—years, in one case. Kehret's parents and brother gradually incorporated all of them into these family gatherings, celebrating birthdays, recording and showing home movies, and supplying treats and makeup. It evolved into a community project, as Kehret recalls: "Friends and neighbors of my family, hearing about the four girls who didn't get much company, loaded my parents with home-baked brownies, animal crackers, and tins of peanuts. Mother added bags of apples and oranges and bunches of bananas. It was a regular supermarket under my bed." This of course undermined that institution's snack policy.[117] Even into the 1950s, some parents found themselves overwhelmed—traumatized by their child's transformation, exhausted by round-the-clock attention, and broken by the financial obligations. Regina Woods, a young polio patient at a Houston hospital, witnessed how parents discarded their four-year-old child who was disabled: "They simply didn't want her anymore."[118] These remained rare cases indeed but nonetheless testify to the fact that infantile paralysis profoundly changed many lives, straining all of the family's resources and sometimes even fracturing emotional bonds.

The family's polio experience also reveals a somewhat different wrinkle in the history of medicine. A science driven by research and technology emerged during the first half of the twentieth century. But this was not a simple linear progression, as it is often portrayed. For better or worse, former alternatives never completely disappeared. Relentless epidemics every summer revived some of them. Furthermore, this virus encouraged the emergence of yet other unorthodox treatments confronting mainstream medicine. Some families decided to act on these choices, confounding the established medical community.

In sum, the lines between the hospital and home blurred, formal education transcended the public school classroom, and parents made important emotional, medical, and financial choices. Some parents deserted their children, either emotionally or financially overwhelmed or embarrassed by their disabilities, while others extended their own infrastructures to include them as at least temporary members of their families. In the end, those affected by infantile paralysis and their parents alike changed in a variety of ways to new, demanding realities. Only schooling, an integral part of twentieth-century childhood, played second fiddle to home life. It represented the next institutional challenge in this journey.

Chapter 6

The Cripples

*I could neither run properly on the springboard
nor jump properly onto the wooden vaulting block . . .*

—Marc Shell

Twelve-year-old Peg Kehret received a bag full of get-well cards and notes from her classmates while in a Minnesota hospital recovering from infantile paralysis in 1949. As she read them, she felt removed from her classmates.

> I had the strange feeling that I was reading about a different lifetime. The other kids were upset about such unimportant things . . . Now none of this mattered. I had faced death. I had lived with excruciating pain and with loneliness and uncertainty about the future. Bad haircuts and lost ball games would never bother me again . . . I put the letters aside, knowing I was changed forever.[1]

Kehret had become the "other," and she was not alone. In the United States, the "annual incidence of poliomyelitis reached a high during several epidemic years in the 1930s and 1940s of more than 10,000 paralytic cases . . . [In] almost half of these the muscle weakness subsided within six months or more and was not the cause of serious disability."[2] This still represented a sobering figure. For many, the child disabled by polio and the iconic "Tiny Tim," Dickens's sweet, young, and vulnerable character, became one and the same.[3] For others, their mere presence produced a sense of revulsion, as we have seen. Those who attempted to cling to their previous, *normal* lives experienced a complex mixture of shame, embarrassment, and overachievement. This virus aroused deep emotions and constructed new, enduring realities. And young women discovered a redefined femininity.

The school, in many ways, served as center stage for this intense social drama. More than any other institution, it exposed children to the public experience of living with the altered self; it glaringly displayed their disabilities.[4] They *had* to resume their education, or so it would seem. State compulsory attendance laws mandated it. Its policies and architecture, as well as educators' and students' perceptions, catapulted them into the disabled world. How, then, did school administrators respond? Teachers? Peers? Did they reflect the feelings of the public at large; that is, a mixture of pity and rejection?

School Days

The schooling experience, both the institution and its social milieu, reified disability. The physical plants themselves presented one obstacle after another to children with disabilities. Administrators focused on efficiency, moving pupils through the system as smoothly and cheaply as possible. Virtually untrained in special needs approaches, teachers felt inadequate when they were confronted with pupils with disabilities. Students viewed their readmitted companions differently, now through the lens of disability. Peer relationships changed as a result; students responded in countless ways to their presence, ranging from pity to insensitivity. The realities of children disabled by polio offer unique insights into the roles of school administrators, teachers' perceptions and actions, and peer reactions; that is, a side of public schooling we have rarely seen.[5]

Public school officials rarely welcomed children with disabilities. Members of the Cambridge, Massachusetts, school committee in 1885 barred John A. Watson from attending school, because of mental and behavioral disabilities that allegedly disrupted the school. The state court ruled in the committee's favor when his parents filed suit. In 1919, the Antigo, Wisconsin, board of education refused to admit Merritt Beattie as a student, a thirteen-year-old child with physical and speech disabilities. School authorities claimed that his appearance both depressed and nauseated his classmates and that his needs demanded too much of his teacher's attention, namely at the cost of his peers. Local and state courts upheld that board's decision when Merritt's father attempted to file an appeal.[6]

Through the first half of the twentieth century, school administrators responded in a variety of ways to students affected by infantile paralysis who wanted to return to school. In the 1940s, as physicians at the Orthopedic Clinic of New Haven Hospital discharged patients, hospital personnel sent letters to their school principal or school nurse, designating part-time or full-time attendance as well as excusing them from physical education class. However, some schools refused to even readmit them. Following six-year-old Clara Yelder's treatment at Tuskegee's Infantile Paralysis Center, the local public school superintendent refused to re-enroll her, thereby ending her formal educational experience. Robert C. Huse felt completely unwelcome: "When I applied for admittance to high school the principal had said he was doubtful it would work . . . It was obvious he did not want the responsibility of my being there." If readmitted, generally speaking, the only building preparations administrators made consisted of relocating all classes to the first floor. Michael W. R. Davis found his neighborhood Louisville school to be completely unresponsive. He had to continue his daily hot pack treatments every morning at home and needed to continue to visit the hospital's physical therapist. His school's principal proved too inflexible to alter the daily schedule in any way for him. His parents instead had to enroll him in a local private school that accommodated his fragmented attendance. By October, the morning hot pack treatments stopped, and he was able to attend a half-day for five days a week. His treatments became less frequent by January, allowing him to attend school on a full-time basis. Susan Richards Shreve had completed fifth grade in 1950, just before her parents drove her to Warm Springs, Georgia, from Washington, DC. The fact that it was a Quaker school proved to be significant, because, she stresses, "unlike the public schools," it accepted "handicapped children." On the other hand, Mia Farrow's school appeared to be quite accommodating. She only attended school for half a day for a semester because of fatigue and then returned full-time the next semester.[7] No consistent school policy existed.

Siblings occasionally paid a price. Shelby Sigmon, age four, contracted poliomyelitis during North Carolina's 1944–45 epidemic. Her sixteen-year-old sister, Clara, visited her daily at the Hickory emergency treatment center. Clara's high school principal, fearful of her being a possible carrier, ordered her to his office and gave her an ultimatum: stop visiting her younger sister or quit school. Clara chose her sister over her formal education.[8]

In the most extreme instances of flexibility, public high school administrators arranged for teachers to send lessons home to students after hospitals had discharged them. Even this was not always the case, however. Regina Woods, already a tenth-grader in her rural Kentucky high school, fell ill at the age of thirteen in September 1952. The school district refused to provide her with home instruction after her lengthy hospitalization. She appealed, but to no avail: "I wrote a letter to the school board, which, I was told, brought tears to the eyes of those in attendance. The press became involved, but authorities refused to budge, saying that there simply was not enough money to finance home instruction." This forced Woods to complete her remaining three years of high school education in an unorthodox manner, earning graduation credits through correspondence courses. These were often advertised on the inside covers of matchbooks. Those interested in pursuing their education in this manner paid a fee and then received and returned lessons and examinations through the postal system.[9]

In sum, while some school leaders completely barred students disabled by this disease, others integrated them into the daily routine but remained intransigent regarding their schedules and removed few, if any, physical barriers. Still others admitted them but segregated them within the building or simply transferred them to separate facilities. When he eventually returned to school, Richard Owen discovered the meaning of such segregation: "Mostly the children who had polio were put off in crippled children's schools. So there was nobody with a visible physical handicap in any school I had ever attended." He alone used braces and crutches that provided awkward mobility.[10] He clearly stood out. Finally, a very few administrators made special arrangements. But this was not the only challenge faced by students with disabilities.

They attempted to resume their formal schooling but recognized that their childhood and adolescent periods had changed in fundamental ways. Simple mobility required incredible effort and consumed considerable time and energy. Transportation to and from school proved cumbersome. After her initial surgical procedure, at the age of six, young Kay Brutger left the hospital largely immobilized in a large and bulky plaster cast. Yet, according to her recollections, she had to somehow continue her schooling: "My mom had to deliver me to and from school in a baby buggy . . . that was quite embarrassing." She faced physical barriers as well: "I had to use crutches to get around the school, and that wasn't easy." But Brutger found sympathetic peers: "The kids never made fun of me and generally included me in what they were doing." After a third surgical procedure that left her in a body cast, the school sent a home teacher in order to continue her education. Once she had recuperated, Brutger completed her senior year of high school by taking a taxi each morning. She took another cab after school to go to the hospital for outpatient physical therapy, after which her father drove her home. A special bus, with a hydraulic lift, literally picked up Ruth E. Frischer and some other high school students, but it took two hours to travel each way in 1950s New York City.[11]

Architects designed public school buildings for students without disabilities. No ramps existed, making the typical facility virtually inaccessible for those who used wheelchairs. Likewise, those structures lacked elevators that could allow them to easily move between floors. When young Robert Huse returned to his primary school during the 1930s, he discovered how the lack of these accommodations made life extremely difficult for him. The custodian carried him up and down the stairs four times a day, while classmates vied to carry his crutches. Huse recognized this as a money-making opportunity, selling this privilege for two cents per crutch. It proved to be highly lucrative for him until his mother discovered his scheme and quashed it. He fell and was injured when his crutches slipped on a wet spot in the hallway. Frustrated, Huse quit school and opted for home tutoring. He progressed much easier, "functioning in a more conducive environment free of structural and social pressures." The situation did not improve for him in his Lowell, Massachusetts, high school. Relying on braces and crutches for mobility, Huse always arrived late for his classes at the three-story facility. Stairs and long distances between classes delayed him, while crowded hallways impeded his progress; invariably this congestion caused a crutch to be accidently kicked out from under him. Out of frustration, he quit after two weeks: "From the beginning, it was apparent it could never work . . . No one checked to see how it was going for me. No one ever offered any suggestions as to how the problems might be solved." His parents transferred him to a small private school; nevertheless, he recalls, "no concessions would be made because of my 'condition.'"[12]

David Kangas had to complete his last two years of high school after leaving the hospital. In an era that lacked mandated adaptations, he too faced many physical impediments. Kangas used a wheelchair, and he recalls how he required a great deal of assistance from his classmates to attend classes: "There were no elevators, so in order to get to the upper floors, a crew of several students would have to grab my chair and lift me up the steps." Kangas, a former high school athlete, felt helpless: "I just had to face up to the fact that it was the only way I was going to get up to those other classes and continue with my schooling. For the most part, the guys who helped me were quite willing to do it, but I sure didn't like it." School administrators rescheduled some classes for him so he could remain on the first floor. They also assigned a student monitor. Finally, he found it extremely difficult to attend that high school's informal functions.[13]

These students battled many other imposing architectural challenges. Richard Owen, who wore a leg brace, found these buildings dangerous at times: "I had to climb a rather long flight of stairs without a railing, which was pretty scary." He continues, "I think it was such a strange event for them because it was unusual for a child, with a physical disability as severe as mine, to be integrated in a regular classroom. I came back to a group of people who had known me, and here I was on two crutches and lugging a fifteen-pound brace with me."[14] Arvid Schwartz recalls that administrators at his four-story high school made no changes whatsoever for him: "We had two minutes between bells and classes, and I was expected to get from the bottom floor to the top floor in the same two minutes as everybody else." Some classmates willingly carried his books.[15] He was lucky, as another student remembers a distinctly different experience: "Every morning I put on my leg braces, took my crutches and walked a mile to school. When I got to the building the boys were waiting for me at the top of a long flight of stone stairs. They would yell and throw garbage at me during the fifteen minutes it took to climb those stairs."[16] The school's physical plant also destroyed any intimacy for students with such disabilities. They often needed assistance to use the toilet at school, since none had been appropriately equipped. This proved to be embarrassing for them, as a designated adult or peer stood nearby, waiting for them to finish.[17]

However, overcoming readmission hurdles, complex transportation arrangements, and architectural obstacles did not necessarily translate into academic success: Whatever fate they faced was ultimately predicated on teachers' attitudes about and expertise with disabilities. And teachers proved, for the most part, to be wholly insensitive and ill equipped. After a serious disciplinary infraction, Shreve's fifth-grade instructor announced to the class, "We all know that Suzie Richards [Shreve] has caused a lot of trouble this year. But we must feel sorry for her because she has a crippled leg." In another case, a teacher assigned a twelve-year-old female student disabled by polio to a chair, leaving her to sit there isolated and neglected all day.[18] No class revealed disability more than physical education, where many faced certain defeat because they usually had to take part in the regular routine and exercises. For Marc Shell, this represented a disaster when it came time for him to perform a gymnastics activity: "I could neither run properly on the springboard nor jump properly onto the wooden vaulting block that my classmates called the pommel horse." As a result, that instructor severely penalized him: "One failing grade was for the physical subject itself (because I did not do the jump) and the other was for my psychological effort (because I had not tried hard enough). I was ashamed of myself."[19] Humiliation in the gymnasium became a common experience.

Children disabled by poliomyelitis had quite uneven education experiences. Obtaining any formal education meant subjecting themselves to the prerogatives of local school authorities, overcoming transportation and architectural barriers, and dealing with ill-prepared classroom instructors. Dumping these students into special classes and schools represented a simple option for educators, washing their hands of the whole mess.

Segregation

Barb Johnson's kindergarten teacher attempted to remove her from contact with *normal* students: "They wanted to put me in special education, and it wasn't special education for kids with physical handicaps. I would have been segregated off into a classroom with mentally handicapped children. I guess they thought that since I was physically handicapped, I must be mentally handicapped as well."[20] Johnson's perception is correct, as disability experts Sharon L. Snyder and David T. Mitchell insist: "Physically disabled people presented the visible markers that presumed inferior intelligence."[21] This constituted a common notion as special education in general, and schooling for children with physical disabilities in particular, unfolded during the first half of the twentieth century.

The latter followed a common pattern, as it began with private endeavors. The Industrial School for Crippled and Deformed Children (later Cotting School) opened in the basement of Boston's St. Andrew's Parish House, accommodating seven children in 1894 as the first private day school for children with physical disabilities in the United States. Its founders based it on European prototypes in Denmark, Germany, Norway, and Sweden and, according to its 1906 report, conceived of its purpose as a "free school to promote the education and special training of the crippled and deformed." This proved necessary since some institution had to compensate for, its official history proclaims, the "cultural and architectural barriers as well as lack of good teacher and administrator training" in the public schools. It used adjustable desks and chairs that moved to different heights and angles. This school also supplied metal and leather apparatuses to allow children to use utensils in order to learn to feed themselves. It grew steadily, and by 1911 the school owned its own building and housed one hundred students while it continued its policy of free tuition, hot lunches, and transportation. The following year it added an open-air classroom, expanding again in 1926 with a new building extension; it doubled enrollment, offering more extensive vocational education programs. Finally, it maintained a racially integrated student body from its inception.

Cotting School functioned as a full-service institution. Every day from 9:00 AM to 4:00 PM, the primary and grammar departments provided age-graded manual training in basketmaking, carpentry, needlework, shoemaking and repair, typesetting and printing, and weaving, as well as prepared them to make cane seating. As soon as they were deemed proficient, they received pay, its 1906 report claimed. This school also provided medical services through the hiring of a full-time nurse. Volunteers from a nearby gymnastics school provided some low-level physical therapy through massages.

A girl disabled by infantile paralysis at age two and barred from the public schools entered Cotting at age sixteen in 1919. She was the first, but other children disabled by this disease followed; they eventually made up a large portion of the enrollment. The Department of Physiotherapy by the 1930s emphasized massages for these students. One staff member was in charge, with the help of fifty assistants, generally female graduate interns from Boston's universities. The school's medical committee also visited "regularly" to monitor the patients' progress. By 1948, the school had installed ascending and descending stairs to help patients learn to walk with their leg braces.[22]

In nineteenth-century Pennsylvania, the separation of children drew on an explicit "benevolent" impulse to do what was best for children with disabilities, as well as an implicit perception based on a conviction of inferiority. These dichotomized attitudes coexisted well into the twentieth century: "The presence of two groups of teachers instead of a single group trained to teach all children seems to reflect the belief that two different groups of children existed. Indeed, parallel systems of education, instead of a single one created to deal with all children, appeared to acknowledge that physical status is a legitimate differentiating criterion." While early twentieth-century observers saw special education as nondiscriminatory, it in fact was discriminatory.

Progressive school reformers moved most children with disabilities from private to public schools. State compulsory attendance laws, a consequence of Progressive education initiatives, forced public school administrators to respond not only to increased enrollments but also to profoundly different types of students. Two reasons, one rational and the other subjective, explain this phenomenon. First, advocates asserted that these students needed special care: "Because their schooling was looked upon as a medical process, handicapped children were frequently considered to be sick. In this circular fashion, designating these children as patients and their education as a therapeutic measure both justified and engendered segregation." Second, separation resulted from the dominant social perception of disability: "At the time, and for many decades thereafter, however, *any* handicapped child could be kept out of an integrated class by the personal beliefs or wishes of school administrators."[23] Personal bias could, and often did, trump the best stated intentions.

The 1916 poliomyelitis epidemic exacerbated this challenge: how to educate unprecedented numbers of "crippled children." According to a 1918 federal report by the Bureau of Education, however, instruction provided to children with disabilities occurred solely in large urban areas and appeared to be somewhat uneven across the spectrum of private and public institutions. As this report noted, students disabled by this virus "constitute the bulk of the enrollment in a class for crippled children, and they usually stay in the special classes for a good many years before they are able to go to regular classes. Many of them are never able to attend school except in special classes for cripples." In Chicago, students disabled by infantile paralysis accounted for 50 percent of the enrollment in such classes. Children disabled by bone tuberculosis represented an additional 25 percent, and those born disabled or who had suffered an accident accounted for the final 25 percent.

School districts undertook a variety of institutional adaptations, albeit limited ones. "From 1910 to 1930 there was a huge spurt . . . in the number and type of special classes that were formed." Boston became a leader in 1941with 141 such offerings. Cities especially created special classrooms and buildings, but only at the elementary level.[24] Parents had to initiate the admissions process, seeking permission to enroll their children in school. The school district's medical department then evaluated each case to determine if the child qualified; the medical staff did not admit all students. Moreover, these education programs, regardless of location, maintained low social and academic expectations. Educators shortened the school day to avoid overtaxing the students and often instituted rest periods, actually mandated for New York City's "children with bone tuberculosis." The curriculum always focused on practical skills, such as bookkeeping, fabricating metal, knitting, making artificial flowers, repairing shoes, sewing, typing, weaving rugs, and woodworking.[25]

Separate school buildings, according to that same 1918 Bureau of Education report, represented another approach to educating children with disabilities. Four such facilities existed in the United States. Only two of these were public: Chicago's Spalding School for Crippled Children and Cleveland's Wilson School. They featured permanent ramps for easy access and exit as well as to facilitate evacuation during a fire, and all classrooms, plus the auditorium, kitchen, nurse's office, and toilets, were located on the first floor. As early as 1924, Spalding had Hubbard tubs to exercise paralyzed polio patients. Chicago eventually created a number of such special schools. For instance, the remodeled Fallon School, with upgraded equipment and an on-duty nurse, housed 107 students during the 1917–18 school year. There, they only learned vocational skills. And the rationale for these institutions shifted, marking a profoundly different outlook. Charity had represented the impetus, as the superintendent stated in his annual report: "Sentimental reasons were responsible for the provisions originally made for the crippled children in the City of Chicago." During the early twentieth century, a new outlook drove support for these institutions. Relying on a human-capital approach, with a combination of vocational education and "physical reconstruction," ensured that they did not "grow up as mendicants" and were "thus saved for lives of usefulness." The newly expanded Spalding School for Crippled Children enrolled 352 children during the 1917–18 school year. According to its annual report, "about one-half of the children are paralyzed as a result of infantile paralysis and approximately one-third have tuberculosis of the bones." In addition to the usual classes for low-level jobs, they also were given "corrective gymnastics."[26]

By the late 1930s, the Chicago public school district offered an array of special schools and classes at the elementary and secondary levels that encompassed outreach efforts as well. Four "elementary schools for crippled children" existed, with children physically disabled by poliomyelitis making up 23 percent of enrolled students, the second largest group. Designed by district officials, the facilities for these children included an "electronically operated steel door in the bus entrance." The facilities were equipped with cots and mattresses, sun lamps, and swimming pools. Physicians visited regularly, while nurses remained on the premises. The curriculum had been adapted for them too, because it was perceived that they would immediately enter the workforce after they left school. To this end, it offered them vocational skills such as cooking classes, electrical wiring, "home mechanics," and plumbing. Moreover, Chicago's public education system provided two "high schools for crippled children" that enrolled 430 students, though attendance proved erratic because of the need for treatments at clinics. These buildings maintained a staff of physiotherapists, while teachers emphasized the usual vocational skills, like bookkeeping and typing. Finally, Chicago founded its first hospital school in 1912. Some twenty-five years later, the district operated three such programs based in existing hospital and convalescent institutions. Twenty traveling teachers worked with children in an additional five hospitals, educating an average of five hundred students a month. They ensured literacy through individualized instruction and remedial lessons. Chicago's public library also delivered books to hospitalized children to read. That public school system thus adapted to the needs of children with disabilities. As the district's superintendent reasoned in 1939, "Hospital schools prevent leakage in education. School activities during a period of hospitalization prevent failure and demotion upon returning to school." This policy seemed to provide instructional continuity. When children were hospitalized, instructors collected and maintained their school records; when a child left the hospital, the instructors returned the records to the school, along with progress reports.[27] Chicago offered children with disabilities typical vocational training, since their futures, in the true American spirit, involved working to avoid being dependent on charitable gifts.

Although it had been renamed the Spalding School for the Physically Impaired, the human-capital principle endured there. Chicago's public education system trained these students so that they did not feel, as the superintendent's report for the 1930–31 school year proclaimed, that the "world owes them a living." These "fine youngsters," the report continued, "are striving to develop themselves in spite of their handicaps." The rationale for Chicago's special schools changed. Although pity originally drove their inception, supplanted by human-capital theory by World War I, some twenty years later, yet another shift was evident, this time driven by a "special philosophy." As the superintendent's annual report for the 1938–39 school year articulated it, "They are taught to accept their handicaps philosophically, to overcome them if possible, to rise above them, and to triumph in spite of them."[28] This indicated an internalization of positive values regarding disability. Any problems that individuals had with coping emotionally, finding a job, or dealing with other social and physical barriers resided only within themselves. This can-do attitude, it was asserted, could overcome any obstacles. By placing such responsibility on the individual, biased attitudes and physical impediments in society could be easily overlooked, which of course failed to address root problems.

But another, more fundamental deterrent existed that subverted this glib creed. In truth, the triumph over the effects of this disease would remain limited because of its physical toll. A 1961 survey of 806 individuals with long-term disabilities caused by polio revealed that "29 percent of them could not feed themselves; 31 percent could feed themselves with assistance devices; 83 percent could not get dressed by themselves; 32 percent could not write; 40 percent could not get from bed to wheelchair without help; nearly 50 percent could not propel a wheelchair by themselves."[29]

In many ways, all of these schools operated as extensions of the hospital. Boston's Industrial School for Crippled and Deformed Children and New York City's Crippled Children's East Side Free School operated as semiprivate institutions; in the latter, the public school district supplied all of the teachers. And those districts had adapted these buildings by installing elevators. Of all of these institutions, New York City's Free School maintained the most elaborate medical staff. This included a visiting orthopedic surgeon, who, with the aid of an assistant surgeon and nurse, held weekly clinics at the school to adjust braces and set plaster casts, among other treatments. A staff of nursemaids also bathed all of the students twice a week. Finally, the school sent members of this medical staff to the children's homes for additional attention. Chicago's Spalding School provided dental and vision care, while Cleveland's Wilson School relied on an "orthopedic nurse" to manage children's care, beginning at hospitals, visiting their homes, monitoring their progress at convalescent centers, and treating them at schools. A "physical culture" instructor visited the Wilson School three times a week to massage the children and oversee their "gymnastic exercises."[30]

Students disabled by infantile paralysis endured segregated schooling from the beginning. Hospital physicians, as they discharged them, usually advised that parents enroll them in a special or handicapped school. To reinforce this notion, some public school authorities, as we have seen, refused to readmit these returning students, assigning them to a special facility that served children with physical disabilities. Segregation continued to expand. "By 1930, sixty-six cities had special classes and/or special schools for handicapped children."[31] Yet the majority of those with orthopedic disabilities remained excluded. "Rehabilitation professionals favored educating them in more 'appropriate' settings such as hospitals. Moreover, public resistance to educating them at all, whether in special or general classes, seems to have intensified during the 1930s. Those allowed entry were often stigmatized."[32]

Segregation exacerbated disability. Administrators and teachers used special classes to purge unwanted students, physically isolating them from their peers. "Children were totally segregated—although in the same building, they entered and left school at different times and were kept apart at recess." Their classrooms were also located in dank basements and converted closets. There, they became the charges of, generally speaking, poorly trained personnel. "Conditions were deplorable; children struggling with different conditions were lumped together, and no real effort was made to teach them." This led to "social rejection and stigmatization." At best, special education classes served primarily a custodial role.[33]

In sum, a clear system of differentiated yet limited educational opportunities unfolded for these students during the first half of the twentieth century, albeit relegated to urban areas. This of course largely ignored the needs of their counterparts who resided in small towns and rural areas. Presuming that they could even attend their local educational institutions, they had to fend for themselves in school environments that offered virtually no assistance. Ron Zemke represented an exception. He attended a rural one-room schoolhouse during his elementary years, and in that intimate setting, neither his teacher nor his peers saw him as a student with disabilities. He played softball at recess by hitting the ball and crawling to first base on his hands and knees, which his classmates found perfectly acceptable.[34]

New Identities

Education transcended the formal administrative structure and instructional practices of public schooling: social attitudes toward children disabled by poliomyelitis created the most serious obstacles. As soon as school administrators in Virginia, Minnesota, learned that thirteen-year-old Charlene Pugleasa had been rushed to the hospital, they removed the contents of her locker to be incinerated and then fumigated it and burned her desk. Naturally, when these students returned, their actual physical presence proved to be embarrassing or created discomfort. Peg Kehret's friends visited her at home after she had been discharged from the rehabilitation facility. She felt more like a curiosity than a chum: "My friends took turns coming, but the visits seemed strained . . . they could not help staring at my walking sticks . . . they wanted to hear what it was like to have polio . . . I felt like a freak in a sideshow, valued only because I was different."[35] In the public realm of disability, the seer and the seen exist. "The dominant mode of looking at disability in this culture is staring." This action, according to disability historian Rosemarie Garland Thomson, shapes "the social relationship that constitutes disability identity and gives meaning to impairment by marking it as aberrant." The gawker is "normal"; the individual with a disability is not. This represents an act of "exclusion from an imagined community of the fully human."[36] Lenny Kriegel, with his braces, summarizes his reintroduction into community life, after returning from a two-year hiatus at a rehabilitation facility, as a "spiritual lynching." People stared continuously on the street, at his synagogue, and in other social settings. "Those eyes hurt—fool, clown, whimperer for their wonder, that's what I was."[37] Physical disabilities conveyed a powerfully negative connotation, one deeply ingrained in human existence; people historically shunned, ridiculed, or isolated such individuals. This, of course, extended to school peers.

Children with disabilities failed to meet the given social standard, one that became especially embedded in the reality of schooling. First, in formal social situations, their physical appearance, from the bulky shape of orthopedic shoes to the pronounced metallic clink of leg braces, signaled that they were different. Second, their inability to participate in socially oriented recess activities like baseball, jump rope, and tag limited their informal peer-interaction opportunities; play thus became an isolated, individual act. Third, peer associations shifted. Pre-polio friends rarely, if ever, remained the same. This transformation proved to be gradual but nonetheless emotionally unpleasant. James, who contracted polio in 1949, discovered a lonely social world when he returned home. His previous chums no longer wanted to visit him. When his mother intervened, it only made matters worse: "Mom bribes them to keep me company and they come for my toys, not for me. When they come to my front yard, they come for the freak show. There is no admission charge to play with the freak. And after you play for a while you can hit the freak in the head with a baseball bat or steal some of his toys. The freak has so many toys no one will notice." Classmates at the "handicapped" schools often became stand-ins. Still, the regular and frequent rhythm of prepubescent as well as adolescent social interactions deteriorated into random and scheduled weekend visits with other children disabled by infantile paralysis who did not necessarily reside in the same neighborhoods.[38]

Divergent experiences unfolded at the primary and secondary levels. Generally speaking, elementary students found a modicum of acceptance and comfort. That school's social world shaped the self-identity of younger children who, because of their youth and naiveté, appeared to be quite oblivious to their disabilities, as did their peers. Some disabled by infantile paralysis became "celebrities," with crutches attracting the playful curiosity of classmates.[39] Seven-year-old Robert Huse's wheelchair became the source of adventures for his friends, whose goal it was to see how many of them it could convey, as he gleefully proclaims: "The wheelchair, it was quickly determined, could hold five, and in a pinch six kids. One over the axle of the smaller back wheel, on each arm, one on the foot rests, and one in the lap of the operator."[40] Joan Headley, who contracted polio at a very young age, represents a unique case, moving from a state of unawareness, or even innocence, to stark realization. In elementary school, she remained totally unaware of her limp. She even stood in line to receive the polio vaccine at her school. She describes her epiphany: "The little boy standing next to me said, 'Why are you taking this?' I looked at him and thought, 'Why shouldn't I?' Then all of a sudden it occurred to me: all this fuss was for something I had had—and it didn't even hit me."[41]

Less tolerance characterized the secondary school setting. That level of education operated more and more, through the first half of the twentieth century, as the time and place for adolescents to shape and ultimately define themselves, sometimes through a painstaking process. Social rejection haunted them; acceptance, as an elusive goal, mocked them. This proved especially difficult for those with disabilities, since "social relations between the disabled and the able-bodied are tense, awkward, and problematic. To further complicate matters," sociologist Robert F. Murphy adds, "the disabled . . . enter the social arena with a skewed perspective. Not only are their bodies altered, but their ways of thinking about themselves and about the persons and objects of the external world become profoundly transformed." Disability toyed with the process of creating their self-identities; they thus entered junior or senior high schools as "damaged selves." Disability moved them from the "center of . . . society to its perimeter . . . They have become aliens, even exiles, in their own lands." Murphy summarizes the impact of disability: "lowered self-esteem; invasion and occupation of thought by physical deficits; a strong undercurrent of anger; and the acquisition of a new total and undesirable identity."[42] Children disabled by infantile paralysis were thus experiencing extreme emotional turmoil. This only intensified as they entered an already insecure teen world where conformity ruled.

And gender perceptions, as social constructs, proved to be highly subjective. "The state explicitly used the education system to teach boys (and girls) what they considered to be appropriate gender roles." This socialization process involved boys competing on the playing fields and girls learning how to cook in the home economics classroom.[43] "Everyone [was] expected to display an appropriate gender identity." Both young men and women defined themselves by their bodies; bodies also served as "vehicles for determining value, which in turn translates into status and prestige." This therefore represented an "interactive process," one that was profoundly altered by disability. And the intersection of gender and disability remains largely unanalyzed.[44] This could not have been more true than in the 1920s, a pivotal point in fashioning modern perceptions of feminine sexuality.

The notion of the flapper framed femininity for subsequent decades; it was an idea that certainly incorporated various developments but nonetheless represented a tipping point. "She was about nineteen, slender and supple, with a spoiled alluring mouth and quick gray eyes full of radiant curiosity. Her feet, stockingless, and adorned rather than clad in blue-satin slippers which swung nonchalantly from her toes, were perched on the arm of a settee adjoining the one she occupied." Later, when she swam, she wore a one-piece bathing suit that "shocked the natives all along the Atlantic coast from Biddeford Pool to St. Augustine," while she easily and confidently dove off of a cliff, executing a "perfect jack-knife." She boasted about her many exploits to a would-be kidnapper: "The only thing I enjoyed was shocking people; wearing something quite impossible and quite charming to a fancy-dress party, going round with the fastest men in New York, and getting into some of the most hellish scrapes imaginable." Thus we are introduced to Ardita Farnam, one of F. Scott Fitzergald's quintessential flappers. He also presents Sally Carrol Happer, who loved winter sports, and Marcia Meadow, who appeared bold and confident in everything she did. Through these characters, as well as others, Fitzgerald creates a composite picture of a different young woman: brazen, comfortable with men, daring, hedonistic, impulsive, independent, passionate, self-centered, and self-assured; she flaunted her sexuality, listened to ragtime music, smoked cigarettes, and took daring risks.[45]

The concept of femininity by the early 1920s had thus been irrevocably transformed. Here was the new woman, liberated if not shocking in her appearance and behavior, wearing "scantier attire which emphasized her boyish, athletic form, just as she used makeup and bobbed and dyed her hair." Sleeveless dresses exposed bare arms; low-cut styles displayed bare backs; and shorter skirts made legs visible, showcased by the new hosiery. All of these had supplanted restrictive and modest, if not downright prudish, Victorian garments and mores. With her limbs much more exposed than those of her proper Victorian sister, femininity now became embedded in the physical form. The flapper had replaced the Gibson girl, who epitomized "maidenly reserve." One fashion commentator, during the early years of the 1900s, noted, "This is the day of the figure . . . The face alone, no matter how pretty, counts for nothing unless the body is as straight and yielding as every young girl's."[46] Jazz music and highly energetic dancing, like the Turkey Trot and later the Charleston, with arms, hips, and legs gyrating and swinging furiously, now dominated. Women were no longer dainty little porcelain dolls to be protected. Exposed skin and sensuous social interactions with men had introduced a new sexuality. As adolescent culture emerged during the 1930s, femininity became a key component as swing music and acrobatic jitterbug dancing grew ever more popular.

But it ran much deeper than this, as historian Angela J. Latham points out: the human body operates as a "social signifier." She applies this concept to her analysis of female bodies during the 1920s, namely how they were displayed. Latham acknowledges that the "fashionable flapper was correctly perceived to present a serious challenge to the tenacious influence of American Victorian traditions of feminine behavior and display" but avoids oversimplification, transcending the stereotypical flapper genre; rather, she builds context through the sexual hegemony of that time. This encompassed popular obsessions about posture during a time when dress styles revealed more of the body. Fashion tastes dictated that restrictive corsets be abandoned; coupled with dancing, this removed any anatomical mysteries, proving to be sensuous in some eyes but downright immoral in others. Short skirts exposed women's legs and feet, causing silk stockings and high-heeled, narrow, and pointed shoes to come into vogue.[47] This experience moreover proved to be universal; it was not isolated to big cities but existed in rural, small-town America as well—east and west, north and south. The concept of femininity and women's bodies became redefined. Dating had replaced courting. And any woman in her late teens and early twenties—the prime matrimony stage—had to be physically attractive to appeal to potential male suitors.[48]

Young women, Latham continues, engaged in both private and public "performances." The former involved ordinary lives during everyday events or social interactions. The unveiling of the one-piece bathing suit at beaches, which displayed the female form unlike any other clothing, best illuminates this experience. It "registered resoundingly in the public consciousness." Public performances occurred through theatrical entertainment before a defined audience. Beauty contests represented a wholesome example, while the Ziegfeld Follies presented a risqué version. The Miss America pageant, which began in 1921 in Atlantic City, quickly became emblematic of the new femininity as attractive women paraded around in their swimsuits. This became a socially approved and popular event. Producers of less "respectable" theatrical venues found that "the display of women, particularly in scanty attire, was lucrative business." This produced the famous icon of the "Ziegfeld Girl."[49]

These new images became ubiquitous through advertisements and magazines but especially on cinema screens. "One survey concluded that females between the ages of eight and nineteen attended the movies on average forty-six times a year in the twenties." Movie plots dwelled on "winning the loved one," a supposed goal of all women. They yearned to escape the drudgery of the work world through a blissful life of marriage and motherhood. The new woman "won her retirement through the promptings of love and trusting submission to her man." The new movie starlets became role models for young women everywhere.[50] Whether beauty revues, chorus girls, or the cinema, the female body became a "cultural icon." Thus, the female body "*inevitably* functions as a site where cultural values are displayed, contested, negotiated, and ultimately transformed."[51]

The female form, Latham asserts, evokes sexuality, as the entertainment world demonstrated. The "commercial display of women's bodies" sparked many censorship campaigns. The private display of the female form encountered a subtle ban. Here self-censorship proved to be powerful, as women who did not conform to what was deemed attractive covered their supposed defects. As long as a woman had sex appeal, she was valued; when she did not project that image, she was devalued. Failing to meet a set sexual model produced, in Latham's words, "undesirable femininity." While these imperfections encompassed "fat" and "thin" women, it would not be a leap of faith to include women with disabilities in this category. Clear and neat categories of femininity therefore grew out of the commercial culture of the 1920s. Those women who failed to meet the standards of desirable femininity became "transgressors and must be punished." After all, as popular culture portrayed, they were not "fully human."[52]

Where did all of this leave a young woman disabled by poliomyelitis? She felt incredibly self-conscious and typically experienced social rejection; she confronted, as Garland Thomson asserts, "multiple identities."[53] After a great deal of painful physical therapy, Jean Johnson learned to walk again. However, she quickly discovered that her male peers no longer perceived her as attractive. Infantile paralysis had stamped her as an untouchable, as she recalls: "In this kind of culture . . . men like perfect women; they like their arms and legs to match. And that was quite a shock to me . . . Right away, you knew where you stood with men and it was just devastating." Dates and school dances proved to be emotionally traumatic for Josephine Walker; she sadly discovered she was imperfect in the eyes of her male peers. The general public generally perceived these young women as sexually "neutered," which of course was not true.[54] Nonetheless, disability made a woman's body appear "asexual and unfeminine."[55]

Based on these adolescent experiences, many young women saw a dark future for themselves, regardless of their previous life goals. Peg Kehret's dreams of becoming a veterinarian or writer evaporated because of the paralysis of her legs. And it threatened her very femininity, as she recalls: "Even the ordinary hope of being a wife and mother was dim; who would want to marry a woman who couldn't go to the bathroom alone?"[56] Disability produced lifelong humiliating consequences and, through her youthful eyes, undoubtedly trumped the intimacy of marriage.

Popular culture, peers, and institutions defined femininity, and the family reinforced this attitude, one that remained strong through the 1950s. When Ruth F. Frischer was fifteen, a boy invited her for dinner at his house. However, he suddenly phoned the day before to cancel. Frischer later recalls what he confided in her: "He told me that in preparing for our dinner, he removed one of the dining-room chairs from the table. His mother asked why, and he replied that I did not need a chair since I was in a wheelchair. Upon hearing this, she forbade him to see me ever again or else she would disown him."[57] The mother did not foresee a bright future for her son with a young woman with disabilities and promptly and imperiously prohibited any further formal social contact.

This outlook could even be found among some parents of young women disabled by poliomyelitis, resulting in tragic emotional consequences. Some of this attitude can be attributed to psychological professionals who embraced the mental hygiene perspective. They admonished parents for coddling their children with disabilities and urged them instead to institute tough love. Ellen Balbar's father, "obsessed" with a rigid sense of "physical beauty," saw her disabled right leg as unattractive and brutally socialized her into feeling unfeminine: "If he saw I was limping he would walk in front of me and imitate my limp to make me stop limping. That was a cruel thing to do . . . I was very aware of it. It also made me self-conscious. In my teen years, I did not date much because of it." Because of paralysis, the calf muscle had atrophied and shrunk in mass. Her father, she recalls, found this *abnormality* unsettling because he "thought no man would ever be attracted to me if I didn't have two normal legs." To correct this situation, he had a prosthesis made. As Balbar describes it, "It was made with felt, covered with leather, and [I] wore it over an elastic stocking and then put a regular stocking over the elastic stocking . . . My father likened it to a woman who has her breast cut off and uses a prosthesis for a breast, so that equated this with sexuality." This took an enormous emotional toll on her: "It . . . made my [physical] handicap something that made me less. It robbed me of my self-esteem." Her brother reinforced this view, telling her that he could not marry a woman "who wasn't perfect or who had a deformity."[58] This trauma proved to be permanent, since she continues to believe that most men felt this way about her.

A multilayered process of desexing unfolded with the social taboo of disability. Emily Donahue, who had become infected at age seven in Ithaca, New York, developed spinal curvature as a result. Her experience was that of a progressive loss of femininity. Adult observations, physical impediments, and peer associations all contributed to the erosion of her sexual self-esteem. One part of this rejection experience followed on the heels of insensitive remarks and treatment by friends, neighbors, and relatives. Donahue recalls that her mother's friend, a nurse, "voiced a concern to me that . . . I was probably never going to have much of a figure. I was not only going to be kind of skewed, but she doubted I'd ever have any breasts." That medical professional's pronouncement contributed to a desexing process that only exacerbated Donahue's self-doubt, already inflicted by her disability. Persistent pain marked another layer, as she elucidates: "When I was ready to go into eleventh grade, there was a brand-new school. I remember it was quite uncomfortable to sit, partly because the fusion had fused my pelvic bones, and I was healing." Such discomfort proved to be a constant personal, internal, and invisible reminder of her differences. Hard desk seats only made it worse. Redefined social relationships characterized yet another measure, as Donahue points out: "I made very close friends with somebody who was just a normal person—she was a cheerleader, a color guard in the band and beautiful. It was the physical side of her that I couldn't even compete with because she was so gorgeous and I was so twisted and awful looking."[59] The presence of attractive, able-bodied females who proudly and publicly displayed their physical skills and social popularity conveyed a sense of deficit to these students, a constant reminder of what was valued. Donahue apparently saw her alter ego in this person—someone she could not be, who did the things she could not do.

Young men fared somewhat better. Moving from able-bodied to disabled did not represent a new historical experience. Wounded war veterans have always existed, especially so in the twentieth century following both world wars. Certainly they "experienced a brief period of favor" as resources shifted "from the female to the male; from the young to the middle-aged; from the civilian to the ex-servicemen." However, within a few short years after those wars, public gratitude and respect faded away. The public saw them as men with disabilities and less as war heroes. They were now part of the civilian population, with no exceptions. They quickly realized how disability modified "masculine images and ideals."[60] Respect was replaced by "pity and fear." These represent "common emotions associated with our response to disability," historian David A. Gerber writes, that "serve to subvert honor and infantilize and feminize the male." Thus, in the absence of war, male disability naturally lapsed into the usual modes, a long historical experience of "compromised manhood." Although veteran and civilian identities became shared in this case, they diverged in some ways. The former maintained a "group consciousness," while the latter individually faced society's challenges. This "group history" of veterans with disabilities "is ultimately a product of [their] interaction with the state." The state served, to one degree or another, as a service provider and "advanced their interests."[61] Civilians with disabilities relied on charities, for the most part, while their veteran counterparts received federal support. "This shift was most effective in economic terms, as wounded ex-servicemen were given priority over disabled children." In sum, neither of these wars "radically improved the position of disabled civilians."[62] Popular culture, peers, and institutions ultimately defined masculinity.

Becoming disabled by polio unleashed a process of social and self redefinition, a "transformative life event."[63] Male sexuality followed a social script, according to researchers Thomas J. Gerschick and Adam S. Miller: The "body is a central foundation of how men define themselves and how they are defined by others." They label this "hegemonic masculinity," encompassing qualities like aggression, competitiveness, courage, independence, physical strength, self-reliance, and toughness. "On the other hand, people with disabilities are perceived to be, and are treated as, weak, pitiful, passive, and dependent." At the turn of the last century, masculinity became defined less by character and more by body type. Lean and muscular, "real men" physically asserted their individuality. This became embodied in aggressive acts like participating in contact sports. Boys welcomed this conflict. As men, they could assert their male prowess in the workplace, as farmers, machinists, steelworkers, or welders, and during recreation on baseball fields, on tennis courts, and in swimming pools. Competitiveness, physical aggression, strength, and toughness defined them.[64] "There is not a clear distinction between the study of men's bodies and masculinity," historian Joanna Bourke asserts.[65]

The media embedded this social benchmark into the public's consciousness, long portraying lean and muscular men who exuded strength and confidence. Through the first half of the twentieth century, as it does now, the media shaped notions of attractiveness, health, and success for young people. Their "self-worth and perceptions of others," media scholar Joe Grixti asserts, "relate to recurring projections of desirability in the media," and "their self-images are inevitably inflected by the commercial imperatives of the entertainment industries and advertising." Grixti concludes that "those who do not fit these 'norms' often come to be seen, and also come to see themselves, as the other."[66] William Zanke, disabled by infantile paralysis since age four and raised in Wheeling, West Virginia, in the 1950s, grew to realize his social limitations:

> Puberty affected my social life; I started becoming self-conscious about limping, and was unclear about what impact that was going to have on dating and just success with women, or was convinced that it rendered me out of the game. In high school it was clear to me that the range of possible dates for me was somewhat limited; inside I knew it had to do with the limp.[67]

Bill Norkunas, who in 1944 contracted polio at age four, in Worcester, Massachusetts, grew up with a disabled leg. In his teens, it created self-doubts, limiting his opportunities for dates: "I always thought, if I didn't have polio, would I have more dates, or would I have been more popular with the girls?"[68]

In sum, masculinity underwent redefinition because of disabilities caused by poliomyelitis, and this created a profound identity crisis. These adolescent males, against the cultural backdrop of the 1940s and 1950s, appeared "weak and effeminate" to their peers, sometimes even becoming susceptible to the pejorative label—at that time—of homosexuality.[69] Gerschick and Miller trace three dominant responses that frame how men with disabilities coped within this social construct. The first involves reformulating the notion of masculinity. Unable to meet given cultural standards, "they distanced themselves from masculine ideals." Through this process, they redefined masculinity; an internal creation supplanted an external construct. Their versions of manhood were based on a personal, highly individualistic set of ideas and, as such, escape generalizations. A second strategy largely adheres to the social definition of masculinity. For adolescents in particular, their malleable gender identities were uncertain to begin with, and disability intensified this tenuousness. These individuals clung to some of their pre-disabled notions of masculinity, like competition, independence, and sexual prowess. Some have referred to it as hypermasculinity. The third response outright rejects hegemonic masculinity. These men "believed that the dominant conception of masculinity was wrong, either in its individual emphasis or as a practice." They embraced a "people-first" outlook, maintaining that intelligence or mental capacity trumped traditional male qualities.[70]

The social scene at the secondary school level, resplendent with innumerable conformities, proved to be a far less tolerant setting than its elementary school counterpart. Neither females nor males felt comfortable with their bodies, but females felt even less so. Fred Davis's insightful 1954–55 ethnographic study found that older students, regardless of gender, responded in a variety of ways, but none of them appeared to be mutually exclusive. These involved, in no particular order, denial, escape, insulation, and overcompensation.[71]

Denial

Some students disabled by poliomyelitis tried to recapture their pre-polio lives. A 1947 study conducted at the Clinic of the Orthopedic Hospital, Los Angeles, analyzed the psychological impact of the disease's aftereffects. It included 437 European American subjects, 203 males and 234 females, who had contracted the virus. At that time, their ages ranged from sixteen to forty-eight: 90 percent of them were younger than thirty years old, with a mean age of twenty-two. They had generally become ill very early, with 60 percent at age five or younger and 92.5 percent under thirty. Fifty percent of the sample had visible physical disabilities. The findings proved sobering: 96 percent of the entire cohort avoided association with peers who were physically disabled. For students in denial, they dissociated themselves from their bodies. Disability defined them—and they did not want to accept that identity.[72] In spite of the kinship they had developed with others while undergoing rehabilitation in the closed world of the convalescent ward, most shunned them in public.

They generally participated in activities as though nothing whatsoever had happened to them, refusing to wear their braces or attempting to ride the school bus, acutely aware, nevertheless, of their differences. Charles Mee, a ninth-grade high school football player, became infected in 1953 at age fourteen in Barrington, Illinois. He hated being "crippled" and plunged into the regular life of the school social scene. His attempts to recover his previous life resulted in varying behaviors, from embarrassment to overachievement. Mee hid his crutches from view when anyone photographed him. Using intellectual acuity as a tool to offset physical disability, he resorted to humiliating students he disliked, verbally bullying them.[73] Michael Davis contracted the disease as he finished seventh grade, during the 1944 Kentucky epidemic. He admits in his memoir to overcompensating in ninth grade when he returned to school. He played soccer, because it did not require the use of his left arm and it earned a varsity letter: "It helped my feelings of physical inferiority and thus terrible shyness with girls."[74] Some purposely followed President Franklin D. Roosevelt's public example. This is what Brenda Serotte, in retrospect, realized what she had done: "All his life Roosevelt denied being a cripple. He acted as if he'd never had polio or else as if it was over and done with. In a few short years I'd act the same."[75]

Nevertheless, these students' attempts to recapture their former social lives could only go so far. Impenetrable barriers existed, no matter their efforts. And simple activities like school dances, as alluded to above, clearly separated them from their able-bodied peers. Gender especially differentiated them in these and other informal interactions, though boys with physical disabilities found it somewhat easier and more socially acceptable to attend school socials, like homecoming celebrations or prom extravaganzas. Mee, a former athlete, donned his white tuxedo and took Suzy, a cheerleader, to the junior prom: "We danced. That is, she moved with me. I had figured out how, with one hand on her waist and my other hand steadying myself by holding my own hip, I could stand and move a few steps without my crutches. She let one arm rest lightly on my shoulder, one hand took me lightly but supportively at the waist, and we moved to the music."[76]

Clearly, some adolescents affected by disability feebly attempted to divorce themselves from their bodies: They embraced what some termed "fake normalcy."[77] Yet in spite of their efforts to resume their previous lives, they had many experiences and received a variety of messages, whether intended or not, that they had become the "other." Many of them responded by purposefully confronting this cultural stereotype.[78]

Flight

Another response involved those students with disabilities who retreated from "normals."[79] Anger, resentment, and a sense of loss, even shame, shaped their outlooks. Their emotional trauma matched the physical catastrophe, and their reality became one of *them versus us*. This polarized world consisted of two distinct cultures: the disabled and the able-bodied. Lorenzo Wilson Milam clearly describes this social dynamic: "Simple relationships became complexly bound up in my physical presence in the room, as if I had been turned into some six-foot tarantula," evoking Kafka's imagery in *The Metamorphosis*. Lenny Kriegel takes it a step further: "The dirty little secret of anyone who's lived with polio—or any severe disability—on intimate terms is that after a while you come to feel a certain contempt for people who haven't."[80]

Many only gradually became aware of this new reality. Zemke felt increasingly left out of his high school's social scene because his childhood friends advanced to varsity sports, while he did not. Richard Owen, stricken at age twelve in 1940, found himself the "only disabled person in a student body of about 3,000." He wore a leg brace. His social life, because of numerous school absences and impaired mobility, proved to be limited: "I had . . . become a slow-moving person, and that was something that was really difficult for me, particularly in high school. I ended up walking alone much of the time."[81] Some dreaded attending school, as another recalls: "Sunday nights I am really anxious. Tomorrow I go to school . . . in school I'm a loner. If I walk very fast and don't look up no one will seem, no one will see my limp. Every Monday is Blue Monday."[82]

As we have seen, many students with disabilities encountered academic challenges and perceived social barriers, whether imposed or self-inflicted. As Gail Bias recalls, "The kids in school used to laugh at me." After a while, however, her classmates accepted her and invited her to play at recess. By the time she reached high school, and even though she had regained some mobility, she avoided social events, like dances, and extracurricular activities, such as cheerleading; she simply felt too self-aware.[83] She moved from reluctant acceptance to total avoidance.

A few experienced a complete emotional collapse. Feeling self-pity and discouragement, as well as general depression, they disassociated themselves from the *normal* world, severing all organizational ties, such as the Boy Scouts and Girl Scouts. Classmates taunted them, cruelly hurling terms like "cripples" or "sissies" at them. Overwhelmed with self-consciousness, some chose self-exile, avoiding educational opportunities and even employment, becoming "prisoners in their own homes."[84] Unable to cope with her disability, Marilynne Rogers attempted to starve herself to death until a doctor intervened. In the most extreme case, two teenage boys who had been high school football stars during the late 1940s became emotionally distraught over the loss of their athletic skills: they would no longer play a sport they loved and jubilantly celebrate their team's victories. That symbol of their masculinity had suddenly disappeared. They faced a new reality dominated by the frustration of physical immobility and the trauma of becoming social outcasts. They committed suicide while undergoing physical therapy at a rehabilitation center.[85]

Insulation

There is no question that poliomyelitis adversely affected the mental health of children and adolescents. The New York Neurological Society, in its 1910 report, reflected the traditional attitude towards disability. It acknowledged the emotional toll wrought by polio and suggested "mental adaptations" to reduce or eradicate feelings of being "morose, reticent and shy" as well as to prevent growing "selfish" because of family indulgences. It glibly declared that a sense of hope provided the only means of overcoming these feelings: "The best training is for him to hear stories of great men who have triumphed over some physical weakness."[86] During the 1930s and 1940s, and somewhat in the same vein, canon dictated that physical disability shaped the emotional and social maturation of adolescents. Developmental psychologists generally believed that they experienced anxiety about their sexual self-image and concomitant social acceptance: "They pointed out that adolescents with sex-inappropriate characteristics had the most difficult time fitting in with their peer groups and consequently exhibited a greater degree of psychopathology and antisocial behavior than those who developed normally. Sometimes the burden of being different could result in severe mental disorder." Being able-bodied therefore dictated a sexual standard; peer conformity would then be achieved. "Physicians and mental hygiene experts worried [that this disease] could cause deep-rooted psychological scars if physical disability prevented successful integration into youth culture." These ideas and practices, regardless of the period, simply placed the burden of disability on the individual, under the guise of scientific research. Physical impediments and peer perceptions did not have to be altered at the schools; instead, young people disabled by poliomyelitis had to adopt a positive demeanor to overcome all of their emotional despair and *perceived* physical and social difficulties.

This produced unintended outcomes, however. Many indeed protected themselves from pitiful stares and condescending attitudes by constructing an accepting and tolerant, but limited, network of friends and acquaintances. Jack Dominik, who became ill in 1925 at three years of age, at first avoided school recess because he could not participate in many physical games. His classmates, rather than tease him, actually helped: "One boy used to walk home with me every day and make sure I got safely across a busy street." Len Jordan contracted polio at age ten in 1945 and, with the acceptance of some classmates, participated to a limited extent in games and sports: "When we'd play kick the can, I would kick it, but somebody else would run for me. That was the same way I played baseball; they'd let me hit, but then someone else would have to run the bases."[87]

"Supercrip"[88]

Post-polio expert Richard L. Bruno found in his 1995 survey that over 30 percent of individuals disabled by this virus classified themselves as "Type A" personalities, "hard-driving, time conscious, competitive, self-denying, perfectionistic, overachieving." They felt driven to overcompensate for their disabilities. Margaret, who fell ill in 1942, boldly states, "Don't let any polio survivor tell you they just want to 'be normal like everyone else.' We want to be better than everyone else just to break even . . . and that may not be enough!"[89]

These students had to find a personal way to "'fit in.'" And gender often prescribed the outcome. Females were expected to compensate for their "physical shortcomings" by adopting an extroverted and charming attitude. A winning personality seemingly replaced sexual attractiveness. Males, now seen as physically "frail," could adapt through artistic or academic excellence. Aesthetic or intellectual achievements substituted for physical prowess. They thus had to individually adjust and at the same time display a socially acceptable demeanor. If not, they were deemed emotionally deficient in addition to being physically disabled.[90]

In school, some purposely made substitutions, shifting from physically demanding activities, like athletics, to more cerebral outlets, like debating. No longer able to participate in high school athletics, Arvid Schwartz became the team manager and recalls that he "suddenly became part of the group." A social outcast in high school, Mary Ann Hoffman experienced this shift: "I remember going to the freshman dance. I was all excited about it, but no one asked me to dance all night! I was just crushed." She transferred to another high school in tenth grade and assumed control of her social world by participating on the student council, editing the yearbook, selling tickets at sports events, going on dates, attending dances, and eventually becoming class valedictorian.[91]

While adults presented few public models for children with disabilities, Roosevelt became the supreme example. His seemingly indomitable attitude inspired many. His perpetually smiling face reflected determination and the will to return to a socially acceptable life. Roosevelt became a hero to many children disabled by polio. "Sometimes, as I wheeled through the [convalescent home's] corridors alone," Lenny Kriegel recalls, "I pronounced his initials, 'F.D.R., F.D.R.,' over and over again, finding the cheap reassurance of worship in the sounds. He was an easy god to worship." The fifteen-year-old Kriegel kept a scrapbook full of newspaper clippings about Roosevelt, but especially his pictures. "He fought my virus with me. And [World War II] itself I began to think of as a war to end all virus." They were comrades in arms: Roosevelt was the general and Kriegel a soldier.[92]

Roosevelt's well-chronicled story offers vital insight into this disability paradox. Although he had become seriously ill and survived the 1918 influenza pandemic, even a scion of wealth could succumb to the poliovirus and paralysis. Born to the politically renowned Roosevelt family, Franklin at age thirty-nine had already been elected to the New York State Senate, served as assistant secretary of the navy in President Woodrow Wilson's administration, and run as the democratic vice presidential candidate during the 1920 election. In late July 1921, physically exhausted after the pressures of political life, he decided to retreat to Campobello, New Brunswick, to join his family. As chair of the Boy Scouts of America, he stopped at the Bear Mountain camp on his way. Located on the Hudson River, it hosted some 2,100 boys from New York and New Jersey. This is where he probably came into contact with that contagion. He joined his family on August 7, 1921. There, he pursued a highly active couple of days fighting a brush fire, sailing, and swimming. He went to bed feeling especially fatigued, with a pain in his lower back, on the night of August 10. The next morning he stumbled into the bathroom to shave, returned to bed, and felt worse as the day progressed. A local physician, who had never seen a case of infantile paralysis, attributed his aches, chills, high fever, and general pain to a summer cold. By August 12, suffering from leg paralysis, Roosevelt was not able to stand. Two days later, as his condition worsened, William W. Keen, a doctor summoned by the family from Bar Harbor, provided a second opinion, declaring that Roosevelt had a spinal blood clot. Keen optimistically declared that he would experience a full recovery. Louis Howe, Roosevelt's close political adviser, privately questioned Keen's analysis while speaking with Roosevelt's wife, Eleanor, and mother, Sara. Eleanor secured Robert W. Lovett, from the Harvard Infantile Paralysis Commission, who arrived on August 24 and rendered his fateful diagnosis. Lovett conveyed an optimistic prognosis to the Roosevelts, and he wrote to George Draper, Roosevelt's physician, that he thought it a mild case and that Roosevelt would, most probably, recover his mobility. Lovett ordered Roosevelt to remain at Campobello to rest. On September 14, Roosevelt returned to his New York City residence, where Draper oversaw his hospitalization.[93]

Lovett directed Roosevelt's therapy. In 1922, he went to Boston to consult with Lovett, who had a custom set of leg and back braces made for him. Roosevelt revisited Lovett in 1923 and devoted the next few years to regaining the use of his legs.

> He tried everything: massage, saltwater baths, ultraviolet light, electric currents, walking on braces with parallel bars at waist height, walking while hanging from parallel bars mounted above his head. He tried horseback riding, and an electric tricycle . . . exercises in cold water . . . He would sweat and strain, pulling himself across the carpet on his stomach. Sitting up he would inch himself backward, dragging along his useless legs.

Nevertheless, all of his good intentions and valiant efforts proved for naught. Once this virus damaged the nervous system, no amount of desire or work would renew it. But Roosevelt refused to accept his condition, becoming obsessed with full recovery. Battling bouts of depression, he managed to recover enough to stand on his feet on occasion, with the help of leg and pelvic braces as well as crutches, projecting a tenuous image of being *normal*.[94]

Roosevelt's response to disability proved to be highly enigmatic, causing two distinct historical interpretations to emerge. Hugh Gregory Gallagher, a historian and disability advocate, argues that Roosevelt led two lives: his political life followed a strict public relations approach, avoiding any media images of him in a wheelchair, a successful effort at preventing the portrayal of a vulnerable political candidate and eventually president; in his private life, he adopted a personal, informal attitude toward his paralysis, revealing deep ambivalence toward it. Gallagher labels this charade a "splendid deception." The president of the United States had to project an image of strength, vigor, and control. Roosevelt, acutely aware of this social reality, protected his political career by completely hiding his disability. The physical norm could not be violated. And all willingly participated in this masquerade. The White House press corps, for the most part, complied with his wishes and censored itself regarding photographs of him in a wheelchair. "If, as happened once or twice, one of its members sought to violate it . . . one or another of the older photographers would 'accidentally' knock the camera to the ground or otherwise block the picture. Should the President himself notice someone in the crowd violating that interdiction, he would point out the offender and the Secret Service would move in, seize the camera, and expose the film." As a result, only four pictures survived with him sitting in a wheelchair. Gallagher further asserts that denial of Roosevelt's disability extended beyond the president and the press corps—it included the American public as well. "The people would pretend that their leader was not crippled, and their leader would do all that he could not to let them see that he was." Highly choreographed public appearances assured that perception.[95]

Disability historians Paul K. Longmore and David Goldberger echo Gallagher. Roosevelt became a symbol of an "overcomer," but only through shrewd manipulation. He achieved a "socially valid identity," they continue, less through rigorous physical therapy and more through "denying and hiding the disabled parts of himself." He not only survived this disease but also seemingly prevailed over disability to become a hero to individuals affected by polio when he won the 1928 gubernatorial election in New York. His stature grew when he became president of the United States in 1932.[96] Roosevelt projected "a new cultural symbol," serving as polio's hero because of his individual triumph and his concrete contributions to fighting, treating, and ultimately finding a cure for this dreaded disease. In this regard, even his public image proved ambiguous. While Roosevelt remained sensitive concerning reports about his disability, he freely served as a national symbol to fight the disease. And with his hectic presidential schedule, he honored his polio tradition, attempting to visit Warm Springs every Thanksgiving.[97]

James Tobin's biography of Roosevelt differs in subtle but important ways. He asserts that Roosevelt's polio infection represented a matter of degree. After Lovett's diagnosis, Eleanor Roosevelt and Louis Howe carefully protected Roosevelt's promising political career by releasing a press announcement that vaguely alluded to an illness. Following his return to New York City for convalescence, Eleanor, Howe, and even Roosevelt's mother, Sara, muddied the media waters, each speculating that he had contracted either a severe cold, rheumatism, or pneumonia. They left it to Draper to provide a definitive, but optimistic, public statement; that is, that Roosevelt had indeed contracted infantile paralysis but would not be permanently paralyzed. As Howe saw it, to protect Roosevelt's lofty political ambitions, the story of a health problem, even a serious one, was preferred to one of disability and the social stigma that accompanied it. The context reinforced this view: "A survey of 600 major U.S. employers in the 1920s found that half would not employ a disabled worker under any circumstance; another 25 percent would think of doing so only if the individual had been disabled while working at the firm." This was what Howe and Roosevelt felt, but on a grander scale: "Virtually everyone equated disability with weakness and incapacity. The cripple was not whole, not a real man. Certainly not a man to be entrusted with power." Roosevelt, Tobin writes, hid the extent of his paralysis so that the public generally did not want to think of him that way: "People knew but didn't know, knew but didn't think about it. Year after year in the 1930s and 1940s, there was a massive, nationwide drive on Roosevelt's birthday to raise money to fight infantile paralysis, with Roosevelt's picture on posters and appeals over his signature. But people didn't think about the president being crippled."[98]

He gave the public a glimpse of his disability in 1924 at the Democratic Party's presidential convention where he nominated Alfred E. Smith as that party's presidential candidate. Wearing back and leg braces, he used a crutch and his son's elbow to inch his way to the podium, which he gripped for stability while he delivered his speech. Attendees saw him as a hero, overcoming adversity. His popularity surged. "In the eyes of onlookers, the crippling had somehow not diminished him but enhanced him. This was no longer merely the fine-looking Harvard boy with the golden name. It was that boy tried and tempered, his face creased with lines, yet somehow joyous." During the 1928 New York gubernatorial race, Roosevelt did not hide his disability; rather, he used it to reveal what he had overcome, as Tobin stresses: "He [showed] himself to be something he had never been seen as before: a fighter and, better yet, an underdog; not a man to pity, not a man to envy, but a man to cheer." It remained an emotional appeal, but it was one that won him that election. Political journalists treated Roosevelt's disability as a positive story, when they even wrote about it. "For American reporters raised on heroic tales of the underdog, it was the mold into which the facts fit naturally . . . It was the good old comeback story," one that Roosevelt and his political advisers used to their advantage. Political opponents, especially anti-Roosevelt Democrats, publicly pointed out his physical disability, and some even hinted at mental deficiencies—a few resorted to syphilis as the cause instead of infantile paralysis. He fought back by defining himself and his disability. Roosevelt ran a vigorous and ambitious presidential campaign in 1932, walking and standing but clearly needing support. He repeatedly portrayed physical strength and defiance at his campaign stops. This was "not a deception but a *performance* in which actor and audience tacitly agreed to go through a drama together."[99] More importantly, though, the mere fact that a historiographic debate exists over Roosevelt's attitude toward his disability places this matter into context. The degree of exposure is what these historians debate. The social (and, in this case, political) stigma remains.

Both interpretations generally agree that Roosevelt privately felt comfortable with his disability. His "cane and crutches and wheelchair became part of the furniture" as he met with military and civilian advisers, politicians, staff members, and friends. He freely used a wheelchair with close aides, most friends, and his entire family. Others rarely saw it. Roosevelt usually entered a room first and flipped from it to a standard chair; as guests were led in, they only saw the president relaxing in a comfortable chair.[100] At Warm Springs, he dropped all pretensions. Out of the eyes of his political enemies and away from public scrutiny, with the White House Press Corps restricted to the perimeter of the compound, he relaxed. Within those safe confines, he accepted his disability, roughhousing with his attendants, "pulling them down on top of him with his powerful arms." He laughed if he fell, unembarrassed by his inability to walk. He frolicked with patients in the swimming pool and felt comfortable crawling on the ground and up the steps to parties being held in any of the cottages. Roosevelt purchased automobiles and had them modified at Warm Springs with hand controls; his last one was a dark blue 1938 Ford touring model. With these, he explored the property to oversee the numerous construction projects. He gained a reputation for driving wildly throughout the countryside, enjoying the lush foliage, transporting residents, and pulling up to chat with them. Roosevelt also organized bridge parties, fish fries, picnics, and sing-alongs to break up the monotonous rehabilitation routine.[101]

Roosevelt, in short, felt at ease separating the disease from the disability. He openly and vigorously fought the former but seemed to sidestep the latter. Roosevelt, as Tobin states, "was not a crusader for the rights of the disabled."[102] He was purely pragmatic in that regard.

Good Old School Days

Simon Flexner, director of the Rockefeller Institute for Medical Research, in a 1911 speech before the National Academy of Sciences, referred to children paralyzed by infantile paralysis as "cripples," a common label at that time and for most of the twentieth century.[103] This designation excluded these children, both implicitly and explicitly, from the norm, assigning them a different place in society's hierarchy. Their experiences therefore reveal in sharp terms how disability was (and remains) socially constructed.[104] Polio itself did less to create disability than the fact that people affected by polio deviated from being socially and educationally acceptable. Infantile paralysis added yet another wrinkle to the disability experience. When we speak of individuals with physical disabilities, we often link this to a condition that began at birth. This was simply not the case. Those disabled by this virus had led able-bodied lives and suddenly had to cope with disabled ones. Not only did this disease contribute to their new self-identity, but their physical and social environment changed it as well. They saw their functionality reduced by the lack of accommodations in public places, especially school buildings. They too often became social outcasts, either through compulsion or by choice. Their peers, who had originally befriended them as non-disabled people, often altered their perceptions and reevaluated their relations. They now saw someone different, and in extreme cases, they saw someone less human. Finally, the physical appearance of students disabled by poliomyelitis conflated their public and personal realities. Disguised as a witch on Halloween during the 1950s, Ruth E. Frischer brutally and unexpectedly became aware, for the first time, of what she had become: "At the second door I rang, a woman answered and opened the door. She proceeded to yell at me, believing that I was masquerading in a wheelchair. She did not even see my witch's costume, she saw only the wheelchair, and thought that I was using it as a Halloween disguise. It was then I came to the realization that some people see only the wheelchair, irrespective of the person sitting in the chair."[105]

We can make three generalizations about the schooling experiences of children disabled by polio. First, the impact on their academic achievement (i.e., learning) remains unclear. We are left to infer patterns from existing sources. By the 1940s, elementary school teachers observed that many of these children, overwhelmed by the sheer amount of schoolwork they had missed and the daunting task of trying to catch up, easily succumbed to any pressure or stress, frequently experiencing emotional meltdowns that were most often marked by crying spells. Nevertheless, this much is sure: Overcompensation tended to be typical, both implicitly and explicitly. Second, social relations shifted profoundly. Physical disability built a wall between them and other students; their physical transformation narrowed their world of possibilities; for example, in athletics, basic mobility, school dances, and sexuality. Third, this virus unleashed an emotional maelstrom. Because they deviated from the accepted physical standard, they felt anger, fear, hurt, and loneliness, among many other sentiments. Some of these manifested through pathological disorders, such as substance abuse and suicide attempts.

In its own time and in limited ways, formal education responded to the demands that infantile paralysis inflicted on children. This became manifested in at least three different ways, often following a common pattern. Since the children were unable to attend school while hospitalized, some educational administrators assigned teachers to instruct them while they were still confined to their beds. In other cases, after being released from the hospital or convalescent home but still limited to home care, district authorities sometimes sent teachers to oversee students' lessons. Finally, when children were strong and mobile enough to attend classes, a few building principals provided limited adaptations. Generally speaking, school personnel perceived them as different, not fitting a prescribed image. The public school system as a whole never attempted to confront the tyranny of disability as a social construct. Instead, it institutionalized it through special education classes and schools, segregating students.

This disease's influence on children proved to be profound. Public images in general, and schooling in particular, defined them. And as historical actors, they responded in many different ways. Many attempted to escape from their sense of helplessness, shame, pity, and deep anger. Others, through their medical, physical, and social experiences, created "a new model for disability." They became the vanguard of the disability rights movement of the 1960s and 1970s.[106]

Chapter 7

Polio's Legacy[1]

Epidemics exacted an especially heavy toll on children, but cultural artifacts like the following nursery rhyme reenact them in playful, and certainly harmless, ways:

> *Ring-a-ring o' roses.*
> *A pocket full of posies,*
> *Hush! Hush! Hush! Hush!*
> *We all fall down.*[2]

This famous little song has entertained generations of young children with endless hours of laughter and silliness, holding hands, spinning in a circle, and crumpling to the ground. Although seemingly benign, it obscures—as well as echoes—a dark and tragic time in Western history. The Great Plague struck London not once but several times over a hundred-year period. "Around one-fifth of London's population perished in each of the plague outbreaks of 1563, 1603, 1625 and 1665, the death toll in 1665 approaching 80,000."[3] These verses neatly capture that story. If a person had a rosy rash, this usually signaled that they had become infected. However, carrying posies of herbs, people believed, shielded them from the contagion. Sneezing marked the "final fatal symptom." And, of course, "we all fall down" clearly refers to inevitable death.[4] Children—especially those who resided in the United Sates—perpetually suffered high morbidity and mortality rates from a variety of infectious diseases, so that, until relatively recent times, illness and death naturally became embedded in their culture.

At the dawn of the twentieth century, many health experts felt supremely confident that emerging modern medical science had given them the tools to combat contagious outbreaks. However, this "illusion of medical certainty" proved to be extremely fragile: Infantile paralysis struck the United States with devastating results, and children accounted for about 80 percent of those infected.[5] This disease exacted an enormous emotional and physical toll for decades. Mark Sauer, who contracted it at age six in 1958, during the last major epidemic in Detroit, sums it up best: "There were many other diseases that were bad for America, but polio broke its heart." It "was the robber of childhood innocence, it was the robber of hope for a generation, several generations of children."[6]

Indeed, the interaction between diseases and culture is profound. Poliomyelitis altered the life courses of tens of thousands of children. It made them pariahs in so many ways. Uninformed and overly cautious public health officials hunted them down and isolated them. Fearful private citizens, in some cases, reverted to vigilante tactics, banishing New York City's children in general, and those ill in particular, from their communities. Public facilities closed. Parent and child relations ruptured as hospitals and rehabilitation institutions assumed—sometimes forcibly—total responsibility for their very lives and well-being. As these young patients progressed from one institution to another, they became resocialized. In the process, often left to their own devices, they developed unique worlds in their wards, creating hierarchies, undermining rigid rules, and retaliating against cruel medical staff members. Physical disability, stemming from this disease, marked them. Race compounded this. Caring for an infected daughter or son at home commonly fell on mothers' shoulders, occasionally breaking them physically and emotionally. In a few cases, the entire family fell apart because of the strain. With no health insurance, households sacrificed their financial futures. And sibling relations teetered. Too many children disabled by polio could not resume their schooling, or found it extremely difficult, or became segregated as they received a second-rate education. The public shunned them and hounded them from public spaces.

American culture responded to infantile paralysis in a variety of ways. Pity led to new organizational structures. The National Foundation for Infantile Paralysis employed advertising campaigns utilizing the new mass media, resorting to highly emotional appeals for support. It built an unprecedented nationwide volunteer structure that mobilized thousands of communities, eventually including African Americans. The foundation empowered women and gave the public a sense of altruism and hope, raising and spending millions of dollars for care and a cure. But fear, if not outright loathing, trumped everything. Local newspapers published the names and addresses of ill children, destroying any privacy. The emerging motion picture industry reified physical disability through its mixed images of Tiny Tim and, more importantly, repulsive monstrosities. Popular movies only portrayed physically desirable women—of course, with their limbs intact. The femininity of young women with physical disabilities became questionable.

While the last children's plague had been overcome, American society began to come to grips with this disease's heritage: Even with the success of Jonas E. Salk's and Albert Sabin's vaccines, "150,000 paralytic polio cases . . . would require treatment for many years to come."[7] Poliomyelitis had made physical disability an integral part of the American experience. The sheer numerical size of the "polio nation"—individuals with physical disabilities—eventually led to initial forays into disability rights.[8] For the longest time, disability represented an individual problem and as such required a largely personal and independent effort to overcome. This hampered the development of a viable disability movement, as activist Hugh Gregory Gallagher points out: "The disabled did not see themselves as a community with shared interests or rights. There was no such thing as 'disability culture.' Most people had never considered that the disabled might have, as a right, access to public facilities such as schools, movies, transportation. Nor had they given thought to the proposition that the disabled should have equal access to employment." This seemingly isolated experience, fed by a naïve public attitude of inspirational tales of overcoming disability, just prolonged a tortured social reality.

Gallagher attributes the breakthrough for the disability movement to three variables that converged by the end of the 1940s. First, the growth in the scope of polio epidemics in the postwar era raised the consciousness of the general public. Newspapers devoted wide coverage to them, while the March of Dimes campaigns purposefully made disability visible through their poster children in order to generate donations. And President Franklin D. Roosevelt, of course, became a national symbol in the campaign against this disease. Second, medical breakthroughs, particularly with antibiotics, extended the life expectancy of individuals with disabilities as never before. Third, massive casualties during World War II forced American society to come to grips, in an unprecedented fashion, with physical disabilities. Roosevelt took the initiative to rehabilitate returning veterans. Congress budgeted funds for training them and developing new mobility equipment. The Veterans Administration led the way by removing physical obstacles, like constructing one-story houses and adapting automobiles.[9]

Nevertheless, individuals paralyzed by infantile paralysis contributed significantly to "community formation" themselves, establishing the "first population of Americans with physical impairments to lobby successfully for disability rights."[10] Simply stated, they served as the vanguard during the 1960s and 1970s. The sizeable epidemics of "1946 (25,000 cases), 1952 (58,000 cases), and 1953 (35,000 cases)" resulted in more individuals with disabilities placed in rehabilitation institutions then ever: "The rehab hospitals may unwittingly have provided common social space that would help to develop social networks of people with similar impairments and similar concerns."[11]

The University of California-Berkeley's initial rejection of Edward Roberts's student application represents a case in point. He had been disabled by poliomyelitis. That university eventually allowed him to enroll in 1962. That seemingly simple action "quietly opened a civil rights movement that would remake the world for disabled people," allowing other students with physical disabilities to register for classes. They and Roberts, who became known as the "Rolling Quads," organized and launched a campaign that altered that university's policies and won a commitment from the local community to convert street curbs to ramps, facilitating wheelchair mobility. They also proved instrumental in changing a university regulation that required students with disabilities to live on campus. With the support of the federal Department of Heath, Education, and Welfare, they established the Physically Disabled Students' Program that provided counseling and support. They found accessible off-campus apartments, repaired wheelchairs, and modified cars and vans. The Rolling Quads christened this the "independent living movement." It soon expanded its scope to include all students with disabilities. In May 1972, they expanded operations once again to include non-students, forming the Center for Independent Living (CIL). Run by individuals with disabilities, it dealt with work issues but focused on efforts to facilitate independent living. Governor Jerry Brown appointed Roberts as director of Californian's state Department of Rehabilitation, where he reformed that department's policies, stressing independent living rather than just rehabilitation services.

Meanwhile, across the continent, the New York City board of education refused to hire Judy Heumann, disabled by polio at 18 months of age, for a teaching position in 1970. She sued that school system for discrimination and took her story to the newspapers. She won that suit and, after receiving similar complaints from others, organized the Disabled in Action (DIA). Unlike Roberts's community efforts, the DIA was "explicitly political," staging protests in Washington, DC, in 1972, reminiscent of the League of the Physically Handicapped's tactics 37 years earlier. At Roberts's request, she moved to Berkeley. There she acted as the CIL's deputy director from 1975 to 1985, "blending her East Coast political activism with the Berkeley disability living services. In California, Heumann, along with Roberts, would continue to rewrite the history of the disabled."[12]

Hugh Gregory Gallagher, likewise paralyzed by infantile paralysis, is known as the father of the Architectural Barriers Act of 1968 and the grandfather of the Americans With Disabilities Act. As a Senate staffer during the 1960s, he witnessed the dawning of many equal rights legislative initiatives and worked in particular on disability rights. He "conceived and drafted what became the Federal Architectural Barriers Act of 1968," which, he asserts, became the "first step on the road to the Americans with Disabilities Act of 1990." Working through Senate offices, Gallagher also proved instrumental in the installation of ramps for the Kennedy Center, the Library of Congress, and the National Gallery of Art, the publication of disabled guides for the various national parks, and the display of signs for accessible bathrooms, and he initiated accommodations for all newly constructed hospitals.[13] Indeed, poliomyelitis had dramatically changed the lives of children and profoundly shaped American culture.

NOTES AND SOURCES

INTRODUCTION

1. Guckin in Julie Silver and Daniel Wilson, *Polio Voices: An Oral History from the American Polio Epidemics and Worldwide Eradication Efforts* (Westport, CT: Praeger, 2007): 32–33.
2. Richard L. Bruno, *The Polio Paradox: Understanding and Treating "Post-Polio Syndrome" and Chronic Fatigue* (New York: Warner Books, 2002): 22–23. Also consult pp. 20, 29, and 36. See as well Harold V. Wyatt, "Poliomyelitis," in Kenneth F. Kiple (ed.), *The Cambridge World History of Human Disease* (Cambridge: University of Cambridge Press, 1999): 942–50; and Russell J. Blattner, "Recent Advances in Clinical Aspects of Poliomyelitis," *Journal of the American Medical Association*, 156 (September 4, 1954): 9–12. For the three types of poliovirus, refer to "Informational Digest for Professional Personnel: 39 Questions and Answers on Polio and the Trial Vaccine," Box 7, Salk Polio Vaccine Manufacture & Distribution (Collection # 90/36/7), UPITT. Consult as well Roland H. Berg, *Polio and Its Problems* (Philadelphia: J. B. Lippincott, 1948): 111–12, 113–15, 119; Paul A. Offit, *The Cutter Incident: How America's First Polio Vaccine Led to the Growing Vaccine Crisis* (New Haven: Yale University Press, 2005): 26; John R. Paul, *A History of Poliomyelitis* (New Haven: Yale University Press, 1971): 5, 8–9, 225; Edmund J. Sass, with George Gottfried and Anthony Sorem, *Polio's Legacy: An Oral History* (Lanham, MD: University Press of America, 1996): 1–2; and Marc Shell, *Polio and Its Aftermath: The Paralysis of Culture* (Cambridge: Harvard University Press, 2005): 44. Gareth Williams, in *Paralyzed with Fear: The Story of Polio* (New York: Palgrave Macmillan, 2013), describes the most recent research into this virus in painstaking detail (81–82, 267–70). Parts of these paragraphs draw on ideas explored in Richard J. Altenbaugh, "Polio, Disability, and American Public Schooling: A Historiographical Exploration," *Educational Research and Perspectives* 31 (December 2004): 137–55.
3. Dr. Alice Turek in Janice Flood Nichols, *Twin Voices: A Memoir of Polio, the Forgotten Killer* (Bloomington, IN: iUniverse, Inc., 2007): 40–41. Refer also to Bruno, *Polio Paradox*, 22. Jason Chu Lee, in "Poliomyelitis in the Lone Star State: A Brief Examination in Rural and Urban Communities" (MA thesis: Texas State University-San Marcos, 2005), provides a clear explanation of this virus in Appendix A, "Polio Pathogenesis"; also see Diane Zemke, *Polio: A Special Ride?* (Minnetonka, MN: Diagnostic Center of Learning Patterns, Inc., 1997): 13–18.
4. Anne Finger, *Elegy for A Disease: A Personal and Cultural History of Polio* (New York: St. Martin's Press, 2006): 5; Anon, "Clinical Diagnosis of Poliomyelitis," *Therapeutic Notes* 92 (July–Aug. 1955): 184.
5. Lawrence K. Altman, "WHO Seeks End of Polio by 2005, Tighter Controls," *Pittsburgh Post-Gazette*, July 30, 2003, section A: 4; "WHO Says Polio Virus

Eliminated in Europe," *Pittsburgh Post-Gazette*, June 22, 2002, section A, p. 2; "WHO Statement on the Meeting of the International Health Regulations Emergency Committee Concerning the International Spread of Wild Poliovirus," May 5, 2014, http://www.who.int/mediacentre/news/statements/2014polio (accessed May 6, 2014); Williams, *Paralyzed with Fear*: 27, 138, 264–65, 293–95.

6. Fred Davis, *Passage through Crisis: Polio Victims and their Families* (Indianapolis, IN: Bobbs-Merrill, 1963): 4–5. Davis, a sociologist, provides a solid analysis of 14 largely European American working-class families—based on occupation and years of schooling—who resided in the Baltimore metropolitan area. His sample included eight boys and six girls, aged four through twelve. This pre-Salk (1954–55) longitudinal study relied on in-depth, open-ended interviews of family members, including the children. Davis also points out "in an 'average' pre-1955 year, the incidence rate among children in this age group living in metropolitan areas of the United States was approximately 50 [per 100,000]." The polio infection rate during the "notorious" 1931 New York and 1947 Berlin outbreaks jumped to 226 and 360 per 100,000, respectively. For additional methodological information, see pp. 3, 182, 183, and 188–90. Refer as well to Harold V. Wyatt, "Poliomyelitis," in Kiple, *The Cambridge World History of Human Disease*: 944–45.

7. "Top 10 Terrible Epidemics," *Time*, http://www.time.com/time/specials' packages'article (accessed October 30, 2010).

8. Bruno, *The Polio Paradox*: 55–56; Carl C. Dauer, "The Changing Age Distribution of Paralytic Poliomyelitis," *Annals of the New York Academy of Sciences* 61 (1955): 954–55.

9. Offit, *The Cutter Incident*: 32.

10. Jane S. Smith, *Patenting the Sun: Polio and the Salk Vaccine* (New York: William Morrow and Co., 1990): 25.

11. Semantic differences exist over terminology and introduce complexity into this study. First, some cited authors, especially contemporary ones, still used labels like "handicapped," "crippled," etc., which project obvious negative connotations. Second, some disability literature generally relies on the phrase "disabled people" as a universal descriptive term to avoid those stereotypes. Third, proponents of "people first" nomenclature prefer the noun phrase "people with disabilities" as most appropriate. People-first language replaces the inherent objectification found within the term "the disabled." The emphasis should be on the person, not on an individual's limitations. In every case, I will rely on people-first language, but when citing primary and secondary sources, some of these less sensitive terms will appear. For a thorough discussion of the meanings assigned to such phrases, see Sharon Barnartt and Richard Scotch, *Disability Protests: Contentious Politics, 1970–1999* (Washington, DC: Gallaudet University Press, 2001): xxiii–xxv; Ann Pointon and Chris Davies (eds.), *Framed: Interrogating Disability in the Media* (London: British Film Institute, 1997): 2–3; Rosemary Garland Thomson, *Extraordinary Bodies: Figuring Physical Disability in American Culture and Literature* (New York: Columbia University Press, 1997): 5–18. Analyses of people-first language can be found in Phil Foreman, "Language and Disability," *Journal of Intellectual and Developmental Disability* (March 2005): 57–59; Carol L. Russell, "How Are Your Person First Skills?" *Council for Exceptional Children* 40 (May/June 2008): 40–43; Kathie Snow, "To Ensure Inclusion, Freedom, and Respect for All, It's Time to Embrace People

First Language," http://www.disabilityisneutral.com (accessed November 6, 2010); Tanya Titchkosky, "Disability: A Rose by Any Other Name? 'People-First' Language in Canadian Society," *Canadian Review of Sociology and Anthropology* 38 (May 2001): 125–37. Fourth, in this study, the label "polio" (and the plural, "polios") will appear because polio literature and, more importantly, some "polios" themselves prefer this terminology: it is not a derisive term. See especially a content analysis of the polio nation newsletters by Jacqueline Foertsch, "'Heads, You Win:' Newsletters and Magazine of the Polio Nation," *Disability Studies Quarterly* 27 (Summer 2007): 5 www.dsq-sds.org, (accessed January 5, 2012). Consult as well Tony Gould, *A Summer Plague: Polo and Its Survivors* (New Haven: Yale University Press, 1995): 43; and Nina Gilden Seavey, Jane S. Smith, and Paul Wagner, *A Paralyzing Fear: The Triumph Over Polio in America* (New York: TV Books, 1998): 10.

12. The literature I refer to here includes Philippe Ariés, *Centuries of Childhood: A Social History of Family Life,* trans. Robert Baldick (New York: Vintage Books, 1962); Wini Breines, *Young, White, and Miserable: Growing Up Female in the Fifties* (Boston: Beacon Press, 1992); Joseph M. Hawes, *Children in Urban Society: Juvenile Delinquency in Nineteenth-Century America* (New York: Oxford University Press, 1971); Joseph M. Hawes, *The Children's Rights Movement: A History of Advocacy and Protection* (Boston: Twayne Publishers, 1991); N. Ray Hiner and Joseph M. Hawes (eds.), *Growing Up in America: Children in Historical Perspective* (Urbana: University of Illinois Press, 1985); Wilma King, *Stolen Childhood: Slave Youth in Nineteenth-Century America* (Bloomington: Indiana University Press, 1995); David Nasaw, *Children of the City: At Work and At Play* (New York: Oxford University Press, 1985); Grace Palladino, *Teenagers: An American History* (New York: Basic Books, 1996); Elliott West, *Growing Up with the Country: Childhood on the Far Western Frontier* (Albuquerque: University of New Mexico Press, 1989); Emmy E. Werner, *Pioneer Children on the Journey West* (Boulder, CO: Westview Press, 1995).

13. Russell Viner and Janet Goldman, "Children's Experiences of Illness," in Roger Cooter and John Pickstone (eds.), *Medicine in the Twentieth Century* (Amsterdam, The Netherlands: Harwood Academic Publishers, 2000): 576; Shell, *Polio and Its Aftermath*: 12.

14. Ernest Freeberg, "'More Important Than a Rabble of Common Kings:' Dr. Howe's Education of Laura Bridgeman," *History of Education Quarterly* 34 (Fall 1994): 305–27; James Axtell, *The School Upon a Hill: Education and Society in Colonial New England* (New York: W. W. Norton & Co., 1971): 73–74; Susan E. Lederer, *Subjected to Science: Human Experimentation in America before the Second World War* (Baltimore: Johns Hopkins University Press, 1995).

15. Paul K. Longmore, *Why I Burned My Book and Other Essays on Disability,* edited by Robert Dawidoff (Philadelphia: Temple University Press, 2003): 11.

16. Robert Dawidoff (ed.), Longmore, *Why I Burned My Book*: vii.

17. Richard J. Altenbaugh, *The American People and Their Education: A Social History* (Englewood Cliffs, NJ: Prentice-Hall/Merrill, 2003); Axtell, *The School Upon a Hill,* 73–74; William H. McNeil, *Plagues and Peoples* (Garden City, NY: Anchor Books, 1976): 186; Werner, *Pioneer Children,* 123–27; Nasaw, *Children of the City*; Viviana A. Zelizar, *Pricing the Priceless Child: The Changing Social Value of Children* (New York: Basic Books, 1985).

18. Bernard Bailyn, *Education in the Forming of American Society* (Chapel Hill: University of North Carolina Press, 1960); Lawrence A. Cremin, *The Wonderful*

World of Ellwood Patterson Cubberley: An Essay on the Historiography of American Education (New York: Teachers College Press, 1965); Lawrence A. Cremin, *Traditions of American Education* (New York: Basic Books, 1977).

19. For the standard and most comprehensive history of special education in the United States, see Margaret A. Winzer, *The History of Special Education: From Isolation to Integration* (Washington, DC: Gallaudet University Press, 1993). Winzer's index makes no reference to disease-induced disabilities in general or poliomyelitis in particular. Garland Thomson's *Extraordinary Bodies* is especially helpful in analyzing special education and disability theory (15).

20. As examples, see Peter Cunningham and Philip Gardner, *Becoming Teachers: Texts and Testimonies, 1907–1950* (London: Woburn Press, 2004); Ian Grosvenor, Martin Lawn, and Kate Rousmaniere (eds.), *Silences and Images: The Social History of the Classroom* (New York: Peter Lang, 1999); Stephen Hussey, "The School Air Raid Shelter: Rethinking Wartime Pedagogies," *History of Education Quarterly* 43 (Winter 2003): 517–39.

21. Altenbaugh, "Polio, Disability, and American Public Schooling." See as well Barnartt and Scotch, *Disability Protests*: 34–35.

22. Paul K. Longmore and Lauri Umansky (eds.), *The New Disability History: American Perspectives* (New York: New York University Press, 2001): 7. Also see Paul K. Longmore and David Goldberger, "The League of the Physically Handicapped and the Great Depression: A Case Study in the New Disability History," *Journal of American History* 87 (December 2000): 921.

23. Roger Cooter and John Pickstone (eds.), *Medicine in the Twentieth Century* (Amsterdam, The Netherlands: Harwood Academic Publishers, 2000): xiii.

24. J. N. Hays, *The Burdens of Disease: Epidemics and Human Response in Western History* (New Brunswick: Rutgers University Press, 1998): 1, 2, 3–4.

25. Charles E. Rosenberg and Janet Golden (eds.), *Framing Disease: Studies in Cultural History* (New Brunswick: Rutgers University Press, 1992): xiii, 227. For specific treatments of such "institutional mediators," see Barbara Bates, "*Quid pro Quo* in Chronic Illness: Tuberculosis in Pennsylvania, 1876–1926" and Ellen Dwyer, "Stories of Epilepsy, 1880–1930," in Rosenberg and Golden (eds.), *Framing Disease*. Refer as well to Finger, *Elegy for A Disease*: 6.

26. Anne Hunnsaker Hawkins, *Reconstructing Illness: Studies in Pathography* (West Lafayette, IN: Purdue University Press, 1993), 78, 86, 87, and 79, respectively. Also consult Rita Charon, *Narrative Medicine: Honoring the Stories of Illness* (New York: Oxford University Press, 2006): 65.

27. James B. Gardner and George Rollie Adams (eds.), *Ordinary People and Everyday Life: Perspectives on the New Social History* (Nashville, TN: American Association for State and Local History, 1983). See also Viner and Goldman, "Children's Experiences of Illness": 575.

28. Elizabeth Bredberg, in "Writing Disability History: Problems, Perspectives and Sources," *Disability and Society* 14 (March 1999), calls for the use of "personal narrative and literary expressions" (191, 192, 197, 198). Finger's *Elegy for A Disease* represents a prime example (10). Also consult Rita Charon, *Narrative Medicine: Honoring the Stories of Illness* (New York: Oxford University Press, 2006): 70; Roger Cooter, "'Framing' the End of the Social History of Medicine," in John H. Warner and Frank Huisman (eds.), *Locating Medical History: The Stories and Their Meanings* (Baltimore: Johns Hopkins University Press, 2004): 310, 327.

29. Hawkins, *Reconstructing Illness*, xii, xi, 1, xii, 2, and 13, respectively. Barbara Bates's analysis in *Bargaining for Life: A Social History of Tuberculosis, 1876–1938*

(Philadelphia: University of Pennsylvania Press, 1992) includes a spectrum of patients' complex life experiences, nicely using their voices to reconstruct them—especially see Chapter 4, "Life as a Patient." The literature that recounts the history of polio rarely taps children's recollections. However, Daniel J. Wilson breaks this tradition. In "A Crippling Fear: Experiencing Polio in the Era of FDR," *Bulletin of the History of Medicine* 72 (1998), he refers to them as "illness narratives" (467). Wilson correctly notes this historiographical lacuna, albeit it is more widespread than he acknowledges: "In focusing on the larger developments in the history of poliomyelitis, historians have largely overlooked the daily struggles of those struck down by the virus" (494). Moreover, he and Julie Silver make a significant effort to address this in their compilation of oral histories in *Polio Voices: An Oral History from the American Polio Epidemics and Worldwide Eradication Efforts* (Westport, CT: Praeger, 2007). Pathography in general builds on a long tradition, though one that has not adequately fulfilled its goal and generated fundamental debate. David Armstrong's 1984 article "The Patient's View," *Social Science and Medicine* 18 (1984): 737–44, painstakingly reviews chronological developments in the medical field regarding the evolution of "case-taking" or "case history" to the "clinical gaze" to the "medical gaze" to "patient attitudes." He concludes with the question, "What is the patient's view?" Throughout his discourse, he asks implicit questions, such as, "Is it what is heard by the physician? Or is it what is said by the patient?" But Armstrong misses the point. He relegates his descriptions of the discourse process to clinical environments: the doctor's office or hospital; that is, public settings. However, the patient's view is not restricted to this alone but includes *private* or *personal* recollections and perceptions. Physical pain and social discomfort constitute the sufferer's reality as much as the public conversation. Roy Porter's more significant and pioneering article, "The Patient's View," *Theory and Society* 14 (1985): 175–98, proposes an unorthodox approach to writing the history of medicine. He suggests diaries as one rich vein to mine, and he stresses uncovering human agency. His analysis also transcends the clinical setting, extending to folk medicine and family care. More recently, Flurin Condrau, in "The Patient's View Meets the Clinical Gaze," *Social History of Medicine* 20 (December 2007): 525–40, provides a comprehensive and critical historiographical analysis of Porter's pioneering work. Condrau generally faults Porter, pointing out that agency represents "more than the patient's view." How did they act on it? Nevertheless, while Porter never elucidates specifics, he does broadly outline the need for agency as well as the use of it. Finally, Shell, in *Polio and Its Aftermath,* asserts, "Historians of medicine have rarely made use of literature written in the polio wards" (119). This is so because they "tend to ignore child-authors . . . but also because they are reluctant to read polio memoirs in particular" (119).

30. Viner and Goldman, "Children's Experiences of Illness:" 577–78. Refer as well to Longmore, *Why I Burned My Book*, pp. 3 and 33, when he states, "Although they often found themselves individually or collectively dominated by nondisabled people, they also frequently acted individually or collectively to alter their social fates."
31. Eric J. Cassell, *The Nature of Suffering and the Goals of Medicine* (New York: Oxford University Press, 2004): 35, 37–38.
32. Jacqueline Foertsch, *Bracing Accounts: The Literature and Culture of Polio in Postwar America* (Teaneck, NJ: Farleigh Dickinson University Press, 2008): 14. An example of a polio novel is Elsie Oakes Barber, *The Trembling Years*

(New York: Macmillan Company, 1949). Charon's *Narrative Medicine*, on the other hand, sees much promise in using autobiographies: "Within this reflective space, one beholds and considers the self in a heightened way, revealing fresh knowledge about its coherent existence" (70).
33. Jerrold Hirsch, "History and a Story of Polio: Using and Abusing Oral History Interviews," *Disability Studies Quarterly* 18 (1998): 264–65.
34. Arthur W. Frank, *The Wounded Storyteller: Body, Illness, and Ethics* (Chicago: University of Chicago Press, 1997): 22 and 1, respectively. Frank adds fascinating insight into the concept of memory: "The interruption that illness is, and the further interruptions that it brings, are disruptions of memory. The disruption is not of remembering; peoples' memories of illness are often remarkable in their precision and duration . . . The past is remembered with such arresting lucidity because it is not being experienced as past; the illness of experiences that are being told are unassimilated fragments that refuse to become past, maintaining the present" (59–60).
35. Sass, Gottfried, and Sorem, *Polio's Legacy*: 16. Refer also to pp. 15, 17–19. See Richard Owen's "Introduction" in this volume as well, pp. ix & x.
36. Hawkins, *Reconstructing Illness*: 12–13. She continues, "Pathography . . . returns the voice of the patient to the world of medicine, a world where that voice is too rarely heard, and it does so in such a way as to assert to the phenomenological, the subjective, and the experiential side of illness. What the voice of the patient tells us can be shocking, enlightening, or surprising." Refer as well to Frank, *The Wounded Storyteller*.
37. Charon, *Narrative Medicine*: ix–x, xii, 9, 12–13. Her stated intent is to improve health care by clinicians as the patient becomes a participant in the treatment process (3–4). Nevertheless, narrative medicine fits nicely into a historical treatment of reconstructing illness, as it centers on patients' views.

CHAPTER 1

1. Referring to the series of polio epidemics as "a plague" represented a contemporary view. Dr. Joseph Goldberger, a famous epidemiologist during the early twentieth century, actually used that word when referring to the 1916 New York City outbreak. See pp. 17–18 of the "Minutes of the Conference of Poliomyelitis, 3 August 1916," Simon Flexner Papers, Rockefeller Institute for Medical Research, Poliomyelitis Cases, microfilm roll 91, RAC. See also a historical analysis of his breakthrough in curing pellagra, prevalent in the South, using vitamin B, in Alan M. Kraut, *Goldberger's War: The Life and Work of a Public Health Crusader* (New York: Hill and Wang, 2003). Finally, refer to Marc Shell, *Polio and Its Aftermath: The Paralysis of Culture* (Cambridge: Harvard University Press, 2005): 16–17.
2. Iona Opie and Peter Opie (eds.), *Oxford Dictionary of Nursery Rhymes* (Oxford: Clarendon Press, 1951): 71–72.
3. Roy Porter, *The Greatest Benefit to Mankind: A Medical History of Humanity* (New York: Norton, 1997): 238. Also refer to pp. 125–126, 237.
4. Opie and Opie, *Oxford Dictionary of Nursery Rhymes*: 71–72.
5. Samuel H. Preston and Michael R. Haines, *Fatal Years: Child Mortality in Late Nineteenth-Century America* (Princeton: University of Princeton Press, 1991): 7, 151, and 99, respectively. Refer also to pp. 2, 131–33, and 165. Preston and Haines, through a quantitative analysis of the 1900 census, grapple with the many variables obfuscating a clear sense of infant and child mortality rates. See

also Gretchen A. Condran and Jennifer Murphy, "Defining and Managing Infant Mortality: A Case Study of Philadelphia, 1870–1920," *Social Science History* 32 (Winter 2008): 488; and Anne Finger, *Elegy for A Disease: A Personal and Cultural History of Polio* (New York: St. Martin's Press, 2006): 149.

6. Preston and Haines, *Fatal Years*: 82, 94, 210, respectively. Refer also to pp. 3–6, 84, 95, 141–46, 165, 176, and 208. See also Vanessa Northington Gamble, *Making a Place for Ourselves: The Black Hospital Movement, 1920–1945* (New York: Oxford University Press, 1995): 47.

7. Naomi Rogers, *Dirt and Disease: Polio Before FDR* (New Brunswick, NJ: Rutgers University Press, 1996): 31.

8. Preston and Haines, *Fatal Years*: 7–8, 10–11, and 13, respectively. See also Gareth Williams, *Paralyzed with Fear: The Story of Polio* (New York: Palgrave Macmillan, 2013): 54.

9. U.S. Department of Education, *Digest of Education Statistics: Historical Summary of Public and Elementary and Secondary Statistics*, www.http:/nces.ed.gov/programs/digest/d05/tables/dt05_032.asp (accessed April 23, 2007).

10. Catherine Rollet, "The Fight Against Mortality in the Past: An International Comparison," in Alain Bideau, Bertrand Desjardins, and Héctor Pérez Brignoli (eds.), *Infant and Child Mortality in the Past* (Oxford: Clarendon Press, 1997): 38, 39, 44–45, 49, 42, 50, and 53, respectively. Refer to pp. 43, and 46–48 as well. See also Condran and Murphy, "Defining and Managing Infant Mortality": 473, 475, 495–98, 499–500; Alexandra Minna Stern and Howard Markel (eds.), *Formative Years: Children's Health in the United States, 1880–2000* (Ann Arbor: University of Michigan Press, 2004): 4–6, 8–9; and Molly Ladd-Taylor, *Raising a Baby the Government Way: Mothers' Letters to the Children's Bureau, 1915–1932* (New Brunswick, NJ: Rutgers University Press, 1986): 25–26.

11. George Alter, "Infant and Child Mortality in the United States and Canada," in Bideau, Desjardins, and Brignoli, *Infant and Child Mortality in the Past*: 105. Determining U.S. infant and child mortality rates is problematic, as Alter notes: "Mortality is one of the most poorly documented problems in the historical demography of North America" (91). Preston and Haines, in *Fatal Years*, make a similar assertion: "Little is known about trends, levels and differentials in American mortality in the nineteenth century. It is not altogether clear when or even whether mortality declined in the United States during the period" (49). This problem exists because prior to 1900, "mortality data were limited to selected cities and states and to the imperfect mortality statistics from the decennial federal censuses from 1850 to 1890 that asked questions on household deaths in the preceding year" (50). Nevertheless, Preston and Haines calculate that "child mortality levels were improving for the United States as a whole in the decades before 1900," which is a trend comparable with other Western countries (73–74). Consult also Thomas M. Daniel, *Captain of Death: The Story of Tuberculosis* (Rochester, NY: University of Rochester Press, 1997):134–36.

12. John R. Paul, *A History of Poliomyelitis* (New Haven: Yale University Press, 1971): 10–11.

13. The quote appears in Paul's *History of Poliomyelitis,*: 45. Refer also to pp. 19, 62–63.

14. "For Deformed Children," *New York Times*, December 9, 1887: 8. See a virtually similar account in "The Orthopedic Hospital," *New York Times*, February 9, 1888: 8; see also "Treating the Crippled Poor: Anniversary of the Orthopedic Dispensary and Hospital," *New York Times*, December 9, 1892: 3; "Puzzling

Child Disease," *New York Times*, August 4, 1899: 3; "Studying Child Paralysis," *New York Times*, August 5, 1899: 2; "More Infantile Paralysis," *New York Times*, August 6, 1899: 2; "New Poliomyelitis Cases," *New York Times*, August 7, 1899: 1; "Infantile Paralysis Kills," *New York Times*, August 16, 1899: 2; "Doctor's Views on Fruit," *New York Times*, August 17, 1899: 12; and "Dr. Sheddy Explains: Says Infantile Paralysis May Be Due to Intestinal Poison," *New York Times*, August 18, 1899: 3.

15. "Flee from Town Epidemic," *New York Times*, August 18, 1907: 4, section 1 (Sunday edition); "Town's Two Epidemics," *New York Times*, August 19, 1907: 1; "Ridgway's Epidemics," *New York Times*, August 23, 1907: 1; "Infantile Paralysis Epidemic: Between 300 and 400 Cases Now Under Treatment in City Hospitals," *New York Times*, September 12, 1907: 7; "Infantile Paralysis," *New York Times*, May 8, 1910: Editorial, p. 12; "Infantile Paralysis," *New York Times*, August 7, 1910: Editorial Section, p. 8 (Sunday edition); "Doctors Fail," *New York Times*, August 9, 1910: 16; "Infantile Paralysis Baffles Doctors: Steadily Grows in Central New England, Where There Are Now 250 Cases—100 Deaths," *New York Times*, September 4, 1910: 9, Section I, (Sunday edition); "658 Infant Paralytics: Disease Spreads Over 45 Pennsylvania Counties—79 Cases in Philadelphia," *New York Times*, September 18, 1910: 1, Section I, (Sunday edition); "Infantile Paralysis," *New York Times*, September 22, 1910: 8, Editorial; "Fight Infantile Paralysis: State Health Board Decides to Quarantine the Disease," *New York Times*, September 23, 1910: 8; "Ravages of New Diseases," *New York Times*, September 25, 1910: 4, Section I (Sunday edition); "Put on Contagious List: Washington Thus Classifies Infantile Paralysis—Cases to be Quarantined," *New York Times*, October 9, 1910: 10, Section C (Sunday edition); "Epidemic of Infantile Paralysis," *New York Times*, November 9, 1910: 8; "Child Paralysis Spreads in the City," *New York Times*, February 4, 1911: 7; "To Curb Infantile Paralysis: State Health Commissioner Porter Asked to Make an Investigation," *New York Times*, February 4, 1911: 5; "State Control of Infantile Paralysis," *New York Times*, March 14, 1911: 13; "Less Infantile Paralysis," *New York Times*, April 21, 1912: 6, Cable and Sporting Sections (Sunday edition); "Infantile Paralysis Once More Epidemic," *New York Times*, July 21, 1912: 7, Section I (Sunday edition); "Call to Fight Paralysis," *New York Times*, August 8, 1912: 7; "Federal Aid to Quell Epidemic," *New York Times*, August 13, 1912: 3; "Disease-Smitten Eskimos," *New York Times*, October 24, 1912: 1 (Front Page); Haven Emerson, *The Epidemic of Poliomyelitis (Infantile Paralysis) in New York City in 1916: Based on the Official Reports of the Bureau of the Department of Health* (1917. Reprint, New York: Arno Press, 1977): Appendix, Table I, "Epidemic of Poliomyelitis Prior to 1916."

16. Emerson, *Epidemic of Poliomyelitis*: 95–96, 100; Robert W. Lovett, *Infantile Paralysis in Vermont, 1894–1922: A Memorial to Charles S. Caverly* (Burlington, VT: Vermont State Department of Health, 1924): 15, 18, 21, 23, 33–37. These two reports originally appeared in the *AMA Proceedings* and *Yale Medical Journal*, reprinted in this memorial. Also see Collective Investigation Committee, *Epidemic Poliomyelitis: Report on the New York Epidemic of 1907* (New York: Journal of Nervous and Mental Disease Publishing Co., 1910): 4; Charles G. Heyd, "Tribute to Haven Emerson, M. D.," *Bulletin of the New York Academy of Medicine* 31 (December 1955): 869–71; C. H. Lavinder, Allen W. Freeman, and Wade H. Frost, *Epidemiologic Studies of Poliomyelitis in New York City and the Northeastern United States during the Year 1916*, U. S. Public Health

Bulletin No. 91 (Washington, DC: Government Printing Office, 1918): 80, 97, 109; Paul, *History of Poliomyelitis*: 79, 80, 85–86; Williams, *Paralyzed with Fear*: 16–17.
17. Williams, *Paralyzed with Fear*: 17.
18. Emerson, *Epidemic of Poliomyelitis*: Appendix, Table III, "Poliomyelitis–Cases and Deaths by Date of Report," pp. 361–63, and Table V, "Case Fatality of Poliomyelitis," p. 366. See also "All Unite to Check Infant Paralysis: Facilities Provided for More Complete Isolation and Better Nursing in Crowded Areas," *New York Times*, June 30, 1916: 8.
19. The Internet Movie Database, http://www.imdb.com/title/tt0054354 (accessed August 15, 2010); Aaron E. Klein, *Trial by Fury: The Polio Vaccine Controversy* (New York: Charles Scribner's Sons, 1972); Stephanie True Peters, *Epidemic! The Battle Against Polio* (New York: Marshall Cavendish, 2005); Shell, *Polio and Its Aftermath*: 196–97; *A Paralyzing Fear: The Story of Polio in America* (PBS Video, 1998); *American Experience: The Polio Crusade* (PBS Video, 2009). Personal accounts cover the gamut and are referenced below.
20. Only a few studies deviate from this pattern. Klein (*Trial by Fury*) and Rogers (*Dirt and Disease*) employ a critical approach and delve into an analysis of the social context. For classic discussions of historical agency, see James B. Gardner and George Rollie Adams (eds.), *Ordinary People and Everyday Life: Perspectives on the New Social History* (Nashville, TN: American Association for State and Local History, 1983), as well as David Montgomery, "History as Human Agency," *Monthly Review* 33 (October 1981): 42–48. Daniel J. Wilson, in "A Crippling Fear: Experiencing Polio in the Era of FDR" (*Bulletin of the History of Medicine* 72 [1998]: 465), correctly points out that most studies tend to gloss over the 1930s, focusing almost exclusively on "Roosevelt, Warm Springs, and the March of Dimes."
21. "Biographies of Disease" is the name of a Greenwood Press series, with Julie K. Silver serving as editor. Wilson's book *Polio* has been published as part of this collection. Refer also to Shell (*Polio and Its Aftermath*), who begins his study with a general historiographical discussion of what he terms the "Polio School" (7–8, 10). He cites Roland H. Berg (*Polio and Its Problems* [Philadelphia: J. B. Lippincott, 1948]) and Bentz Plagmann (*My Place to Stand* [New York: Farrar, Straus & Co., 1949]), who focus on this form (3). In the former case, Berg clearly states this in the first sentence of his introduction: "This is the biography of a disease" (ix). Plagmann, meanwhile, tweaks this by referring to "a biography of an illness" (vii).
22. Paul's venerable *History of Poliomyelitis*, Oshinsky's Pulitzer Prize-winning contribution *Polio: An American Story*, Wilson's *Polio*, and Williams's *Paralyzed with Fear* nicely illustrate this interpretative approach. Jason Chu Lee, in "Poliomyelitis in the Lone Star State: A Brief Examination in Rural and Urban Communities" (MA thesis: Texas State University-San Marcos, 2005), notes a threefold historiography: memoirs represent the first, followed by medical texts focusing on treatment as well as historical treatments (13); while Heather Green Wooten, in *The Polio Years in Texas: Battling a Terrifying Unknown* (College Station: Texas A&M University Press, 2009), presents a brief summary of some standard works and then analyzes those that approach this as cultural history (5–6).
23. See, as examples, Jeffrey Kluger, *Splendid Solution: Jonas Salk and the Conquest of Polio* (New York: G. P. Putnum's, 2004) and Jane S. Smith, *Patenting the Sun: Polio and the Salk Vaccine* (New York: William Morrow and Co., 1990). This

is not an uncommon approach, as illustrated by Hal Hellman, *Great Feuds in Medicine: Ten of the Liveliest Disputes Ever* (New York: John Wiley & Sons, 2001) and Sheryl Persson, *Smallpox, Syphilis and Salvation: Medical Breakthroughs that Changed the World* (Wolloesbi, Australia: Exisle Publishing Limited, 2009). Young adult literature especially includes this genre: see, for example, Stephanie Sammartino McPherson, *Jonas Salk: Conquering Polio* (Minneapolis: Lerner Publications, 2002).

24. Turnley Walker, in *Roosevelt and the Warm Springs Story* (New York: A. A. Wyn, Inc., 1953), provides a warm tale of the emotional relationship between FDR and Warm Springs. Stephanie E. Macceca's *Wilma Rudolph: Against All Odds* (Huntington, CA: Teacher Created Materials, 2011) serves as an example of children's nonfiction. This inspirational tone is compactly captured by Wikipedia, the wildly popular online encyclopedia, which lists over one hundred polio survivors—including entrepreneurs, movie stars, musicians, professional athletes, television personalities, and writers—who not only overcame their illness but also achieved notoriety and success in their fields of endeavor (http://en.wikipedia.org/wiki/List_of_poliomyelitis_survivors, accessed November 3, 2010).

25. Examples of this institutional emphasis include a wonderful collection of photographs in Victor Cohn's *Four Billion Dimes* (Minneapolis, MN: Minneapolis Star and Tribune, 1955) and in David W. Rose, *Images of America: March of Dimes* (Charleston, SC: Arcadia Publishing, 2003).

26. Examples of autobiographies include Hugh Gregory Gallagher, *Black Bird Fly Away: Disabled in an Able-Bodied World* (Arlington, VA: Vandamere Press, 1998); Charles L. Mee, *A Nearly Normal Life* (Boston: Little, Brown & Co., 1999); Lorenzo Wilson Milam, *The Cripple Liberation Front Marching Band Blues* (San Diego, CA: Mho & Mho Works, 1987); and Regina Woods, *Tales from Inside the Iron Lung (and How I Got Out of It)*, with a forward by David E. Rogers, M. D. (Philadelphia: University of Pennsylvania Press, 1994). Memoirs include Thomas M. Daniel and Frederick C. Robbins (eds.), *Polio* (Rochester, NY: University of Rochester Press, 1997) and Peg Kehret, *Small Steps: The Year I Got Polio* (Morton Grove, IL: Albert Whitman and Company, 1996). Finally, collections of oral histories can be found in Gould, *A Summer Plague*; Edmund J. Sass, George Gottfried, and Anthony Sorem, *Polio's Legacy: An Oral History* (Lanham, MD: University Press of America, 1996); Nina Gilden Seavey, Jane S. Smith, and Paul Wagner, *A Paralyzing Fear: The Triumph Over Polio in America* (New York: TV Books, 1998); and Julie Silver and Daniel J. Wilson, *Polio Voices: An Oral History from the American Polio Epidemics and Worldwide Eradication Efforts* (Westport, CT: Praeger, 2007). This is by no means an exhaustive list of each category. Oral histories and interviews of individuals paralyzed by polio prove to be invaluable as historic artifacts. However, it appears, from in-depth study, that their autobiographies or memoirs express deeper emotions, revealing the raw inner struggles. Mee's *A Nearly Normal Life* and Milam's *The Cripple Liberation Front Marching Band Blues* serve as powerful examples of the latter case. They seem to be more authentic. Why? Could it be that the interviewer, either through the editing process or by generating a particular response from the narrator—that is, by the mere fact of being present—unwittingly operates as a filter? I thank Philip Gardner for his keen insights into this process.

27. Daniel J. Wilson, *Living with Polio: The Epidemic and Its Survivors* (Chicago: University of Chicago Press, 2005). Counting this book with his work *Polio* and his coedited collection with Silver, *Polio Voices*, Wilson has been highly prolific.

28. Roy Porter, "The Patient's View," *Theory and Society* 14 (1985): 194. A notable example of this genre is Bates, *Bargaining for Life.*
29. Porter, "The Patient's View:" 182, 175, 194, and 192, respectively.
30. "25 More Deaths from Paralysis," *New York Times,* July 5, 1916: 1.
31. Rockefeller Foundation Minutes, July 14, 1916: 4074; September 26, 1916: 4089; October 10, 1916: 4095–4096, folder #275, "Infantile Paralysis, 1916-1918," box 25, series 200, RG 1.1, projects, Rockefeller Foundation Archives, RAC.
32. New York City Department of Health, *Infantile Paralysis (Poliomyelitis): Information for the Public* (New York: Bureau of Preventable Diseases, 1916), NYCMA. See, for example, "Paralysis Experts Named by Emerson," *New York Times,* July 29, 1916: 16.
33. Mitchel and Emerson are quoted in "Paralysis Takes Lives of 32 More," *New York Times,* July 12, 1916: 1. Refer also to "Noted Scientists Organize to Curb Infant Paralysis," *New York Times,* July 13, 1916: 3.
34. *Report of the Department of Health of the City of Chicago for the Years of 1911 to 1918 Inclusive* (CPL): 223, 193, 208, 204–205, and 207, respectively. See also pp. 192–94 and 201.
35. Emerson, *The Epidemic of Poliomyelitis:* 11–12.
36. Thomas M. Rivers, *Reflections on a Life in Medicine and Science: An Oral History Prepared by Saul Benison* (Cambridge: Massachusetts Institute of Technology, 1967): 292–94; Kluger, *Splendid Solution:* 189.
37. Wooten, *The Polio Years in Texas:* 75.
38. *President's Birthday Magazine* 1, #3 (1938): 64 (folder 113, "Medical Interests—Georgia Warm Springs Foundation, 1928-1954, box 14, RG 2, Medical Interests series, Office of the Messrs). (OMR) Rockefeller, Rockefeller Family Archives, RAC.
39. Emerson, *The Epidemic of Poliomyelitis:* 109. He reports these statistics on pp. 102–103, 105–109, and 364.
40. *Report of the Department of Health of the City of Chicago for the Years of 1907, 1908, 1909, 1910* (Chicago: Department of Health, 1911): 166; *Report of the Department of Health of the City of Chicago for the Years of 1911 to 1918 Inclusive* (CPL): 151, 153, 168.
41. Peter Haggett, *The Geographical Structure of Epidemics* (New York: Oxford University Press, 2000): 2; Paul, *A History of Poliomyelitis:* 92; Department of Health of the State of New Jersey, *Fortieth Annual Report: 1916 Report of the Bureau of Vital Statistics* (Trenton, NJ: State Gazette Publishing Co., 1917): 5–6. Also see pp. 4, 51, and 60; Roland H. Berg, *Polio and Its Problems* (Philadelphia: J. B. Lippincott, 1948): 9; Ivan Wickman, *Acute Poliomyelitis* (1913. Reprinted New York: Johnson Reprint Corporation, 1970): 99; Williams, *Paralyzed with Fear:* 13, 15; Board of Health of the State of New Jersey, *Thirty-Sixth Annual Report: 1912 Report of the Bureau of Vital Statistics* (Union Hill, NJ: Dispatch Printing Company, 1913), http://www.gfsmithlib1umdnj.edu/stockton/NJ1916A.pdf (accessed February 13, 2011).
42. *Report of the Department of Health of the City of Chicago for the Years 1926 to 1930 Inclusive* (Chicago: Chicago Printers, Inc., 1931): 126–27. Refer also to *Report of the Department of Health of the City of Chicago for the Years 1919, 1920, and 1921* (Chicago: Kenfeld-Leach Co., 1923): 96. See p. 95 for additional statistics. See also *Report of the Department of Health of the City of Chicago for the Years 1923, 1924, and 1925* (Chicago: James T. Igoe Co., 1926): 138–39; *Annual*

Report of the Board of Health of the City of Chicago for 1933 (Chicago: 1934): 37; *Annual Report of the Board of Health of the City of Chicago for 1939* (Chicago: 1940), CPL: 9, 68. Stephen E. Mawdsley's "Polio and Prejudice: Charles Hudson Bynum and the Racial Politics of the National Foundation for Infantile Paralysis, 1938-1954" (MA thesis, University of Alberta, 2008) capably dispels the myth of African American immunity.

43. Gallagher, *Black Bird Fly Away*: 91. See also "Minutes of the Conference of Poliomyelitis, 3 August 1916," pp. 11–12 (Flexner Papers, RAC); and Ralph K. Ghormley, "History of Treatment of Poliomyelitis," *Journal of the Iowa State Medical Society* 37 (August 1947): 348.
44. Mee, *A Nearly Normal Life*: 5; Oshinsky, *Polio*:161; Seavey, Smith, and Wagner, *A Paralyzing Fear*: 170. Annual statistics proved to be notoriously unreliable because misdiagnoses may have indicated polio when it did not exist, or overlooked it because of flu-like symptoms.
45. Daniel J. Wilson, *Polio* (Santa Barbara, CA: Greenwood Press, 2009): 14. Refer also to Arthur Allen, *Vaccine: The Controversial Story of Medicine's Greatest Lifesaver* (New York: W. W. Norton Company, 2007): 169; and Rogers, *Dirt and Disease,*: 31.
46. *Report of the Department of Health of the City of Chicago for the Years of 1911 to 1918 Inclusive* (CPL): 154, 167; *Poliomyelitis 1955: Annual Statistical Review* (New York: National Foundation for Infantile Paralysis, Inc.), folder 1, National Foundation for Infantile Paralysis, Joseph Stokes, Jr., Papers, APS; Oshinsky, *Polio*: 162; Alice A. Grant, "Medical Social Work in an Epidemic of Poliomyelitis," *Journal of Pediatrics* 24 (June 1944): 692.
47. Klein, *Trial by Fury*: 7. Also consult Iezzoni, *Influenza 1918*: 180–82; and Shell, *Polio and Its Aftermath*: 143.
48. Gould, *A Summer Plague*: 20.
49. Haggett, *Geographical Structure of Epidemics*: 101–02 and 110, respectively. Also see Markel, *Quarantine!*: 2–3.
50. Howard Markel, *Quarantine! East European Jewish Immigrants and the New York City Epidemics of 1892* (Baltimore: Johns Hopkins University Press, 1997): 145. See also pp. 4–5.
51. Condran and Murphy, "Defining and Managing Infant Mortality:" 491–92.
52. New York City Department of Health, *Circular of Information Regarding Procedure in Poliomyelitis: Information for Field Workers* (New York: NYCDH, 1916): 5, 3, 7–8, and 6, respectively (NYCMA). Richard L. Bruno, *The Polio Paradox: Understanding and Treating "Post-Polio Syndrome" and Chronic Fatigue* (New York: Warner Books, 2002): 61. Berg nicely summarizes the 1916 New York City epidemic in Chapter 1 of *Polio and Its Problems*, describing the quarantine and attempts to circumvent it.
53. "Threaten to Wreck Paralysis Hospital," *New York Times*, August 27, 1916: Section 1, p. 12. Refer also to "Row Over Hospital Still On: Armed Guards Watch Crowds About Woodmere Institute," *New York Times*, August 28, 1916: 7; and Kluger, *Splendid Solution*: 21–23. For other such incidences, see "Bar Excursionists' Landing," *New York Times*, July 10, 1916: 19; "Brooklyn Girl Refugee Dies," *New York Times*, July 10, 1916: 18; and "Noted Scientists Organize to Curb Infant Paralysis," *New York Times*, July 13, 1916: 3.
54. Emerson, *The Epidemic of Poliomyelitis*: 11; Klein, *Trial by Fury*: 6; Mee, *A Nearly Normal Life*: 5 and 51–52; Seavey, Smith, and Wagner, *A Paralyzing Fear*: 20–21; "Mayor Mobilizes City's Employees in Paralysis War," *New York Times*, July 10, 1916: 1.

55. The quotes, in order, are from "Paralysis Grows," *New York Times,* August 3, 1916: 7, and "Connecticut's Fear for Children," *New York Times,* August 4, 1916: 8.
56. *Report of the Department of Health of the City of Chicago for the Years of 1911 to 1918 Inclusive* (CPL): 223, 186, 190, 200, and 201 respectively. Refer also to pp. 187, 189, 191, 192, and 222.
57. Dept. of Health of the State of New Jersey, *Fortieth Annual Report*: 4; also see p. 49 (http://www.gfsmithlib1umdnj.edu/stockton/NJ1916A.pdf, accessed February 13, 2011).
58. Faith Baldwin, "Not Everyone Can Dance," *President's Birthday Magazine,* 1, #3 (1938): 15, folder 113, box 14, RG 2, Series: Medical Interests, OMR, Rockefeller Family Archives, RAC. Finger, *Elegy for A Disease*: 154; Mee, *A Nearly Normal Life*: 43.
59. Chaim Potok, *In the Beginning* (Greenwich, CT: Fawcett Publications, Inc., 1975): 36.
60. Baldwin, "Not Everyone Can Dance": 64. The italics appear in the original text.
61. *Flexner Papers,* RAC; Hays, *The Burdens of Disease*: 247, 264, 265.
62. Haggett, *Geographical Structure of Epidemics*: 93–95. Refer in particular to Figure 3.10 on p. 94. See also Shell, *Polio and Its Aftermath*: 212. During the height of New York City's 1916 polio epidemic, the American Automobile Association encouraged car drivers to take tours of the New York countryside as well as visit other states. See "Motoring Feasible Despite Quarantine," *New York Times,* August 23, 1916: 22.
63. Haggett, *Geographical Structure of Epidemics*: 102, 104–05.

CHAPTER 2

1. Hoffman in Edmund J. Sass, with George Gottfried and Anthony Sorem, *Polio's Legacy: An Oral History* (Lanham, MD: University Press of America, 1996): 134. Refer as well to p. 138.
2. Sass, Gottfried, and Sorem, *Polio's Legacy*: 30; George Draper, *Acute Poliomyelitis* (Philadelphia: P. Blakiston's Son & Co., 1927): 62–63.
3. Gurney in Sass, Gottfried, and Sorem, *Polio's Legacy*: 22; Davis's narrative is part of a collection in Thomas M. Daniel and Frederick C. Robbins (eds.), *Polio* (Rochester, NY: University of Rochester Press, 1997): 31. See also Philip Lewin, *Infantile Paralysis: Anterior Poliomyelitis* (Philadelphia: W. B. Saunders Co., 1941): 118; Mia Farrow, *What Falls Away: A Memoir* (New York: Nan A. Talese, 1997): 1; Alice Sink, *The Grit Behind the Miracle: A True Story of the Determination and Hard Work Behind an Emergency Infantile Paralysis Hospital, 1944-1945, Hickory, North Carolina* (Lanham, MD: University Press of America, 1998): 41.
4. Liza Dawson, "The Salk Polio Vaccine Trial of 1954: Risks, Randomization and Public Involvement," *Clinical Trials* 1 (2004): 122–30. The nurse is quoted on p. 123. See also Michael W. R. Davis's recollections in Daniel and Robbins, *Polio*: 30–31; Sink, *The Grit Behind the Miracle*: 41.
5. Eiben in Daniel and Robbins, *Polio*: 97. Also refer to p. 99, as well as to comments by Dr. Martha Lipson Lepow in Daniel and Robbins, *Polio*: 140. See also Helen McNellis and Jerry McNellis, *"Don't Pick Him Up": Our Family's Experience with Polio* (Beaver Falls, PA: BrainTrain Press, 2011): 65.
6. Charles E. Rosenberg, *The Care of Strangers: The Rise of America's Hospital System* (Baltimore: Johns Hopkins University Press, 1987): 292.

7. Farrow, *What Falls Away*: 3–4. Emphasis is in the original text. Richard L. Bruno uses this same quote in *The Polio Paradox: Understanding and Treating "Post-Polio Syndrome" and Chronic Fatigue* (New York: Warner Books, 2002): p. 61.
8. Finger, *Elegy for A Disease*: 55. Some very young children have no memory of being hospitalized. For example, Ron Zemke, who contracted polio at 17 months of age in 1945, has no recollection whatsoever of the three years he spent in acute and convalescent care, because of the physical and emotional trauma. See Diane Zemke, *Polio: A Special Ride?* (Minnetonka, MN: Diagnostic Center of Learning Patterns, Inc., 1997): 8, 10, 18.
9. Bruno, *The Polio Paradox*: 61.
10. Lynne M. Dunphy, "'The Steel Cocoon:' Tales of the Nurses and Patients of the Iron Lung, 1929–5," *Nursing History Review*, 9 (2001): 16. Refer also to William S. Langford, "Physical Illness and Convalescence: Their Meaning to the Child," *Journal of Pediatrics* 33 (1948): 247–48; Marc Shell, *Polio and Its Aftermath: The Paralysis of Culture* (Cambridge: Harvard University Press, 2005): 68–69.
11. Rita Charon, *Narrative Medicine: Honoring the Stories of Illness* (New York: Oxford University Press, 2006): 14 and 21, respectively. Consult p. 17 as well.
12. Dunphy, "The Steel Cocoon'": 14. See also Charles L. Mee, *A Nearly Normal Life* (Boston: Little, Brown & Co., 1999): 26; Finger, *Elegy for a Disease*: 57.
13. Davis in Daniel and Robbins, *Polio*: 32.
14. This boy's quote appears in Fred Davis, *Passage through Crisis: Polio Victims and Their Families* (Indianapolis, IN: Bobbs-Merrill, 1963): 52.
15. Boyer in Nina Gilden Seavey, Jane S. Smith, and Paul Wagner, *A Paralyzing Fear: The Triumph Over Polio in America* (New York: TV Books, 1998): 77–78. Refer also to p., 126. See also Davis, *Passage through Crisis*: 69; and the recollections of Gail Bias in Sass, Gottfried, and Sorem, *Polio's Legacy*: 78.
16. Gareth Williams, *Paralyzed with Fear: The Story of Polio* (New York: Palgrave Macmillan, 2013): 141.
17. Jeffrey Kluger, *Splendid Solution: Jonas Salk and the Conquest of Polio* (New York: G. P. Putnam's, 2004): 155–56.
18. Hoffman in Sass, Gottfried, and Sorem, *Polio's Legacy*: 135–37. See also Henry O. Kendall and Florence P. Kendall, *Care during the Recovery Period in Paralytic Poliomyelitis*, U.S. Public Health Service. Bulletin No. 242 (Washington, DC: Government Printing Office, 1939): 1; Lewin, *Infantile Paralysis*: 118–19; Dr. Alice Turek's narrative in Janice Flood Nichols, *Twin Voices: A Memoir of Polio, the Forgotten Killer* (Bloomington, IN: iUniverse, Inc., 2007): 40.
19. Robert W. Lovett, *The Treatment of Infantile Paralysis* (Philadelphia: P. Blakiston's Son & Co., 1917): 12.
20. Hugh Gregory Gallagher, *Black Bird Fly Away: Disabled in an Able-Bodied World* (Arlington, VA: Vandamere Press, 1998): 22–24.
21. Peg Kehret, *Small Steps: The Year I Got Polio* (Morton Grove, IL: 1996): 18, 20, 22.
22. Mee, *A Nearly Normal Life*: 20. See also pp. 17–18. See also Kehret, *Small Steps*: 34–35; Davis in Daniel and Robbins, *Polio*: 29–30. Finally, refer to Lorenzo Wilson Milam, in chapters 1 and 2 of *The Cripple Liberation Front Marching Band Blues* (San Diego, CA: Mho & Mho Works, 1987), who provides vivid descriptions of the physical impact of a polio infection, as does Gallagher in Seavey, Smith, and Wagner, *A Paralyzing Fear*: 52–53.
23. Gallagher, *Black Bird Fly Away*: 54. See also pp. 46–47.
24. For the nurse's perspective, see Carmelita Calderwood, "Nursing Care in Poliomyelitis: Orthopedic Nursing Care of Patients in the Acute Stage of Poliomyelitis,"

American Journal of Nursing 40 (June 1940): 630. Consult p. 628 for her directions on how to turn a bedridden polio patient.
25. Gallagher, *Black Bird Fly Away*: 29–30.
26. Flexner is quoted in "Infantile Paralysis a Scourge and Puzzle," *New York Times*, July 9, 1916, Magazine Section, p. 14.
27. Leonard Kriegel, *Falling into Life* (San Francisco: North Point Press, 1991): 152. Brenda Serotte, in *The Fortune Teller's Kiss* (Lincoln: University of Nebraska Press, 2006), refers to this experience in similar terms: a "way station between life and death" (83).
28. Tracie C. Harrison and Alexa Stuifbergen, "A Hermeneutic Phenomenological Analysis of Aging with a Childhood Onset Disability," *Health Care for Women International* 26 (September 2005): 736.
29. Farrow, *What Falls Away*: 4–5.
30. Gallagher, *Black Bird Fly Away*: 38. He describes this desperate struggle earlier (p. 33) in existential terms. See as well Leonard Kriegel, *The Long Walk Home: An Adventure in Survival* (New York: Appleton-Century, 1964): 12–13; Mee, *A Nearly Normal Life*: 21; Flood Nichols, *Twin Voices*: 52, 56, 62, and 65; Russell Viner and Janet Goldman, "Children's Experiences of Illness," in Roger Cooter and John Pickstone (eds.), *Medicine in the Twentieth Century* (Australia: Harwood Academic Publishers, 2000): 576.
31. Samuel H. Preston and Michael R. Haines, *Fatal Years: Child Mortality in Late Nineteenth-Century America* (Princeton: University of Princeton Press, 1991): 30.
32. Viviana A. Zelizer, *Pricing the Priceless Child: The Changing Social Value of Children* (New York: Basic Books, 1985): 23. See also Philippe Ariés, *The Hour of Our Death: The Classic History of Western Attitudes Toward Death Over the Last One Thousand Years*, translated by Helen Weaver (New York: Barnes & Noble Books, 1981): 447.
33. Ariés, *Hour of Our Death*: 597. Also, see p. 536. See also Zelizer, *Pricing the Priceless Child*: 25–26.
34. Zelizer, *Pricing the Priceless Child*: 25–26; Ariés, *Hour of Our Death*: 460.
35. Heather Green Wooten, *The Polio Years in Texas: Battling a Terrifying Unknown* (College Station: Texas A&M University Press, 2009): 82–83. Also refer to Rosenberg, *The Care of Strangers*: 40.
36. Edith Powell and John F. Hume, *A Black Oasis: Tuskegee Institute's Fight Against Infantile Paralysis, 1941–1975* (copyright, 2008): 29; Sink, *The Grit Behind the Miracle*: 73–75.
37. Bobby Johnson in Wooten, *The Polio Years in Texas*: 82. Also refer to pp. 27, 39, and 83. See also Powell and Hume, *A Black Oasis*: 35.
38. The information in these paragraphs is from Stephen E. Mawdsley, "Polio and Prejudice: Charles Hudson Bynum and the Racial Politics of the National Foundation for Infantile Paralysis, 1938–1954" (MA thesis, University of Alberta, 2008): 17 and 16, respectively. See as well pp. 13 and 15. Refer also to Vanessa Northington Gamble, *Making a Place for Ourselves: The Black Hospital Movement, 1920–1945* (New York: Oxford University Press, 1995): 44; "Medical News," *Journal of the American Medical Association* 113 (July 1939): 340; McNellis and McNellis, *"Don't Pick Him Up"*: 33–34; Powell and Hume. *A Black Oasis*: 101.
39. Dunphy, "Steel Cocoon'": 6. Consult also Calderwood, "Nursing Care in Poliomyelitis": 624; Kehret, *Small Steps*: 41–43; Jason Chu Lee, "Poliomyelitis in the Lone Star State: A Brief Examination in Rural and Urban Communities" (MA thesis, Texas State University-San Marcos, 2005): 62; Mary Grimley Mason, *Life*

Prints: A Memoir of Healing and Discovery (New York: Feminist Press, 2000): 6; Mee, *A Nearly Normal Life*: 14, 15–16, 24, 28, and 29.
40. John R. Paul uses the term "pest house" in *A History of Poliomyelitis* (New Haven: Yale University Press, 1971): 223. See also pp. 212, 216, 217, 222, and 224.
41. Kehret, *Small Steps*: 33–34. Bruno, *The Polio Paradox*: 66.
42. Tisdale is quoted on p. 6 and the Minnesota physician on p. 21 in Dunphy, "Steel Cocoon." Refer as well to pp. 6, 18, 20, and 22. See also Alice A. Grant, "Medical Social Work in an Epidemic of Poliomyelitis," *Journal of Pediatrics* 24 (June 1944): 696.
43. Lee, "Poliomyelitis in the Lone Star State": 87.
44. Woody Baird, "Tennessee Woman Who Spent Life in Iron Lung Dies at Age 61," *Pittsburgh Post-Gazette*, Section A, May 29, 2008, p. 8.
45. Gallagher, *Black Bird Fly Away*: 30–31. Also consult Shell, *Polio and Its Aftermath*: 173; Lee, "Poliomyelitis in the Lone Star State": 80–81.
46. Earl C. Elkins and K. G. Wakim, "The Present Concept of Treatment of Poliomyelitis," *Journal of the Iowa State Medical Society* 37 (August 1947): 358.
47. Elkins and Wakim, "Present Concept of Treatment of Poliomyelitis": 358; Dunphy, "The Steel Cocoon'": 6.
48. David J. Rothman, "The Iron Lung and Democratic Medicine," in David J. Rothman (ed.), *Beginnings Count: The Technological Imperative in American Health Care* (New York: Oxford University Press, 1997): 45. Consult p. 46 as well. See also Mee, *A Nearly Normal Life*: 75.
49. Dunphy, "The Steel Cocoon'": 6; Eiben in Daniel and Robbins, *Polio*: 106; James H. Maxwell, "The Iron Lung: Halfway Technology or Necessary Step?" *Milbank Quarterly* 64 (1986): 10–11; Paul, *History of Poliomyelitis*: 331; Rothman, "The Iron Lung and Democratic Medicine": 45–46 and 48.
50. Bruno, *The Polio Paradox*: 56.
51. John E. Affeldt, "Recent Advances in the Treatment of Poliomyelitis." *Journal of the American Medical Association* 156 (September 1954): 12; Bruno, *The Polio Paradox*: 63; Eiben in Daniel and Robbins, *Polio*: 106.
52. Regina Woods, *Tales from Inside the Iron Lung (and How I Got Out of It)*, with a forward by David E. Rogers, MD (Philadelphia: University of Pennsylvania Press, 1994): 6. Lynne M. Dunphy also uses this term on p. 13 in "'The Steel Cocoon': Tales of the Nurses and Patients of the Iron Lung, 1929–55" (*Nursing History Review* 9, 2001). See also Lewin, *Infantile Paralysis*: 130 and 134. The foremost guide, in booklet form, that covered every aspect of nursing care for polios was from the National Organization for Public Health Nursing (NOPHN) and the National League of Nursing Education (NLNE), "Nursing for the Poliomyelitis Patient" (New York: NOPHN & NLNE, 1948): 45–47, 49, and 56. See also Anon., "Landmark Perspective: The Iron Lung," *Journal of the American Medical Association* 255 (March 1986): 1177; Maxwell, "The Iron Lung": 7–9; Naomi Rogers, *Dirt and Disease: Polio Before FDR* (New Brunswick, NJ: Rutgers University Press, 1996): 176; Rothman, "The Iron Lung and Democratic Medicine": 43.
53. Dunphy, "The Steel Cocoon": 25; Gustav J. Beck, George C. Graham, and Alvan L. Barach, "Effect of Physical Methods on the Mechanics of Breathing in Poliomyelitis," *Annals of Internal Medicine* 43 (September 1955): 551, 564.
54. Eiben in Daniel and Robbins, *Polio*: 106; Lewin, *Infantile Paralysis*: 130.
55. Daniel in Daniel and Robbins, *Polio*: 90; Lewin, *Infantile Paralysis*: 130; Woods, *Tales from Inside the Iron Lung*: 125.

NOTES AND SOURCES

56. Greenberg in Julie Silver and Daniel Wilson, *Polio Voices: An Oral History from the American Polio Epidemics and Worldwide Eradication Efforts* (Westport, CT: Praeger, 2007): 56; NOPHN & NLNE, "Nursing for the Poliomyelitis Patient," 47–48, 50–53, 55–56, 58; Louis Sternburg and Dorothy Sternburg, *View from the Seesaw* (New York: Dodd, Mead & Company, 1986): 20.
57. Lawrence Alexander, as told to Adam Barnett, *The Iron Cradle: My Fight Against Polio* (New York: Thomas Y. Crowell Co., 1954): 65–66; Lee, "Poliomyelitis in the Lone Star State": 61; Juanita Howell in Seavey, Smith, and Wagner, *A Paralyzing Fear*: 26, 147, and 151; NOPHN & NLNE, "Nursing for the Poliomyelitis Patient:" 49.
58. Gallagher, *Black Bird Fly Away*: 32; Mee, *A Nearly Normal Life*: 73.
59. Williams, *Paralyzed with Fear*: 158.
60. Kehret, *Small Steps*: 30–31.
61. Eiben in Daniel and Robbins, *Polio*: 104.
62. Tafil in Seavey, Smith, and Wagner, *A Paralyzing Fear*: 38. Also see p. 36.
63. Woods, *Tales from Inside the Iron Lung*, pp. 5, 6, and 7; Alexander, *The Iron Cradle*: 33; Dunphy, "Steel Cocoon": 13.
64. Daniel J. Wilson, "Braces, Wheelchairs, and Iron Lungs: The Paralyzed Body and the Machinery of Rehabilitation in the Polio Epidemics," *Journal of Medical Humanities* 26 (Fall 2005): 182.
65. This nurse is quoted on p. 19 of Dunphy, "Steel Cocoon."
66. Woods, *Tales from Inside the Iron Lung*: 6.
67. Woods, *Tales from Inside the Iron Lung*: 6. Rogers's experience is recounted in Seavey, Smith, and Wagner, *A Paralyzing Fear*: 27–28. Sass, Gottfried, and Sorem (*Polio's Legacy*) and Seavey et al. (*A Paralyzing Fear*) cite Rogers's oral history, but they spell her first name differently. The former spells it "Marilynne," while the latter uses "Marilyn." I will use the longer version.
68. Dunphy, "Steel Cocoon": 7.
69. Wooten, *Polio Years in Texas*: 108. Refer as well to pp. 107 and 113. See also Eiben in Daniel, *Polio*: 108–111 and 114.
70. Wooten, *Polio Years in Texas*: 108–09.
71. Sternburg and Sternburg, *View from the Seesaw*: 21. For information about the NFIP's iron lung policies, refer to Paul, *History of Poliomyelitis*, pp. 331–32 and 334; and Mee, *A Nearly Normal Life*, p. 2.
72. Wooten, *Polio Years in Texas*: 110.
73. Woods, *Tales from Inside the Iron Lung*: 125; Robert Baker, *Before Bioethics: A History of American Medical Ethics from the Colonial Period to the Bioethics Revolution* (New York: Oxford University Press, 2013): 59.
74. Alexander, *The Iron Cradle*: 62 and 119–20; Barker in Silver and Wilson, *Polio Voices*: 29; Seavey, Smith, and Wagner, *A Paralyzing Fear*: 140–41; Sternburg and Sternburg, *View from the Seesaw*: 39 and 46; John Troan, *Passport to Adventure: Or, How a Typewriter from Santa Led to an Exciting Lifetime Journey* (Pittsburgh, PA: Geyer Printing, 2000): 191–92; Woods, *Tales from Inside the Iron Lung*: 60; Jessie Wright Papers, 1925–1970, Record Group 7/1, box No. 2, folder No. 1–Medical Staff-newspaper clippings, 1946 and 1949, WIA.
75. Boyer in Seavey, Smith, and Wagner, *A Paralyzing Fear*: 78.
76. Davis in Daniel and Robbins, *Polio*: 32–33. Shell, *Polio and Its Aftermath*: 125.
77. Eiben in Daniel and Robbins, *Polio*: 106.
78. Greenberg in Silver and Wilson, *Polio Voices*: 56. Milam describes the tracheotomy procedure in *Cripple Liberation Front Marching Band Blues*, pp. 5–6;

see chapters 1 and 2 in general. Also see Sass, Gottfried, and Sorem, *Polio's Legacy*: 145.
79. Daniel in Daniel and Robbins, *Polio*: 84–85. See also p. 79.
80. J. N. Hays, *The Burdens of Disease: Epidemics and Human Response in Western History* (New Brunswick: Rutgers University Press, 1998): 265; Lewin, *Infantile Paralysis*: 327–28; Francis W. Peabody, George Draper, and A. A. Duchey, "A Clinical Study of Acute Poliomyelitis," monograph of the Rockefeller Institute for Medical Research, No. 4, 1912, reprint of Vol. 61 (New York: RIMR, 1913): 54, 57–58, 69; RAC *Report of the Department of Health of the City of Chicago for the Years of 1911 to 1918 Inclusive* (Chicago: Department of Health, 1919): 174 (CPL); *Annual Report of the Board of Health of the City of Chicago for 1933* (Chicago: 1934): 38 (CPL).
81. The quote appears on p. 64 in Paul, *History of Poliomyelitis*. Refer as well to pp. 62, 65, and 67.
82. Lewin, *Infantile Paralysis*: 165; Kendall and Kendall, *Care during the Recovery Period in Paralytic Poliomyelitis*: 8 and 10; John F. Landon and Lawrence W. Smith, *Poliomyelitis: A Handbook for Physicians and Medical Students* (New York: Macmillan Company, 1934): 218–220.
83. NOPHN and NLNE, "Nursing for the Poliomyelitis Patient": 69–70; Gould, *A Summer Plague*: 93, 94–95, and 99; Lewin, *Infantile Paralysis*: 138, 157, and 191; Paul, *History of Poliomyelitis*: 338–40; Seavey, Smith, and Wagner, *A Paralyzing Fear*: 102–03; Sass, Gottfried, and Sorem, *Polio's Legacy*: 21; Daniel J. Wilson, *Living with Polio: The Epidemic and Its Survivors* (Chicago: University of Chicago Press, 2005): 52.
84. Paul, *History of Poliomyelitis*: 339–40; Turnley Walker, *Roosevelt and the Warm Springs Story* (New York: A. A. Wyn, Inc., 1953): 242, 244.
85. Lovett, *The Treatment of Infantile Paralysis*: 50, 53–54, and 59; Lewin, *Infantile Paralysis*: 138.
86. Lewin, *Infantile Paralysis*: 143; consult pp. 138–39 and 131–42 as well. See also Kendall and Kendall, *Care during the Recovery Period in Paralytic Poliomyelitis*: 1–2 and 5–8.
87. The first two quotes are from Lewin, *Infantile Paralysis* (p. 145), while the third is from Lovett, *The Treatment of Infantile Paralysis* (pp. 100–101). See also pp. 50, 54, 59, and 87–88 in Lovett.
88. H. W. Frauenthal, "The Treatment of Infantile Paralysis Based on the Present Epidemic," *Journal of Electrotherapeutics and Radiology* 34 (October 1916): 507. He vehemently opposed plaster casting based on his experiences treating patients during the 1916 epidemic, arguing that atrophy and poor casting, which appeared common, hindered paralysis recovery.
89. Susan Richards Shreve, *Warm Springs: Traces of a Childhood at FDR's Polio Haven* (Boston: Houghton Mifflin Company, 2007): 62–63.
90. Paul, *History of Poliomyelitis*: 340.
91. Janet Golden and Naomi Rogers, "Nurse Irene Shea Studies the 'Kenny Method' of Treatment of Infantile Paralysis, 1942–1943," *Nursing History Review* 18 (2010): 191. See also "Kenny Paralysis Treatment Approved by U.S. Medicine," *New York Times*, December 5, 1941, 1 and 26; Victor Cohn, *Sister Kenny: The Woman Who Challenged the Doctors* (Minneapolis: University of Minnesota Press, 1976): 69–70; Naomi Rogers, *Polio Wars: Sister Kenny and the Golden Age of American Medicine* (New York: Oxford University Press, 2014): x, 3.

92. Cohn, *Sister Kenny*: 97; see also pp. 4, 87–94, 99–100, 107, and 119–20. See also Elizabeth Kenny Papers, MHS; Elizabeth Kenny, *The Treatment of Infantile Paralysis in the Acute Stage* (Minneapolis: Bruce Publishing Co., 1941): xiv; Elizabeth Kenny, *My Battle and Victory* (London: Robert Hale, Ltd., 1955): 15–16; Finger, *Elegy for A Disease:* 93–96; Gould, *A Summer Plague*, 86–89; Paul, *History of Poliomyelitis:* 339–41; Rogers, *Polio Wars:* 5–6 and 9–11; Sass, Gottfried, and Sorem, *Polio's Legacy:* 9.
93. Kenny, *My Battle and Victory:* 18–19; see p. 16 as well. See also Cohn, *Sister Kenny:* 126–28 and 161; Victor Cohn, *Four Billion Dimes* (Minneapolis, MN: Minneapolis Star and Tribune, 1955): 61, 65; Gould, *A Summer Plague:* 95–96; Steven E. Koop, *We Hold this Treasure: The Story of Gillette Children's Hospital* (Afton, MN: Afton Historical Society Press, 1998): 93; Rogers, *Polio Wars:* 16–17; Sass, Gottfried, and Sorem, *Polio's Legacy:* 9–10.
94. Koop, *We Hold this Treasure:* 80. Refer as well to pp. 78–79, 81, and 93–94.
95. Rogers, *Polio Wars:* 18.
96. Rogers, *Polio Wars:* 20.
97. Rogers, *Polio Wars:* 22–23 and 90, respectively; see also pp. 92 and 153. See also Wallace H. Cole, John F. Pohl, and Miland E. Knapp, *The Kenny Method of Treatment for Infantile Paralysis* (New York: NFIP, 1942).
98. Gurney in Sass, Gottfried, and Sorem, *Polio's Legacy:* 21, 24–26, and 27; also consult p. 10. See also Lewin, *Infantile Paralysis:* 132 and 137; Porter, *Greatest Benefit to Mankind:* 695; Rogers, *Polio Wars:* 21; Wilson, *Living with Polio:* 76.
99. Kenny, *My Battle and Victory:* 36; also refer to pp. 116–17. See also Bruno, *Polio's Paradox:* 72; Cohn, *Sister Kenny:* 129–33, 144–45, and 150; Gould, *A Summer Plague:* 96–98; Koop, *We Hold This Treasure:* 94–96; Rogers, *Polio Wars:* 20–21; Sass, Gottfried, and Sorem, *Polio's Legacy:* 10; "Kenny Paralysis Treatment Approved by U.S. Medicine," *New York Times*, December 5, 1941: 1 and 26; Kenny to Gudakunst, December 14, 1941 (MHS); MOD, Kenny to Gudakunst, December 24, 1942 (MHS); Medical Records Programs; Series 8: Grants and Appropriations; Approved Grants, 1941–1942.
100. Gullickson in Sass, Gottfried, and Sorem, *Polio's Legacy:* 40 and 42–45. Emphasis is in the original. For a similar experience, see Finger, *Elegy for a Disease*, 92.
101. Peg Kehret, *Small Steps: The Year I Got Polio* (Morton Grove, IL: 1996): 52–53.
102. Naomi Rogers, "American Medicine and the Politics of Filmmaking: *Sister Kenny*," in Leslie J. Reagan, Nancy Tomes, and Paula A. Treichler (eds.), *Medicine's Moving Pictures: Medicine, Health, and Bodies in American Film and Television* (Rochester, NY: University of Rochester Press, 2007): 202, 214, and 218, respectively; also consult p. 206. See also MOD, Approved Grants, 1943, series 8: Grants and Appropriations, Medical Records Programs. Bruno, in *Polio Paradox*, uses the term "Kenny Technicians" on p. 72. See also Cohn, *Sister Kenny:* 157 and 170; Golden and Rogers, "Nurse Irene Shea:" 190 and 192; Gould, *A Summer Plague:* 110; Kenny, *My Battle and Victory:* 26, 27–28, and 30; Koop, *We Hold This Treasure:* 95; Rogers, *Polio Wars:* xv and 99; Heather Green Wooten, *The Polio Years in Texas: Battling a Terrifying Unknown* (College Station: Texas A&M University Press, 2009): 60–61; "Kenny Paralysis Treatment Approved by U.S. Medicine," *New York Times*, December 5, 1941, 1 and 26; George Draper, "No Specific Cure," *New York Times*, April 12, 1942, Section E: 9; "Miss Kenny's Paralysis Theory Verified by Tests, Doctors Say," *New York Times*, July 17 1942: 17.

103. Cohn, *Sister Kenny*: 151; "Kenny Technician Training Course for Registered Nurses," Box 4, Administrative, 1920–1960, Folder 34, Kenny Institute and Foundation, 1944–1952, Sheltering Arms Records, 1882–1983 (SWHA); Gudakunst to Kenny, January 12, 1943 (MHS); MOD, Medical Programs Records, Series 8: Grants and Appropriations, Approved Grants, 1943; "To Teach Kenny Method," *New York Times*, January 20, 1943: p. 19; "Sister Kenny Visits Jersey City," *New York Times*, January 27, 1943: p. 10; "Sister Kenny to Speak," *New York Times*, February 4, 1943: 25; "Sister Kenny Lectures," *New York Times*, February 5, 1943: 13; "Teaching Kenny Method," *New York Times*, June 21, 1943: 13; Rogers, *Polio Wars*: 91.
104. "Crosby Names Chairman for Paralysis Fund," *New York Herald Tribune*, Oct. 14, 1945, folder 118, "Medical Interests—Sister Kenny Foundation, 1944–60," box 15, RG 2, Medical Interests series, Office of the Messrs. Rockefeller (OMR), Rockefeller Family Archives, RAC. See also Cohn, *Sister Kenny*: 146, 169–70, and 201–04; Golden and Rogers, "Nurse Irene Shea": 192, 204, 208, 216, and 224; Paul, *History of Poliomyelitis*: 340; John F. Pohl, in collaboration with Sister Elizabeth Kenny, *The Kenny Concept of Infantile Paralysis and Its Treatment* (Minneapolis: Bruce Publishing Co., 1943). For a contemporary review of this book, refer to M. F. Ashley Montagu's article in the Book Review section of *The New York Times,* July 18, 1943. Consult also "RKO Acquires Right to Make Life of Sister Elizabeth Kenny, Australian Nurse," *New York Times*, September 5, 1942, p. 9; "Rochester Degree for Sister Kenny," *New York Times* (Amusements section), May 3, 1943: 12; "N.Y.U. Class of 3,607 Is to Be Graduated," *New York Times*, June 9, 1943: 10; Rogers, *Polio Wars*: 106 and 375.
105. Rogers, *Polio Wars*: 209 and 360–61.
106. Davis in Daniel and Robbins, *Polio*: 34. For the Shannon Hospital experience, consult Lee, "Poliomyelitis in the Lone Star State": 59.
107. Owen in Sass, Gottfried, and Sorem, *Polio's Legacy*: 30; also see p. 34; See also Susan Richard Shreve, *Warm Springs: Traces of a Childhood at FDR's Polio Haven* (Boston: Houghton Mifflin Company, 2007): 39–43; "Girl Walks Again in Kenny Cure Test," *New York Times*, October 27, 1942: 30; "Paralysis Victim Cured," *New York Times*, November 24, 1942: 21.
108. McCarroll is quoted in Maurice L. Laurence, "Hits Kenny Method in Poliomyelitis" (*New York Times*, October 31, 1942: 9.
109. Finger, *Elegy for a Disease*: 97–98.
110. Marilyn Moffat, "The History of Physical Therapy Practice in the United States," *Journal of Physical Therapy Education* 17 (Winter 2003): 17. See also Golden and Rogers, "Nurse Irene Shea": 202; Gould, *A Summer Plague*: 103.
111. Bruno, *Polio Paradox*: 72–73; Kenny to Gudakunst (February 15, 1943), Gudakunst to Ober (February 16, 1943), Gudakunst to Kenny (May 10, 1943), Kenny to Gudakunst (May 11, 1943), Elizabeth Kenny Papers, box 2, Correspondence, Gudakunst, Dr. Don W., 1941–1944 (MHS); Kenny to O'Connor (February 19, 1942), Elizabeth Kenny Papers, box 2, Correspondence, O'Connor, Basil, 1940–1941 (MHS); Kenny to O'Connor (June 28, 1943), box 2, Correspondence, O'Connor, Basil, 1943–1947 (MHS); "The Story of the Kenny Method," Sheltering Arms Records, 1882–1983, Box 4, Administrative, 1920–1960, Folder 34, Kenny Institute and Foundation, 1944–1952 (SWHA). Likewise, refer to Cohn, *Sister Kenny*: 158 and 173; Rogers, *Polio Wars*: 109–110; and Seavey, Smith, and Wagner, *A Paralyzing Fear*: 103.

Notes and Sources 213

112. Rogers in Sass, Gottfried, and Sorem, *Polio's Legacy*, pp. 56–57. See also Cohn, *Sister Kenny*: 161–62 and 175; Golden and Rogers, "Nurse Irene Shea": 202; Rogers, *Dirt and Disease*: 176; Rogers, *Polio Wars*: 87.
113. Rogers, *Polio Wars*: 204 and 206, respectively. Also refer to pp. 202–3, 205, and 270.
114. Rogers, *Polio Wars*: 217. Consult also pp. 213, 217, 218, 220, and 221–22.
115. Cohn, *Sister Kenny*: 207; Rogers, *Polio Wars*: 202 and 224; Letter from Dr. Don W. Gudakunst (Medical Director, NFIP) to Marvin L. Kline (President, Elizabeth Kenny Institute, Inc.), July 27, 1944, Elizabeth Kenny Papers, box 1, Formal Correspondence, 1942–52 (MHS); Cusack to Kline, March 16, 1945, box 1, Formal Correspondence, 1942–52 (MHS); "And They Shall Walk," Sister Kenny Foundation Pamphlet, folder 118, "Medical Interests—Sister Kenny Foundation, 1944–60," box 15, Medical Interests series, RG 2, OMR, Rockefeller Family Archives (RAC); "Kenny Campaign Fund," Sheltering Arms Records, 1882–1983, box 4, Administrative, 1920–1960, folder 34, Kenny Institute and Foundation, 1944–1952 (SWHA); Rogers, *Dirt and Disease*: 176; Paul, *History of Poliomyelitis*: 344; "Heads Drive on Paralysis," *New York Times*, December 10, 1946: 41; "Sister Kenny Clinic Planned for City," *New York Times*, February 19, 1947: 7; "Sister Kenny Takes Stand in Court Here," February 6, 1948: 27; "Paralysis Clinic for East," *New York Times*, February 27, 1948: 23; "Sister Kenny Gives Counsel on Polio," *New York Times*, December 17, 1948: 34; "Post Office Promises to Unsnarl Tangle Caused by 2 Rival Drives for Polio Funds," *New York Time*, September 16, 1949: 25; "Polio Seminar Planned," *New York Times*, October 2, 1949: 65; "Jersey Kenny Clinic May Have to Close," *New York Times*, October 6, 1949: 33; "Sister Kenny Data Will Go to World," *New York Times*, February 11, 1950: 19; "Will Begin Polio Drive," *New York Times*, August 20, 1950: 65.
116. Cohn, *Sister Kenny*: 171. Also refer to pp. 172–73, 189, and 226.
117. Cohn, *Sister Kenny:* 208; also consult pp. 206 and 234. See also Cohn, *Four Billion Dimes*: 95–97; Aaron E. Klein, *Trial by Fury: The Polio Vaccine Controversy* (New York: Charles Scribner's Sons, 1972): 69; News Release from the Second International Poliomyelitis Conference of the International Poliomyelitis Congress, 8/28/51, and News Release from the Second International Poliomyelitis Conference of the International Poliomyelitis Congress, 9/5/51 (Copenhagen), box 7, file folder, International Poliomyelitis Congress (Collection # 90/36/7), Jonas Salk Papers (UPITT); "Kenny Fund Tells of Growth Needs," *New York Times*, September 15, 1949: 30; "Sister Kenny Here," *New York Times*, August 23, 1951: 1; "Sister Kenny Arrives Here," *New York Times*, September 11, 1951: 19.
118. Cohn, *Sister Kenny*: 224, 233, 236–38, 251, and 256–57; Rogers, *Polio Wars*: 372–73 and 381; Sass, Gottfried, and Sorem, *Polio's Legacy*: 10; "Sister Kenny in Australia," *New York Times*, February 21, 1951: 8; "Sister Kenny Dies In Her Sleep at 66," *New York Times*, November 30, 1952: 1, 85; "Sister Kenny," *New York Times*, December 1, 1952: 22; "Typsin, Like That Flown to Australia for Sister Kenny, Dissolves Some Blood Clots," *New York Times*, December 7, 1952: E9.
119. Lewin, *Infantile Paralysis*: 162–63. Refer also to pp. 136, 158–59, and 177–78.
120. Lewin, *Infantile Paralysis*: 165 and 187, respectively.
121. L. McCarty Fairchild, "Some Psychological Factors Observed in Poliomyelitis Patients," *American Journal of Physical Medicine* 31 (1952): 277, 278, and 279, respectively.
122. Rogers in Sass, Gottfried, and Sorem, *Polio's Legacy*: 58.

Chapter 3

1. "Arrest in Hundreds to Check Infant Paralysis," *New York Times*, July 11, 1916: 1, 4; George Draper, "No Specific Cure," *New York Times*, April 12, 1942 (Section E): 9.
2. Amy L. Fairchild, Ronald Bayer, and James Colgrove, *Searching Eyes: Privacy, the State, and Disease Surveillance in America* (Berkeley: University of California Press, 2007): 144–45. Consult pp. 51–53 and 54 as well.
3. "Defense League of 21,000 Citizens Fights Paralysis," *New York Times*, July 9, 1916: 14; "Arrest in Hundreds to Check Infant Paralysis," *New York Times*, July 11, 1916: 1, 4. For Ager, see "Dr. Ager's Appeal Met," *New York Times*, August 9, 1916: 10.
4. "Paralysis Cripples a Problem for City," *New York Times*, July 31, 1916: 18.
5. The first quote is from "Paralysis Cripples a Problem for City," *New York Times*, July 31, 1916: 18; the second is from "Paralysis Forecast Cut by 1,000 Cases," *New York Times*, September 4, 1916: 14; the third is from "Paralysis Cripples Flock to Hospitals," *New York Times*, September 24, 1916, Section 1, p. 16.
6. "55 Die of Paralysis in This City in a Day," *New York Times*, August 2, 1916: 4; "To Sustain the Brace Fund," *New York Times*, August 10, 1916: 8; "Contributors Send Gifts of $246 through New York Times," *New York Times*, August 15, 1916: 18.
7. "Asks $100,000 Fund For Cripples' Care," *New York Times*, September 3, 1916 (Section 1): 16; "Defense League of 21,000 Citizens Fights Paralysis, *New York Times,* July 9, 1916: 14; "Brace Fund Nears $40,000," *New York Times*, September 21, 1916: 24.
8. These four quotes can be found, in order, in the following sources: "New York Schools May Open Sept. 25," *New York Times*, August 17, 1916: 6; "To Sustain the Brace Fund," *New York Times*, August 10, 1916: 8; "Emerson Defends Opening of School," *New York Times*, October 1, 1916 (Section 1): 19; "Paralysis Figures Rise in Manhattan," *New York Times*, July 26, 1916: 5. Consult also "Day Shows Drop in Infantile Paralysis," *New York Times*, July 21, 1916: 18; "See Paralysis Curb in Cooler Weather," *New York Times*, August 12, 1916: 16; Cynthia A. Connolly, *Saving Sickly Children: The Tuberculosis Preventorium in American Life, 1909–1970* (New Brunswick, NJ: Rutgers University Press, 2008): 31–33.
9. Rockefeller Foundation Minutes, "After Care of Infantile Paralysis Cases, New York Committee on After Care of Infantile Paralysis Cases," October 10, 1916, p. 4096; Foundation Minutes, "State Charities Aid Association," October 30, 1916, p. 4106; Foundation Minutes, March 6, 1917, p. 5034; Foundation Minutes, April 3, 1917, p. 5040; Foundation Minutes, November 16, 1916, p. 4109 (folder 275: "Infantile Paralysis, 1916–1918," box 25, series 200, Record Group 1.1, Projects, Rockefeller Foundation Archives). Refer especially to "Proposed Method of Organizing Orthopedic Treatment of Infantile Paralysis Cases in New York City," p. 4, folder 277, "Infantile Paralysis—New York Committee on After-Care, July 1916," Rockefeller Foundation Archives (RAC). See also "Ask Rockefellers for Paralysis Aid," *New York Times*, August 6, 1916 (Section 1): 15; Haven Emerson, *The Epidemic of Poliomyelitis (Infantile Paralysis) in New York City in 1916: Based on the Official Reports of the Bureau of the Department of Health* (1917; reprint, New York: Arno Press, 1977): 36–37; Gareth Williams, *Paralyzed with Fear: The Story of Polio* (New York: Palgrave Macmillan, 2013): 276.

10. "Want Blood of 1,000 in Paralysis Fight," *New York Times*, August 25, 1916: 18. See also "To Aid Paralysis's Cripples," *New York Times*, July 13, 1916: 3; "Paralysis Gains Only in Manhattan," *New York Times*, July 20, 1916: 11; "Fears Paralysis Will Flare Again," *New York Times*, August 20, 1916: 12; "Brace Fund Total $18,925," *New York Times*, August 29, 1916: 20; "Asks $100,000 Fund for Cripples' Care," *New York Times*, September 3, 1916 (Section 1): 16; "Paralysis Up Again," *New York Times*, September 8, 1916: 18; "Cripples' Fund Now $36,924," *New York Times*, September 14, 1916: 10; "Brace Fund Nears $40,000," *New York Times*, September 21, 1916: 24.

11. Greene to Wald, August 13, 1916; Greene to Wald, November 20, 1916; "Suggested Order of Procedure for Conference of Orthopedic Surgeons, August 5, 1916"; "List of Physicians, Public Officials and Others Attending the Conference on Infantile Paralysis"; John D. Rockefeller Jr. (JDR Jr.) to Greene, August 21, 1916 (box 25, series 200, RG 1.1, Projects, Rockefeller Foundation Archives, RAC). See also Doris Fleischer and Frieda Zames, *The Disability Rights Movement: From Charity to Confrontation* (Philadelphia: Temple University Press, 2001): 10.

12. Rockefeller Foundation Minutes, May 22, 1918, pp. 6075–6076; Riley to Embree, February 13, 1919 (folder 282, "Infantile Paralysis—New York Committee on After Care, 1919–21"); Greene to Wald, August 13, 1916; Greene to Wald, November 20, 1916; "Suggested Order of Procedure for Conference of Orthopedic Surgeons, August 5, 1916"; "List of Physicians, Public Officials and Others Attending the Conference on Infantile Paralysis"; JDR Jr. to Greene, August 21, 1916; Rockefeller Foundation Minutes, October 10, 1916, p. 4094; January 16, 1919, pp. 19003–19004 (folder 277, "Infantile Paralysis–New York Committee on After-Care, July 1916"); Riley to Embree, December 18, 1918 (folder 281, "Infantile Paralysis–NY Committee on After Care, 1918," box 25, series 200, RG 1.1, Projects, Rockefeller Foundation Archives, RAC).

13. Connolly, *Saving Sickly Children*: 34–37.

14. A large volume of the minutes for the 1916 meetings of the Rockefeller Foundation indicates a three-pronged response to New York City's epidemic (box 25, series 200, RG 1.1, Projects, Rockefeller Foundation Archives, RAC). See also Rockefeller Foundation Minutes, July 14 1916 and January 23, 1918 (folder 275, "Infantile Paralysis, 1916–1918").

15. Barbara Bates, *Bargaining for Life: A Social History of Tuberculosis, 1876–1938* (Philadelphia: University of Pennsylvania Press, 1992): 252 and 255, respectively; see also pp. 22 and 254. Also see Connolly, *Saving Sickly Children*: 2 and 79–80; Aaron E. Klein, *Trial by Fury: The Polio Vaccine Controversy* (New York: Charles Scribner's Sons, 1972): 13.

16. Nancy Tomes, *The Gospel of Germs: Men, Women, and the Microbe in American Life* (Cambridge: Harvard University Press, 1998): 114 and 118, respectively; see also pp. 115–17, 119, 121–27, 132, and 134. Refer also to Thomas M. Daniel, *Captain of Death: The Story of Tuberculosis* (Rochester, NY: University of Rochester Press, 1997): 44–45. His informative timeline is on pp. 239–42. See also Bates, *Bargaining for Life*: 128.

17. Daniel, *Captain of Death*, 45. Additional information can be found on p. 47.

18. Paul A. Offit, *The Cutter Incident: How America's First Polio Vaccine Led to the Growing Vaccine Crisis* (New Haven: Yale University Press, 2005): 58.

19. James Colgrove, *State of Immunity: The Politics of Vaccination in Twentieth-Century America* (Berkeley, CA: University of California Press, 2006): 81–82, 89;

Evelynn Maxine Hammonds, *Childhood's Deadly Scourge: The Campaign to Control Diphtheria in New York City, 1880–1930* (Baltimore: Johns Hopkins University Press, 1999): 90–92; Samuel H. Preston and Michael R. Haines, *Fatal Years: Child Mortality in Late Nineteenth-Century America* (Princeton: University of Princeton Press, 1991): 18–19.

20. Hammonds, *Childhood's Deadly Scourge*: 216; refer also to pp. 212–13. See also Colgrove, *State of Immunity*: 89.
21. Janet Mace Valenza, *Taking the Waters in Texas: Springs, Spas, and Fountains of Youth* (Austin: University of Texas Press, 2000): 204 and 20, respectively; also consult pp. 3, 5, 8–9, 13, and 25. See also Bates, *Bargaining for Life*: 30; Dr. Paul Haertl, "Notes from Europe," *Polio Chronicle* November 1932 (Vol. 2, no. 4): 1 (RWSIR); Marc Shell, *Polio and Its Aftermath: The Paralysis of Culture* (Cambridge: Harvard University Press, 2005): 99–100. See Chapter 6 in Williams, *Paralyzed with Fear*, for a succinct description of the organizational histories of Georgia Warm Springs, the President's Ball, and the NFIP, as well as the roles of Roosevelt and O'Connor.
22. Bates, *Bargaining for Life*: 39 and 75–77. For clarification, sanitariums served as places for convalescence, not for special treatments, while sanatoriums offered recovery therapies for tuberculosis patients (185). Bates thoroughly describes the early development of philanthropic public and private tuberculosis institutions in Pennsylvania in Chapter 9, "Economy, Charity, and the State," and Chapter 10, "The Private Sanatoriums." Also consult Richard Carter, *The Gentle Legions: National Voluntary Health Organizations in America* (New Brunswick, NJ: Transaction Publishers, 1992): 5, 63–64, 68, 71; Connolly, *Saving Sickly Children*: 41.
23. Turnley Walker, *Roosevelt and the Warm Springs Story* (New York: A. A. Wyn, Inc., 1953): 156, 201; see also pp. 118–19 and 142. Also see Clebourn Gregory, "Franklin Roosevelt Will Swim to Health," *Atlanta Journal*, October 26, 1924: 7; Frank Freidel, *Franklin D. Roosevelt: The Ordeal* (Boston: Little, Brown and Company, 1954): 193–98; Hugh Gregory Gallagher, *FDR's Splendid Deception: The Moving Story of Roosevelt's Massive Disability–and the Intense Efforts to Conceal It from the Public* (Arlington, VA: Vandamere Press, 1999): 1–3, 45–46, 48–50, 53, 155, 157; Tony Gould, *A Summer Plague: Polio and its Survivors* (New Haven: Yale University Press, 1995): 46, 48, 50–52; Shell, *Polio and Its Aftermath*: 183–83; David L. Sills, *The Volunteers: Means and Ends in a National Organization* (1957; reprint, New York: Arno Press, 1980): 42, 45; James Tobin, *The Man He Became: How FDR Defied Polio to Win the Presidency* (New York: Simon & Schuster, 2013): 204, 219.
24. Carter, *The Gentle Legions*: 107 and 115. Refer also to "Correspondence beginning May 15, 1928," Basil O'Connor to JDR Jr., November 3, 1933, "Invitation to Mrs. John D. Rockefeller Jr. to the Birthday Ball for the President of the United States for the benefit of Warm Springs Foundation, to be held 30 January 1934"; and "Different Parties" and "Celebration in New York," *President's Birthday Magazine* 1, no. 3 (1938): 19, 32–33, folder 113, box 14, Medical Interests series, RG 2, Office of the Messrs. Rockefeller (OMR), Rockefeller Family Archives, RAC; Arthur Allen, *Vaccine: The Controversial Story of Medicine's Greatest Lifesaver* (New York: W. W. Norton Company, 2007): 164–65; Victor Cohn, *Four Billion Dimes* (Minneapolis, MN: Minneapolis Star and Tribune, 1955): 36–38, 40–41, 43, 51; Offit, *The Cutter Incident*: 20; Sills, *The Volunteers*: 42–44; Tobin, *The Man He Became*: 221 and 251; Walker, *Roosevelt and the Warm Springs Story*: 218–19, 223–25, 227, 229–31, 238, and 252.

25. Williams, *Paralyzed with Fear*: 134; "'To Unify the Fight:' A New National Foundation for Infantile Paralysis," folder 117, box 14, Medical Interests series, RG 2, Rockefeller Family Archives, OMR, RAC. Also see Cohn, *Four Billion Dimes*: 52; Gallagher, *FDR's Splendid Deception*: 150; Stephen E. Mawdsley, "Polio and Prejudice: Charles Hudson Bynum and the Racial Politics of the National Foundation for Infantile Paralysis, 1938–1954" (MA thesis, University of Alberta, 2008): 65; Naomi Rogers, *Dirt and Disease: Polio Before FDR* (New Brunswick, NJ: Rutgers University Press, 1996): 170; David W. Rose, *Images of America: March of Dimes* (Charleston, SC: Arcadia Publishing, 2003): 79.

26. *President's Birthday Magazine* 1, no. 3 (1938): 25–28, 32–37, 40, 42, 44, 46, 48, 50, 51, 52, 54, 55, 56, 69 (folder 113, box 14, Medical Interests series, RG 2, OMR, Rockefeller Family Archives, RAC); Sills, *The Volunteers*: 7, 45–46, and 240.

27. Nancy Tomes, "Celebrity Diseases," in Leslie J. Reagan, Nancy Tomes, and Paula A. Treichler (eds.), *Medicine's Moving Pictures: Medicine, Health, and Bodies in American Film and Television* (Rochester, NY: University of Rochester Press, 2007): 37, 41, 48.

28. "'To Unify the Fight:' A New National Foundation for Infantile Paralysis," folder 117, box 14, Medical Interests series, RG 2, OMR, Rockefeller Family Archives, RAC (italics in the original). Susan Sontag, in *Illness As Metaphor and AIDS and Its Metaphors* (New York: Picador, 1989), has wrongly written that polio is "unmetaphorical" (127); yet, as we see from the NFIP's warlike rhetoric, this is not the case. Shell, in *Polio and Its Aftermath*, likewise disagrees with her assertion (186–87).

29. Shell, *Polio and Its Aftermath*: 142. The italics are in the original. See p. 201 as well. Also consult Mawdsley, "Polio and Prejudice": 5.

30. Carter, *The Gentle Legions*: 112. See also Rogers, *Dirt and Disease*: 170–71; Walker, *Roosevelt and the Warm Springs Story*: 254. For a fascinating treatment of this topic, see Chapter 5, "Handi-Capitation and Cinema Business," in Shell, *Polio and Its Aftermath*.

31. Carter, *Gentle Legions*: 95–96. And, of course, refer to Mawdsley, "Polio and Prejudice": 5–6 and 34–35.

32. Allan M. Brandt, "Polio, Politics, Publicity, and Duplicity: Ethical Aspects in the Development of the Salk Vaccine," *International Journal of Health Services* 8 (1978): 258; National Foundation for Infantile Paralysis, The Philadelphia Chapter—Year 1953: 3–4, 6 (Folder 2: National Foundation for Infantile Paralysis, Joseph Stokes, Jr., Papers, APS).

33. Mawdsley, "Polio and Prejudice": 25–26 and 29–30, respectively. See also Sills, *The Volunteers*: 118–23.

34. Mawdsley, "Polio and Prejudice": 34, 35–36, and 41, respectively; refer as well to pp. 29 and 37–41. See also Naomi Rogers, "Race and the Politics of Polio: Warm Springs, Tuskegee, and the March of Dimes," *American Journal of Public Health* 97 (May 2007): 791–92; Heather Green Wooten, *The Polio Years in Texas: Battling a Terrifying Unknown* (College Station: Texas A&M University Press, 2009): 98.

35. Mawdsley, "Polio and Prejudice": 46 and 58, respectively. Refer to Chapter 2, "Charles H. Bynum, National Policy, and Foundation Headquarters, 1944–1954," for a full and detailed accounting of his goals, strategies, and accomplishments.

36. Rogers, "Race and the Politics of Polio": 793.

37. Charles L. Mee, *A Nearly Normal Life* (Boston: Little, Brown & Co., 1999): 39. Consult also Rogers, *Dirt and Disease*: 172; Shell, *Polio and Its Aftermath*: 145.
38. David M. Oshinsky, *Polio: An American Story* (New York: Oxford University Press, 2005): 82.
39. Nina Gilden Seavey, Jane S. Smith, and Paul Wagner, *A Paralyzing Fear: The Triumph Over Polio in America* (New York: TV Books, 1998): 74.
40. Massey and Boyer in Seavey, Smith, and Wagner, *A Paralyzing Fear*: 92; see also pp. 78–80. Also see Lorenzo W. Milam, *The Cripple Liberation Front Marching Band Blues* (San Diego, CA: Mho & Mho Works, 1987): 54–55.
41. Mawdsley, "Polio and Prejudice": 62.
42. Mawdsley, "Polio and Prejudice": 63, 65, 66, and 67, respectively. Also consult pp. 62 and 64.
43. Brenda Serotte, *The Fortune Teller's Kiss* (Lincoln: University of Nebraska Press, 2006): 76–77; J. N. Hays, *The Burdens of Disease: Epidemics and Human Response in Western History* (New Brunswick: Rutgers University Press, 1998): 266; Martin F. Norden, *The Cinema of Isolation: A History of Physical Disability in the Movies* (New Brunswick, NJ: Rutgers University Press, 1994): 68–72; Daniel J. Wilson, *Living with Polio: The Epidemic and Its Survivors* (Chicago: University of Chicago Press, 2005): 16–17.
44. Serotte, *The Fortune Teller's Kiss*: 180.
45. Milam, *The Cripple Liberation Front Marching Band Blues*, 54–55.
46. Leonard Kriegel, *Falling into Life* (San Francisco: North Point Press, 1991): 67.
47. Marshall in Julie Silver and Daniel J. Wilson, *Polio Voices: An Oral History from the American Polio Epidemics and Worldwide Eradication Efforts* (Westport, CT: Praeger, 2007): 52–53; Anne Finger, *Elegy for A Disease: A Personal and Cultural History of Polio* (New York: St. Martin's Press, 2006): 109.
48. Joseph P. Shapiro, *No Pity: People with Disabilities Forging a New Civil Rights Movement* (New York: Three Rivers Press, 1994): 12–13.
49. Rosemarie Garland Thomson, "Seeing the Disabled: Visual Rhetorics of Disability in Popular Photography," in Paul K. Longmore and Lauri Umansky (eds.), *The New Disability History: American Perspectives* (New York: New York University Press, 2001): 339–40, 341, 342, 355; the indented quote is on p. 356. Fred Davis, in *Passage through Crisis: Polio Victims and Their Families* (Indianapolis, IN: Bobbs-Merrill, 1963), reinforces Garland Thomson's point: "Polio, unlike any other disease, evoked a strong, emotional public response. It came to occupy a pre-eminent—according to some, an exaggerated—place in the awareness, sympathy, and philanthropy of the American people. By the time of the development of the Salk vaccine it had emerged in popular thought as more than a sometimes crippling disease of children; it was regarded as a powerful symbol of blind, devastating, and uncontrollable misfortune whose victims were specially entitled to the support of good will of the community" (6). Roger Cooter, in "The Disabled Body" (in Roger Cooter and John Pickstone [eds.], *Medicine in the Twentieth Century* [Australia: Harwood Academic Publishers, 2000]), expresses similar sentiments: "The crippled child who could be encouraged to stand or walk without a crutch provided a model of self-help; glowing representations of crippled children triumphing over their handicaps provided an idealization of what (without state aid) individuals could do for themselves" (370–71). See also Paul K. Longmore and David Goldberger, "The League of the Physically Handicapped and the Great Depression: A Case Study in the New Disability History," *Journal of American History* 87 (December 2000): 896; Shapiro, *No Pity*: 12.

50. Rose, *Images of America*: 42; Fleischer and Zames, *The Disability Rights Movement*: 10.
51. Philip Lewin, *Infantile Paralysis: Anterior Poliomyelitis* (Philadelphia: W. B. Saunders Co., 1941): 326. No attribution.
52. Flexner is quoted in "Infantile Paralysis a Scourge and Puzzle," *New York Times*, July 9, 1916 (Sunday Edition), Magazine Section, p. 14.
53. Charles L. Lowman and Morton A. Seidenfeld, "A Preliminary Report of the Psychosocial Effects of Poliomyelitis," *Journal of Consulting Psychology* 11 (1947): 30–31. These same researchers acknowledge that the NFIP maintained a higher figure: 50 percent of those infected by polio had a major physical disability (31).
54. Kriegel, *Falling into Life*: xii–xiii. Also see Leonard Kriegel, "Uncle Tom and Tiny Tim: Some Reflections on the Cripple As Negro," *American Scholar* (Summer 1969): 414–15.
55. Garland Thomson, "Seeing the Disabled": 348, 346, and 347, respectively. Also refer to Daniel J. Wilson, "A Crippling Fear: Experiencing Polio in the Era of FDR," *Bulletin of the History of Medicine* 72 (1998): 487.
56. Mee, *A Nearly Normal Life*: 175.
57. Catherine J. Kudlick, "Disability History: Why We Need Another 'Other,'" *American Historical Review* (June 2003), http://www.historycooperative.org?journals/ahr/108.3/kudlick.html (accessed April 29, 2004) (Kudlick, paragraph #2, p. 1); (Kudlick, paragraph #3, p. 3); (Kudlick, paragraph #15, p. 6); (Kudlick, paragraph #22, p. 8).
58. These three quotes are from Sharon Barnartt and Richard Scotch, *Disability Protests: Contentious Politics, 1970–1999* (Washington, DC: Gallaudet University Press, 2001): xxiii. See also Cooter, "The Disabled Body": 369.
59. Rosemarie Garland Thomson, *Extraordinary Bodies: Figuring Physical Disability in American Culture and Literature* (New York: Columbia University Press, 1997): 6, 13–14, 22–23; Fleischer and Zames, *The Disability Rights Movement*: xv; Ruth O'Brien, *Crippled Justice: The History of Modern Disability Policy in the Workplace* (Chicago: University of Chicago Press, 2001): 1–2.
60. Douglas C. Baynton, "Disability and the Justification of Inequality in American History," in Paul K. Longmore and Lauri Umansky (eds.), *The New Disability History: American Perspectives* (New York: New York University Press, 2001): 35, 36. Emphasis is in the original text.
61. Garland Thomson, *Extraordinary Bodies*: 5, 6, 9–10, 11, and 136; Kriegel, *Falling into Life*: 125.
62. Marilynnne Rogers in Edmund J. Sass, George Gottfried, and Anthony Sorem, *Polio's Legacy: An Oral History* (Lanham, MD: University Press of America, 1996): 59.
63. See Claire H. Liachowitz, *Disability as a Social Construct: Legislative Roots* (Philadelphia: University of Pennsylvania Press, 1988), for a systematic analysis of the relationship between public policy and disability. The quote is on p. 1.
64. Susan M. Schweik, *The Ugly Laws: Disability in Public* (New York: New York University Press, 2009): 1–5 and 184, respectively. Refer to pp. 94–97 as well.
65. Liachowitz, *Disability as a Social Construct*: 41 and 83, respectively.
66. Davis, *Passage through Crisis*: 138. Davis provides a useful analytical framework, organized through the experiences of younger and older children disabled by polio. Also consult Mee, *A Nearly Normal Life*: 119–20.
67. Hugh Gregory Gallagher, *Black Bird Fly Away: Disabled in an Able-Bodied World* (Arlington, VA: Vandamere Press, 1998): 28; Robert Bogdan, *Freak*

Show: Presenting Human Oddities for Amusement and Profit (Chicago: University of Chicago Press, 1988): 6.
68. Shell, *Polio and Its Aftermath*: 15.
69. Gallagher, *Black Bird Fly Away*: 9.
70. Connolly, *Saving Sickly Children*: 9 and 2, respectively.
71. Edith Reeves Solenberger, *Public School Classes for Crippled Children*. Department of the Interior, Bureau of Education, Bulletin No. 10 (Washington, DC: Government Printing Office, 1918): iii, 2.
72. Charles E. Rosenberg, *The Care of Strangers: The Rise of America's Hospital System* (Baltimore: Johns Hopkins University Press, 1987): 150; Solenberger, *Public School Classes for Crippled Children*: 5, 29, and 33–36.
73. Rosenberg, *The Care of Strangers*: 316–17; see also pp. 318 and 321. Also see Leonard Kriegel, *The Long Walk Home: An Adventure in Survival* (New York: Appleton-Century, 1964): 138.
74. Gallagher, *Black Bird Fly Away*: 29.
75. Gallagher, *Black Bird Fly Away*: 29; also consult pp. 30–32. See also Oliver H. Bartine, "History of the New York Society for the Relief of the Ruptured and Crippled Children" (*American Journal of Care for Cripples* 3, 1916), in William R. F. Phillips and Janet Rosenberg (eds.), *The Origins of Modern Treatment and Education of Physically Handicapped Children* (New York: Arno Press, 1980): 59, 62; "The Medical Department," *Hospital School Journal* 11 (March–April 1923): 6.
76. Jason Chu Lee, "Poliomyelitis in the Lone Star State: A Brief Examination in Rural and Urban Communities" (MA thesis, Texas State University-San Marcos, 2005): 44, 76–79, 80, 83–84, 92–93, 113; Wooten, *The Polio Years in Texas*: 3, 107, and 113.
77. Solenberger, *Public School Classes for Crippled Children*: 78; also refer to pp. 7, 8–9, 31–32, 35, 55, 71–72, and 74–75. See also "The Medical Department," *Hospital School Journal* 11 (March-April 1923): 5. Nomenclature appeared opaque, since the labels "convalescent," "home," "hospital," "recuperation," and "rehabilitation" were often used interchangeably in their names.
78. Brad Byrom, "A Pupil and a Patient: Hospital Schools in Progressive America," in Paul K. Longmore and Lauri Umansky (eds.), *The New Disability History: American Perspectives* (New York: New York University Press, 2001): 136.
79. The information in the preceding four paragraphs can be found in Steven E. Koop, *We Hold this Treasure: The Story of Gillette Children's Hospital* (Afton, MN: Afton Historical Society Press, 1998): 6–7, 8–10, 14–17, 19, 22–23, 28, 30–33, 37–38, 40, 50–52, 54, 69, and 98.
80. Helen McNellis and Jerry McNellis, *"Don't Pick Him Up": Our Family's Experience with Polio* (Beaver Falls, PA: BrainTrain Press, 2011): 24, 15, 18–19, and 16, respectively. See also p. 20.
81. Francis R. Harbison, *D. T. Watson of Counsel* (Pittsburgh, PA: Davis & Warde, 1945): 289 and 291, respectively. Refer also to pp. 27, 37, 48, 55, 67–68, and 287–88. Watson's complete will is reprinted on pp. 288–91.
82. Jeffrey Kluger, *Splendid Solution: Jonas Salk and the Conquest of Polio* (New York: G. P. Putnam's Sons, 2004): 156; consult page 170 as well. See also Lawrence Alexander, as told to Adam Barnett, *The Iron Cradle: My Fight Against Polio* (New York: Thomas Y. Crowell Co., 1954): 126; Peg Kehret, *Small Steps: The Year I Got Polio* (Morton Grove, IL: 1996): 109, 119; Jane S. Smith, *Patenting the Sun: Polio and the Salk Vaccine* (New York: William Morrow and Co., 1990): 140; Louis Sternburg and Dorothy Sternburg, *View from the Seesaw*

(New York: Dodd, Mead & Company, 1986): 50; Dee Van Balen, *The Closing Door* (Pittsburgh, PA: CreateSpace, 2010): 6; WIA.
83. Jessie Wright Papers, 1925–1970, Record Group 7/1, WIA; Worthington to O'Connor, September 24, 1945, and Worthington to Van Riper, March 4, 1947 (MOD); Medical Programs Records, Series 5: Committees, 1938–1995, Physical Therapy Training Standards Committee, 1945–1947.
84. Kehret, *Small Steps*: 123–24.
85. Background information contained in these five paragraphs draws on Box OS4, Scrapbook from polio treatment period circa 1942–1953, Sheltering Arms Records, 1882–1983, SWHA.
86. Patrick J. Bird, *A Rough Road* (Amazon.com: 2012): 196–97. See also pp. i, ii, 5, 23, 55, 98–99, 113, and 181–83.
87. This mother is quoted by Davis, *Passage through Crisis*, on p. 73. Consult pp. 70 and 72 as well.
88. Richard L. Bruno, *The Polio Paradox: Understanding and Treating "Post-Polio Syndrome" and Chronic Fatigue* (New York: Warner Books, 2002): 76–77.
89. Robert L. Osgood, *For "Children Who Vary from the Normal Type": Special Education in Boston, 1838–1930* (Washington, DC: Gallaudet University Press, 2000): 43. See pp. 46 and 49 as well.
90. Solenberger, *Public School Classes for Crippled Children*: 31–32, 37–38, 56, and 73; Douglas C. McMurtrie, "A Study of the Character and Present Status of Provisions for Crippled Children in the United States," *American Journal of Care for Cripples* 2 (1916): 24–38, reprinted in William R. F. Phillips & Janet Rosenberg (eds.), *The Origins of Modern Treatment and Education of Physically Handicapped Children* (New York: Arno Press, 1980): 34–35. Also refer to Elliot White, "The Inception and Development of an Institute for Negro Crippled Children," pp. 171–74 in that same publication.
91. Pennsylvania Department of Public Welfare, Office of Mental Retardation, "Annual and Biennial Reports of State Institutions for Feeble-Minded of Western Pennsylvania": 1; "A Brilliant Assemblage: The School for Feeble Minded Formally Opened," *Oil City Derrick*, September 24, 1897, Pennsylvania Department of Public Welfare, Record Group 23, Box 2: Administrative File (Harry Shapiro), 1955–58; Correspondence, State Hospital, 1955; General Correspondence, 1955, PSA.
92. *Report of the State Institution for Feeble-Minded of Western Pennsylvania* (Oil City, PA: Derrick Publishing Co., 1916): 8, 19, 49; Box Title: "Annual and Biennial Reports of State Institutions for Feeble-Minded of Western Pennsylvania," Subgroup: Office of Mental Retardation, Department of Public Welfare Record Group-23, PSA.
93. Pennsylvania Department of Welfare, Office of Comptroller, Record Group Number 23, Box 25, "Audits of Institutions, Feeble-Minded, Polk State School, 1927–47," "Records of the Dept. of Public Welfare, Audits of Institutions, Polk State School, 1927–1930": 82; Pennsylvania Department of Public Welfare, Office of Mental Retardation, "Annual and Biennial Reports of State Institutions for Feeble-Minded of Western Pennsylvania," *Report of the State Institution for Feeble-Minded of Western Pennsylvania*: 11, 19, 29. PSA Kluger, *Splendid Solution*: 167–70; "Polk State School," http://www.asylumprojects.org/index.php?title=Polk_State_School (accessed February 22, 2011).
94. Walker to Barr, December 2, 1955; Shapiro to Forker; "Polk State School Newsletter, August 1955"; Pennsylvania Department of Public Welfare, Secretary of

Welfare, Record Group 23, Box 2: Administrative File (Harry Shapiro), 1955–58; Correspondence, State Hospital, 1955; General Correspondence, 1955. Folder: Administrative File, Shapiro, 1955–1958, PSA.
95. Mee, *A Nearly Normal Life*: 175. Rogers's and Gallagher's recollections can be found in Seavey, Smith, and Wagner, *A Paralyzing Fear*, 32 and 55, respectively. Gurney's oral history is quoted in Sass, Gottfried, and Sorem, *Polio's Legacy*: 28. See also Susan Richards Shreve, *Warm Springs: Traces of a Childhood at FDR's Polio Haven* (Boston: Houghton Mifflin Company, 2007): 142. The final statement is quoted on p. 83 in Bruno, *The Polio Paradox*.
96. Mee, *A Nearly Normal Life*: 76. Mee, p. 131, felt like a "Negro," watching a world he could never realize. See Ralph Ellison, *Invisible Man* (New York: Vintage Books, 1952). For Leonard Kriegel, in "Uncle Tom and Tiny Tim: Some Reflections on the Cripple As Negro," *American Scholar* (Summer 1969): 414, "Uncle Tom and Tiny Tim are brothers under the skin." The sight of a person disabled by polio embarrassed people; they simply did not want to see a "cripple." Their presence, he continues on pp. 416–17, made people uncomfortable: "For the cripple, the black man is a model because he is on intimate terms with terror that does not recognize his existence . . . He is in the process of discovering what he is, and he has known for a long time what the society conceives him to be . . . What he has been forced to learn is how to live on the outside looking in."
97. Garland Thomson, "Seeing the Disabled:" 348.
98. Kriegel, *The Long Walk Home*: 131–32.

Chapter 4

1. Fred Davis, *Passage through Crisis: Polio Victims and Their Families* (Indianapolis, IN: Bobbs-Merrill, 1963): 77–79.
2. Robert W. Lovett, *Infantile Paralysis in Vermont, 1894–1922: A Memorial to Charles S. Caverly* (Burlington, VT: Vermont State Department of Health, 1924): 275–76, 282, 200, 285, and 196, respectively; see also pp. 195, 199, 277, 279–81, and 284–85. Also consult Roland H. Berg, *Polio and Its Problems* (Philadelphia: J. B. Lippincott, 1948): 9–10; Collective Investigation Committee, *Epidemic Poliomyelitis: Report on the New York Epidemic of 1907* (New York: Journal of Nervous and Mental Disease Publishing Co., 1910): 107–119; Tracie C. Harrison and Alexa Stuifbergen, "A Hermeneutic Phenomenological Analysis of Aging with a Childhood Onset Disability," *Health Care for Women International* 26 (September 2005): 736; "The Medical Department," *Hospital School Journal* 11 (March–April 1923): 6; John R. Paul, *A History of Poliomyelitis* (New Haven: Yale University Press, 1971): 336.
3. Henry O. Kendall and Florence P. Kendall, *Care during the Recovery Period in Paralytic Poliomyelitis*, U.S. Public Health Service Bulletin No. 242 (Washington, DC: Government Printing Office, 1939): 8; Heather Green Wooten, *The Polio Years in Texas: Battling a Terrifying Unknown* (College Station: Texas A&M University Press, 2009): 159.
4. Kendall and Kendall, *Care during the Recovery Period in Paralytic Poliomyelitis*: 10 and 19, respectively; also consult pp. 12–14, 16, and 24–25. See also John F. Landon and Lawrence W. Smith, *Poliomyelitis: A Handbook for Physicians and Medical Students* (New York: Macmillan Company, 1934): 212–16, 220–23.
5. Philip Lewin, *Infantile Paralysis: Anterior Poliomyelitis* (Philadelphia: W. B. Saunders Co., 1941): 168 and 166, respectively. See also Leonard Kriegel, *Falling into Life* (San Francisco: North Point Press, 1991): 4.

6. Daniel J. Wilson, *Living with Polio: The Epidemic and Its Survivors* (Chicago: University of Chicago Press, 2005): 191–92.
7. Brad Byrom, "A Pupil and a Patient: Hospital Schools in Progressive America," in Paul K. Longmore and Lauri Umansky (eds.), *The New Disability History: American Perspectives* (New York: New York University Press, 2001): 133–34; Lewin, *Infantile Paralysis*: 168–69; Jessica Scheer and Mark L. Luborsky, "The Cultural Context of Polio Biographies," *Orthopedics* 14 (November 1991): 1173; Susan M. Schweik, *The Ugly Laws: Disability in Public* (New York: New York University Press, 2009): 254.
8. Boche is quoted by Steven E. Koop, *We Hold This Treasure: The Story of Gillette Children's Hospital* (Afton, MN: Afton Historical Society Press, 1998): 107–108.
9. Leonard Kriegel, *The Long Walk Home: An Adventure in Survival* (New York: Appleton-Century, 1964): 33. Also see Kriegel's *Flying Solo: Reimagining Manhood, Courage, and Loss* (Boston: Beacon Press, 1998): 1.
10. Hugh Gregory Gallagher, *Black Bird Fly Away: Disabled in an Able-Bodied World* (Arlington, VA: Vandamere Press, 1998): 47; Laura K. Smith, Dorothy M. Iddings, Eva-Marie Pfeiffer, and William A. Spencer, "Physical Therapy in the Poliomyelitis Respiratory Patient," *Physiotherapy* 41 (February 1955): 44–46.
11. W. Howlett Kelleher and R. K. Parida, "Glossopharyngeal Breathing: Its Value in Respiratory Muscle Paralysis of Poliomyelitis," *British Medical Journal* 23 (September 1957): 741; see also pp. 741–42. Also see John E. Affeldt, "Recent Advances in the Treatment of Poliomyelitis," *Journal of the American Medical Association* 156 (September 1954): 13; Smith et al., "Physical Therapy in the Poliomyelitis Respiratory Patient": 49–50.
12. Becker in Tony Gould, *A Summer Plague: Polio and Its Survivors* (New Haven: Yale University Press, 1995): 289–290.
13. Rogers in Edmund J. Sass, George Gottfried, and Anthony Sorem, *Polio's Legacy: An Oral History* (Lanham, MD: University Press of America, 1996): 55–56. Rogers still requires the use of her iron lung each night (53). For general nursing care information as well as additional weaning experiences, see especially National Organization for Public Health Nursing (NOPHN) and National League of Nursing Education (NLNE), "Nursing for the Poliomyelitis Patient" (New York: NOPHN & NLNE, 1948): 57, 59; Lawrence Alexander, as told to Adam Barnett, *The Iron Cradle: My Fight Against Polio* (New York: Thomas Y. Crowell Co., 1954): 48–50; Jason Chu Lee, "Poliomyelitis in the Lone Star State: A Brief Examination in Rural and Urban Communities" (MA thesis, Texas State University-San Marcos, 2005): 86; Lewin, *Infantile Paralysis*: 133.
14. Smith et al., "Physical Therapy in the Poliomyelitis Respiratory Patient": 50–51.
15. Marilyn Moffat, "The History of Physical Therapy Practice in the United States," *Journal of Physical Therapy Education* 17 (Winter 2003): 15–16; "After-Treatment of Child Paralysis Victims," *New York Times*, August 27, 1916 (Magazine Section): 17; Ruth O'Brien, *Crippled Justice: The History of Modern Disability Policy in the Workplace* (Chicago: University of Chicago Press, 2001): xi, 41, 64–65.
16. Robert C. Huse, *Getting There: Growing Up with Polio in the 30's* (Bloomington, IN: 1stBooks: 2002): 92, 93, and 6, respectively; please refer to pp. 94–95 as well. See also Koop, *We Hold This Treasure*: 120.
17. Richard L. Bruno, *The Polio Paradox: Understanding and Treating "Post-Polio Syndrome" and Chronic Fatigue* (New York: Warner Books, 2002): 69, 71. The patients' excerpts are quoted on p. 70.
18. *Polio Chronicle*, November 1933, Vol. 3, #1: 8; *Polio Chronicle*, May 1933, Vol. 2, #10: 8, RWSIR. Refer also to Rogers in Sass, Gottfried, and Sorem, *Polio's*

Legacy: 58; Daniel J. Wilson, "Braces, Wheelchairs, and Iron Lungs: The Paralyzed Body and the Machinery of Rehabilitation in the Polio Epidemics," *Journal of Medical Humanities* 26 (Fall 2005): 174, 184–85.
19. Kriegel, *The Long Walk Home*: 52 and 62, respectively; consult p. 59 as well. See also Kriegel, *Flying Solo*: 31–32.
20. Peg Kehret, *Small Steps: The Year I Got Polio* (Morton Grove, IL: 1996): 104–05. Also see pp. 79 and 124.
21. Helen McNellis and Jerry McNellis, *"Don't Pick Him Up": Our Family's Experience with Polio* (Beaver Falls, PA: BrainTrain Press, 2011): 19 and 23, respectively.
22. Kriegel, *The Long Walk Home*: 77–81, 85–87, and 93. Kriegel relates this episode in somewhat less detail in *Falling into Life*: 12–13.
23. Alice R. Thrall, "Observations from a Wheel Chair," *Polio Chronicle*, June 1933, Vol. 2, #11: 6. RWSIR. Refer also to Robert F. Murphy, *The Body Silent: The Different World of the Disabled* (New York: W. W. Norton, 1990): 93.
24. Kriegel, *Flying Solo*: 32. See also pp. 38–41.
25. Kehret, *Small Steps*: 130 and 121, respectively.
26. These three quotes come from two different sources. Kriegel makes the Frankenstein allusion in *Falling into Life*: 9. His second comment is from *The Long Walk Home*: 75. The third quote comes from *Falling into Life*: 14; also see p. 176.
27. H. A. Robinson, J. E. Finesinger, and J. S. Bierman, "Psychiatric Considerations in the Adjustment of Patients with Poliomyelitis," *New England Journal of Medicine* 254 (May 1956): 976, 978.
28. Wilson, "Braces, Wheelchairs, and Iron Lungs": 187–88; Harrison and Stuifbergen, "A Hermeneutic Phenomenological Analysis of Aging with a Childhood Onset Disability": 737.
29. Dee Van Balen, *The Closing Door* (Pittsburgh, PA: CreateSpace, 2010): 42. Van Balen also refers to this problem on p. 14. See also Mary Grimley Mason, *Life Prints: A Memoir of Healing and Discovery* (New York: Feminist Press, 2000): 23.
30. Joel D. Howell, "Hospitals," in Roger Cooter and John Pickstone (eds.), *Medicine in the Twentieth Century* (Australia: Harwood Academic Publishers, 2000): 506; Lynette Iezzoni, *Influenza 1918: The Worst Epidemic in American History* (New York: TV Books, 1999): 118.
31. Alfred H. Tubbey and Robert Jones, *Modern Methods in the Surgery of Paralysis, with Special Reference to Muscle-Grafting, Tendon-Transplantation and Arthrodesis* (New York: Macmillan & Co., 1903): 73–73 and 171, respectively. Refer also to pp. 99, 185, and 186 (NYAM).
32. Massachusetts State Board of Health, *The Occurrence of Infantile Paralysis in Massachusetts in 1909*: 94. Bruno reviews many of these procedures on pp. 96–97 of *The Polio Paradox*. See also Hugh Gregory Gallagher, *FDR's Splendid Deception: The Moving Story of Roosevelt's Massive Disability—and the Intense Efforts to Conceal It from the Public* (Arlington, VA: Vandamere Press, 1999): 31; Marc Shell, *Polio and Its Aftermath: The Paralysis of Culture* (Cambridge: Harvard University Press, 2005): 166.
33. Massachusetts State Board of Health, *The Occurrence of Infantile Paralysis in Massachusetts in 1909* (Boston: Wright & Potter Printing Co., 1910): 95 and 94, respectively; also see p. 96 (NYAM).
34. Lovett, *Treatment of Infantile Paralysis*: 84–5, 96, 109, 115, and 117–19, respectively; see also pp. 97–98 and 103. See also Berg, *Polio and Its Problems*: 124; Gould, *A Summer Plague*: 24–25; Landon and Smith, *Poliomyelitis*: 228–29; Lovett, "A Plan of Treatment in Infantile Paralysis," in *Infantile Paralysis in*

Vermont: 264, 266–67, and 271; Paul, *History of Poliomyelitis*: 337–38; Gareth Williams, *Paralyzed with Fear: The Story of Polio* (New York: Palgrave Macmillan, 2013): 146.
35. Lewin, *Infantile Paralysis*: 209–11. Refer to seven-year-old Ron Zemke's experience in Diane Zemke, *Polio: A Special Ride?* (Minnetonka, MN: Diagnostic Center of Learning Patterns, Inc., 1997): 20.
36. NOPHN and NLNE, "Nursing for the Poliomyelitis Patient": 78–80.
37. Bruno, *Polio Paradox*: 95. Refer also to pp. 98.
38. Susan Richard Shreve, *Warm Springs: Traces of a Childhood at FDR's Polio Haven* (Boston: Houghton Mifflin Company, 2007): 160; refer also to pp. 4, 11, and 73. See also Massachusetts State Board of Health, *The Occurrence of Infantile Paralysis in Massachusetts in 1909*: 96.
39. Anne Finger, *Elegy for a Disease: A Personal and Cultural History of Polio* (New York: St. Martin's Press, 2006): 84–85, 86–87, and 89, respectively.
40. "A Radical Improvement in Ether Anesthesia," *Journal of the Indiana State Medical Association* 5 (October 1912): 446–47.
41. Bruno quotes Moira on p. 98 of *Polio Paradox*. Also see Shreve, *Warm Springs*: 11.
42. Bias in Sass, Gottfried, and Sorem, *Polio's Legacy*: 78-80. See also pp. 83–84.
43. Brutger in Sass, Gottfried, and Sorem, *Polio's Legacy*: 71 and 72–75.
44. Williams, *Paralyzed with Fear*: 144.
45. Daniel J. Wilson, "Covenants of Work and Grace: Themes of Recovery and Redemption in Polio Narratives," *Literature and Medicine* 13 (Spring 1994): 31. Consult p. 33 as well.
46. Kriegel, *Long Walk Home*: 130–32; also refer to pp. 88–89. See also Kriegel, *Falling Into Life*: viii and xv. Wilson cites Kriegel in "Covenants of Work and Grace," on pp. 26–27. Wilson also provides insights into post-rehabilitation on pp. 35–37.
47. That physician is quoted on p. 14 in Lynne M. Dunphy, "'The Steel Cocoon': Tales of the Nurses and Patients of the Iron Lung, 1929–55." *Nursing History Review* 9 (2001). See also Daniel J. Wilson, *Polio* (Santa Barbara, CA: Greenwood Press, 2009): 78.
48. Richard Owen, "Introduction," in Sass, Gottfried, and Sorem, *Polio's Legacy*: vii–viii; Bruno, *Polio Paradox*: 97.
49. Wooten, *The Polio Years in Texas*: 159. Van Balen, *The Closing Door*: 2.
50. Dunphy, "The Steel Cocoon'": 16 and 24; William S. Langford, "Physical Illness and Convalescence: Their Meaning to the Child," *Journal of Pediatrics* 33 (1948): 246.
51. These three paragraphs draw on data from and analyses by Davis, *Passage through Crisis*: 69, 70, 75, 76, 77, and 78–79; the mother is quoted on p. 77. Also see Kehret, *Small Steps*: 82–83; Charles L. Mee, *A Nearly Normal Life* (Boston: Little, Brown & Co., 1999): 36.
52. Schwartz is quoted on p. 147 and Rogers on pp. 56–57 in Sass, Gottfried, and Sorem, *Polio's Legacy*; see also pp. 80 and 128–29. Mee, in *A Nearly Normal Life*: 34, recalls the boy in the wheelchair, while "Leadfoot" appears in Shreve, *Warm Springs*: 83. Her second quote is on p. 174.
53. Huse, *Getting There*: 89 and 91, respectively. Also refer to p. 93.
54. Kehret, *Small Steps*: 62 and 104; Mee, *A Nearly Normal Life*: 34.
55. Quoted in Bruno, *The Polio Paradox*: 78–79.
56. Headley in Gould, *A Summer Plague*: 277. Refer also to Paul K. Longmore, *Why I Burned My Book and Other Essays on Disability* (Philadelphia: Temple University

Press, 2003): 9; Mee, *A Nearly Normal Life*: 34; Shell, *Polio and Its Aftermath*: 118–19.
57. Lee, "Poliomyelitis in the Lone Star State": 92. Refer also to Louis Sternburg and Dorothy Sternburg, *View from the Seesaw* (New York: Dodd, Mead & Company, 1986): 46.
58. "To Teach Sick Children; Lessons for 500 Infantile Paralysis Victims While in Hospital," *New York Times*, September 5, 1920: 6; Rogers, pp. 56–57 and Schwartz, p. 147, in Sass, Gottfried, and Sorem, *Polio's Legacy*. For additional background, refer to Kehret, *Small Steps*: 124–25; Lee, "Poliomyelitis in the Lone Star State": 93.
59. Kehret, *Small Steps*: 132. See also p. 100.
60. Wooten, *The Polio Years in Texas*: 160. Wooten quotes Gonzalez on that page as well.
61. Sharon Barnartt and Richard Scotch, *Disability Protests: Contentious Politics, 1970–1999* (Washington, DC: Gallaudet University Press, 2001): 34–35.
62. Barnartt and Scotch, *Disability Protests*: 45.
63. Charles Dickens, *A Christmas Carol and Other Christmas Stories* (New York: Signet Classic, 1984): 88, 89. Refer also to pp. 87 and 90–92.
64. Barnartt and Scotch, *Disability Protests*: 46. See also Longmore, *Why I Burned My Book*: 2.
65. Rosemarie Garland Thomson, *Extraordinary Bodies: Figuring Physical Disability in American Culture and Literature* (New York: Columbia University Press, 1997): 46. Consult also Shell, *Polio and Its Aftermath*: 145.
66. Barnartt and Scotch, *Disability Protests*: 46.
67. Thomson, *Extraordinary Bodies*: 25, 27, and 50.
68. Martin F. Norden, *The Cinema of Isolation: A History of Physical Disability in the Movies* (New Brunswick, NJ: Rutgers University Press, 1994): 3.
69. Sharon L. Snyder and David T. Mitchell, *Cultural Locations of Disability* (Chicago: University of Chicago Press, 2006): 156.
70. Paul K. Longmore and David Goldberger, "The League of the Physically Handicapped and the Great Depression: A Case Study in the New Disability History," *Journal of American History* 87 (December 2000): 893. I chose the movie industry in this context because its rise during the first half of the twentieth century coincided with the American polio epidemics. See especially Shell, *Polio and Its Aftermath*, in Chapter 4, "Paralytic Polio and Moving Pictures." He provides a superb analysis in this chapter dealing with "stasis and kinesis."
71. Norden, *Cinema of Isolation*: 52–53 and 54. For a similar analysis, see Snyder and Mitchell, *Cultural Locations of Disability*, pp. 156–57.
72. Longmore and Goldberger, "League of the Physically Handicapped and the Great Depression": 895–896.
73. Robert Bogdan, *Freak Show: Presenting Human Oddities for Amusement and Profit* (Chicago: University of Chicago Press, 1988): ix, 6, 11–12, and 277–78, respectively. Consult also pp. 19–20 and 29–67.
74. This summary is based on my viewing of the film *Freaks*, originally produced by MGM Studios in 1932 and now listed as part of the Turner Classic Movies collection. Also refer to Joan Hawkins, "'One of Us': Tod Browning's *Freaks*," in Rosemarie Garland Thomson (ed.), *Freakery: Cultural Spectacles of the Extraordinary Body* (New York: New York University Press, 1996): 265; "Freaks," Wikipedia, http://en.wikipedia.org/w/index.php?title=Freaks (accessed April 23, 2006).
75. Norden, *Cinema of Isolation*: 115–120, 123, and 133.

76. Longmore and Goldberger, "League of the Physically Handicapped and the Great Depression": 896. Refer also to Rosemary Garland Thomson, "Seeing the Disabled: Visual Rhetorics of Disability in Popular Photograph," in *The New Disability History:* 335–74.
77. Longmore and Goldberger, "The League of the Physically Handicapped and the Great Depression": 893–894; Schweik, *The Ugly Laws*: 97.
78. Sass, Gottfried, and Sorem *Polio's Legacy:* xv. This study not only thematically analyzes the impact of polio on people's lives but also provides 35 oral histories to personally illustrate the various topics.
79. Davis in Thomas M. Daniel and Frederick C. Robbins (eds.), *Polio* (Rochester, NY: University of Rochester Press, 1997): 37–38.
80. Davis, *Passage through Crisis:* 163–64. Refer also to pp. 3, 151, 157–59, 182, 183, and 188–190.
81. Fay S. Copellman, "Follow-Up of One Hundred Children with Poliomyelitis," *The Family* 25 (December 1944): 292; also consult pp. 289–90 and 294. See also Alice A. Grant, "Medical Social Work in an Epidemic of Poliomyelitis," *Journal of Pediatrics* 24 (June 1944): 701.
82. DeHayes to Altenburg, March 1, 1946; "Review of Significant Contributions to the Psychiatric Aspects of Poliomyelitis"; Seidenfeld to Van Riper, October 4, 1946; NFIP press release: NFIP on Psychological Impact of Polio, October 21, 1948; Seidenfeld to O'Connor, "Overall Ten Year Picture of Psychological Services," October 25, 1948, Series 14: Poliomyelitis, Psychological Services, 1946–1951; Morton A. Seidenfeld, "The Physical Therapist and Her Role in the Psychological Care of the Poliomyelitis Patient," *Physiotherapy Review* 27 (July–Aug. 1947); Morton A. Seidenfeld, "Psychological Considerations in Poliomyelitis Care," *American Journal of Nursing* 47 (June 1947) MOD; Medical Programs Records; Series 14: Poliomyelitis; Psychological Services, 1947.
83. Mason, *Life Prints*: xi.
84. Longmore and Umansky, *The New Disability History*: 8.
85. Longmore and Goldberger, "The League of the Physically Handicapped and the Great Depression": 897. Gallagher, in *FDR's Splendid Deception*, provides a superb analysis of Roosevelt's complex character and how he reconciled the personal reality of polio (i.e., vulnerability) with his public image (i.e., a strong and robust leader).
86. Longmore and Goldberger, "League of the Physically Handicapped and the Great Depression": 900, 892, 900, 902, and 904, respectively; consult also pp. 888, 891, 897, 901, 905–8, 916–17, and 919. Barnartt and Scotch (*Disability Studies*, p. 13), Doris Zames Fleischer and Frieda Zames (*The Disability Rights Movement: From Charity to Confrontation* [Philadelphia: Temple University Press, 2001]: 6–7), and Shell (*Polio and Its Aftermath*: 201) allude to this episode. Longmore, in *Why I Burned My Book*, expands his notion of individual and collective struggles to redefine the "social identities of people with disabilities" (p. 3).
87. Richard J. Altenbaugh, *The American People and their Education: A Social History* (Upper Saddle River, NJ: Pearson, 2003): 228, 232.
88. Roger Cooter, "The Disabled Body," in Cooter and Pickstone (eds.), *Medicine in the Twentieth Century*: 373; Margaret Winzer, *The History of Special Education: From Isolation to Integration* (Washington, DC: Gallaudet University Press, 1993): 176–79, 187, 317, 323.
89. Joe F. Sullivan, "Editorial," *Hospital School Journal* 8 (September–October 1919): 1.

90. These two paragraphs draw on descriptions by Lovett, *Infantile Paralysis in Vermont*: 286, 287, 289, and 290. The italics in the first paragraph are mine.
91. "Infantile Paralysis—New York Committee on After-Care, July 1916," "Proposed Method of Organizing Orthopedic Treatment of Infantile Paralysis Cases in New York City": 4, folder 277, box 25, series 200, RG 1.1, Projects, Rockefeller Foundation Archives (RAC).
92. The Seaside Hospital in Brooklyn, reports dated February 17, 1917, and May 31, 1917, "Infantile Paralysis—Brooklyn Bureau of Charities, 1916–1918," folder 276, box 25, series 200, RG 1.1, Projects, Rockefeller Foundation Archives (RAC).
93. Byrom, "A Pupil and a Patient": 139–40.
94. Henry H. Kessler, *The Crippled and the Disabled: Rehabilitation of the Physically Handicapped in the United States* (1935, reprinted New York: Arno Press, 1980): 52–53; consult p. 40 as well. See also Ruth O'Brien, *Crippled Justice: The History of Modern Disability Policy in the Workplace* (Chicago: University of Chicago Press, 2001): 42.
95. Byrom, "A Pupil and a Patient": 135, 143, and 145; also refer to pp. 133 and 142. See also Thomson, *Extraordinary Bodies*: 46.
96. Landon and Smith, *Poliomyelitis*, 227–28.
97. Kessler, *Crippled and the Disabled*: 32. Refer also to pp. 35–36 and 43.
98. Howard A. Rusk, *A World to Care For: The Autobiography of Howard A. Rusk, M.D.* (New York: Random House, 1972): 58 and 28–29, respectively; also consult pp. 106 and 180–81. See also O'Brien, *Crippled Justice*: 41.
99. Naomi Rogers, *Polio Wars: Sister Kenny and the Golden Age of American Medicine* (New York: Oxford University Press, 2014): 42–43. Consult also pp. 172–73.
100. Rusk, *A World to Care For*: 98 and 99–100, respectively; Refer also to pp. 12–14, 19–23, and 27. See also O'Brien, *Crippled Justice*: 8–10, 22, 27–30, 31, and 43–45.
101. Brenda Serotte, *The Fortune Teller's Kiss* (Lincoln: University of Nebraska Press, 2006): 166, 129, 167, 168, and 169, respectively. Italics are in the original text. Also see pp. 6, 63, 115, and 157.
102. Rusk, *A World to Care For*: 188.
103. Joseph P. Shapiro, *No Pity: People with Disabilities Forging a New Civil Rights Movement* (New York: Three Rivers Press, 1994): 63.
104. Howard A. Rusk and Eugene J. Taylor, *Living with A Disability: At Home—At Work—At Play* (Garden City, NY: Blakiston Company, 1953): 7; O'Brien, *Crippled Justice*: 50.
105. Howard A. Rusk, *Rehabilitation Medicine: A Textbook on Physical Medicine and Rehabilitation* (St. Louis, MO: C. V. Mosby Company, 1964): 475. Refer also to p. 25.
106. Shapiro, *No Pity*: 15.
107. Helen Holt and Frances McGaan, "A Polio's Paradise," *Polio Chronicle*, May 1933, Vol. 2, #10: 6. RWSIR.
108. Shreve, *Warm Springs*: 44–45; Mason, *Life Prints*: 8; Bentz Plagemann, *My Place to Stand* (New York: Farrar, Straus & Co., 1949): 35–36, 141–42.
109. Grimley Mason, *Life Prints*: 8. Consult also pp. xi, 5–6, and 9.
110. Lorenzo Wilson Milam, *The Cripple Liberation Front Marching Band Blues* (San Diego, CA: Mho & Mho Works, 1987): 83. See pp. 77 and 80–83 for a more elaborate description. Refer also to Hugh Gallagher in Nina Gilden Seavey, Jane S. Smith, and Paul Wagner, *A Paralyzing Fear: The Triumph Over Polio in America* (New York: TV Books, 1998), for a very similar description (p. 57); and to Plagemann, *My Place to Stand*: 161–65.

111. Shreve, *Warm Springs*: 19, 132, and 50, respectively. See also pp. 131–33.
112. "Do You Drive, Polio?" *Polio Chronicle* (January 1933): 4; Wallace C. Douglas and O. H. Caldwell, "The Electric Eye," *Polio Chronicle* (October 1932): 3; "Going Up," *Polio Chronicle* (December 1932): 6. (All from RWSIR.)
113. Jacqueline Foertsch, "'Heads, You Win': Newsletters and Magazine of the Polio Nation," *Disability Studies Quarterly* 27 (Summer 2007): 3–7 (www.dsq-sds.org, accessed January 5, 2012).
114. Edith Powell and John F. Hume, *A Black Oasis: Tuskegee Institute's Fight Against Infantile Paralysis, 1941–1975* (copyright, 2008): 1; consult as also pp. 6–7 and 45. See also Stephen E. Mawdsley, "Polio and Prejudice: Charles Hudson Bynaum and the Racial Politics of the National Foundation for Infantile Paralysis, 1938–1954" (MA thesis, University of Alberta, 2008): 17.
115. "The Georgia Warm Springs Foundation" (New York: Georgia Warm Springs Foundation, c. 1929): 18, folder 113, "Medical Interests—Georgia Warm Springs Foundation, 1928–1954," box 14, Medical Interests series, RG 2, Office of the Messrs. Rockefeller, Rockefeller Family Archives (RAC). Paul H. Harmon, in "The Racial Incidence of Poliomyelitis in the United States with Special Reference to the Negro," *Journal of Infectious Diseases* 58 (May–June 1936), taps statistics from eleven state and two municipal health departments covering all regions (but predominantly focused on the South) to conclude that the "incidence of poliomyelitis in whites . . . is from two to four times that in negroes." Mortality rates, though, remained similar (336).
116. Mawdsley, "Polio and Prejudice:" 17–18; Powell and Hume, *A Black Oasis*: 29.
117. Wooten, *The Polio Years in Texas*: 46.
118. Gould, *A Summer Plague*: 80 and 189–191, respectively. See p. 78 as well. Note too Dr. John Hume's narrative in Seavey, Smith, and Wagner, *A Paralyzing Fear*: 157–58.
119. MOD, Medical Programs Records, Series 8: Grants and Appropriations, Approved Grants, 1941–1942.
120. Mawdsley, "Polio and Prejudice": 18 and 20, respectively; also refer to pp. 19 and 22. See also Vanessa Northington Gamble, *Making a Place for Ourselves: The Black Hospital Movement, 1920–1945* (New York: Oxford University Press, 1995): 40, 109; "Medical News," *Journal of the American Medical Association* 113 (July 1939): 340; "National Foundation for Infantile Paralysis," *American Journal of Public Health* 31 (1941): 1023; "News on the Polio Front," *American Journal of Public Health* 36 (1946): 179.
121. Gamble, *Making a Place for Ourselves*: 109 and 123, respectively; also refer to pp. 106, 124–25, and 128. James Anderson, through his body of work, has thoroughly analyzed Rosenwald Fund and GEB policies in Southern African American education, especially in *The Education of Blacks in the South, 1860–1935* (Chapel Hill: University of North Carolina Press, 1988).
122. Powell and Hume, *A Black Oasis*: 17. See also pp. 18, 74, and 152.
123. Yelder in Seavey, Smith, and Wagner, *A Paralyzing Fear*: 153–54 and 156; National Foundation for Infantile Paralysis (NFIP), *The Tuskegee Institute Infantile Paralysis Center* (New York: NFIP, 1942): 4–9 (NYAM). Also see Gould, *A Summer Plague*: 81 and 83; Powell and Hume, *A Black Oasis*: 37, 46, 50–51, 54, 56, 67, 69, 70, 78–79, and 81; Mawdsley, "Polio and Prejudice": 20 and 22–25; Naomi Rogers, "Race and the Politics of Polio: Warm Springs, Tuskegee, and the March of Dimes," *American Journal of Public Health* 97 (May 2007): 791–92.
124. Mawdsley, "Polio and Prejudice": 20–21.

125. Rogers, "Race and the Politics of Polio": 784. Rogers, also on p. 784, reinforces Mawdsley's accommodationist approach to segregationist policies.
126. Wooten, *The Polio Years in Texas*: 55; consult pp. 52–54 as well. See also Mawdsley, "Polio and Prejudice": 17.
127. Kriegel, *Long Walk Home*: 118 and 121–22, respectively. See also pp. 49–51 and 117.
128. Durr in Julie Silver and Daniel Wilson, *Polio Voices: An Oral History from the American Polio Epidemics and Worldwide Eradication Efforts* (Westport, CT: Praeger, 2007): 65.

Chapter 5

1. Franz Kafka, *The Metamorphosis*, translated and edited by Stanley Corngold (New York: Bantam Books, 1972): 3 and 40, respectively. *The Metamorphosis* is not at all removed from disability in general and the polio experience in particular. Sociologist Robert F. Murphy, in *The Body Silent: The Different World of the Disabled* (New York: W. W. Norton, 1990), uses it as a metaphor (85). Hugh Gregory Gallagher's autobiographical account—earlier described in Chapter 2, "Many Yellow Caskets"—of awakening to find himself paralyzed stunningly parallels Gregor Samsa's experience. Later Gallagher literally alludes to Kafka's *Metamorphosis*, but in a wholly different sense from that used in Chapter 2. Leonard Kriegel, in *Falling into Life* (San Francisco: North Point Press, 1991), has an entire chapter, "In Kafka's House," likening disability to a Kafkaesque experience: "In Kafka's house, I remind myself, all are welcome" (193). I first encountered Kafka's work as an undergraduate student and immediately fell in love with his surreal world, and I continue to seek refuge in it. As I began my research for this study, images of *The Metamorphosis* quickly and continually came to mind. I was therefore fascinated to discover that other writers, some of them disabled by polio, validated my association. Note Gallagher's chapter titled "Gregor, The Cockroach" for his adaptation. See Hugh Gregory Gallagher, *Black Bird Fly Away: Disabled in an Able-Bodied World* (Arlington, VA: Vandamere Press, 1998): 22–24, 41, 189–95.
2. Corngold's analysis serves as preface for this edition of *The Metamorphosis*. His quoted comments are on pp. xxii and xix, respectively. This volume contains reprints of critical essays that explore a variety of interpretations.
3. Gallagher's writings are extant. The quote in this passage can be found in Nina Gilden Seavey, Jane S. Smith, and Paul Wagner, *A Paralyzing Fear: The Triumph Over Polio in America* (New York: TV Books, 1998): 58. See also his fascinating historical analysis of how Roosevelt coped with polio: Hugh Gregory Gallagher, *FDR's Splendid Deception: The Moving Story of Roosevelt's Massive Disability—and the Intense Efforts to Conceal It from the Public* (Arlington, VA: Vandamere Press, 1999).
4. Arthur Allen, *Vaccine: The Controversial Story of Medicine's Greatest Lifesaver* (New York: W. W. Norton Company, 2007): 169. For the cited statistics, see Max J. Fox and John Chamberlain, "Four Fatal Cases of Bulbar Poliomyelitis in One Family," *Journal of the American Medical Association* 151 (March 28, 1953): 1099–1101. The tone of this article was purely clinical, dispassionately describing symptoms, treatments, and deaths. See also *Report of the Department of Health of the City of Chicago for the Years of 1911 to 1918 Inclusive* (Chicago: Department of Health, 1919): 174 (CPL).

Notes and Sources

5. "$10,000 to Save Children: Losing Daughter, St. Louis Physician Offers Big Sum for Cure of Others," *New York Times*, September 3, 1912, p. 1.
6. "$1,234 More for Cripples," *New York Times*, August 17, 1916: 6.
7. Wade H. Frost, *Epidemiologic Studies of Acute Anterior Poliomyelitis*, Treasury Department, United States Public Health Service, Hygienic Laboratory Bulletin No. 90, October 1913 (Washington, DC: Government Printing Office, 1913): 73–74; "$10,000 to Save Children: Losing Daughter, St. Louis Physician Offers Big Sum for Cure of Others," *New York Times*, September 3, 1912: 1; Fox and Chamberlain, "Four Fatal Cases of Bulbar Poliomyelitis in One Family," 1099–1101; Rosenwald in Julie Silver and Daniel Wilson, *Polio Voices: An Oral History from the American Polio Epidemics and Worldwide Eradication Efforts* (Westport, CT: Praeger, 2007): 48–49.
8. Charles L. Mee, *A Nearly Normal Life* (Boston: Little, Brown & Co., 1999): 119–20.
9. Stephanie Coontz, *The Way We Never Were: American Families and the Nostalgia Trap* (New York: Basic Books, 1992): 72. Refer also to John Demos, *Past, Present, and Personal: The Family and the Life Course in American History* (New York: Oxford University Press, 1986): 5; Robert Wells, "Family History and Demographic Transition," in Michael Gordon (ed.), *The American Family in Social-Historical Perspective* (New York: St. Martin's Press, 1978): 525; Linda Gordon, *Heroes of Their Own Lives: The Politics and History of Family Violence* (Urbana: University of Illinois Press, 2002): 146–58.
10. Saul Benison, "Poliomyelitis and the Rockefeller Institute: Social Effects and Institutional Response," *Journal of the History of Medicine* 29 (January 1974): 84.
11. Gallagher, *FDR's Splendid Deception*: 29. Refer also to Tony Gould, *A Summer Plague: Polio and its Survivors* (New Haven: Yale University Press, 1995): 46. Richard L. Bruno (*The Polio Paradox: Understanding and Treating "Post-Polio Syndrome" and Chronic Fatigue* [New York: Warner Books, 2002]) found similar experiences in his 1995 survey of individuals disabled by polio (88).
12. Alice Sink, *The Grit Behind the Miracle: A True Story of the Determination and Hard Work Behind an Emergency Infantile Paralysis Hospital, 194–1945, Hickory, North Carolina* (Lanham, MD: University Press of America, 1998): 24–25, 29–37; Roland H. Berg, *Polio and Its Problems* (Philadelphia: J. B. Lippincott, 1948): 120–21; Alice A. Grant, "Medical Social Work in an Epidemic of Poliomyelitis" *Journal of Pediatrics* 24 (June 1944): 695.
13. Marc Shell, *Polio and Its Aftermath: The Paralysis of Culture* (Cambridge: Harvard University Press, 2005): 78.
14. Brenda Serotte, *The Fortune Teller's Kiss* (Lincoln: University of Nebraska Press, 2006): 75–77.
15. "Noted Scientists Organize to Curb Infant Paralysis," *New York Times*, July 13, 1916: 3; "Oyster Bay Revolts Over Poliomyelitis," *New York Times*, August 29, 1916: 1; "Oyster Bay Lifts Poliomyelitis Ban," *New York Times*, September 6, 1916: 20; "Expects Epidemic to End in 2 Weeks," *New York Times*, September 7, 1916: 22; "Mother of Patient Missing, Disappears with Son after Baby Is Taken to Hospital," *New York Times*, September 5, 1916: 20; "Parents Resist Policemen," *New York Times*, September 9, 1916: 6; "Mob Riots Over Paralysis," *New York Times*, September 3, 1916: 16; Guenter B. Risse, "Revolt Against Quarantine: Community Responses to the 1916 Polio Epidemic, Oyster Bay, New York," *Transactions and Studies of the College of Physicians of Philadelphia* 14 (March 1992): 37–40.

16. Fred Davis, *Passage through Crisis: Polio Victims and Their Families* (Indianapolis, IN: Bobbs-Merrill, 1963), 35, 37–38, and 39, respectively. Shell's (*Polio and Its Aftermath*) entire chapter entitled "In the Family" represents an excellent literary analysis of the impact of polio on the household, and that impact proved profound; see especially p. 67. See also Gareth Williams, *Paralyzed with Fear: The Story of Polio* (New York: Palgrave Macmillan, 2013): 63–65.
17. Anne is quoted by Bruno, *The Polio Paradox*: 63.
18. Davis, *Passage through Crisis*. The father is quoted on p. 41. Refer as well to pp. 33, 35, and 37–38. Silver and Wilson, in *Polio Voices*, assert that polio left an indelible mark: the family was never the same. See p. 62 for their discussion.
19. O'Connor in Silver and Wilson, *Polio Voices*: 72–73.
20. Bruno, in *The Polio Paradox*, quotes two respondents to his survey on pp. 86–87; refer also to pp. 66, 87–88, and 189. Silver and Wilson also have accounts in their extensive oral history collection, *Polio Voices*; Cote's experience can be found on pp. 63–64 and Meehan's on p. 73. Also, for context on family violence, see Gordon, *Heroes of Their Own Lives*: 174.
21. Peg Kehret, *Small Steps: The Year I Got Polio* Morton Grove, IL: Albert Whitman and Company, 1996): 29; Davis in Thomas M. Daniel and Frederick C. Robbins (eds.), *Polio* (Rochester, NY: University of Rochester Press, 1997): 29; Susan Richards Shreve, *Warm Springs: Traces of a Childhood at FDR's Polio Haven* (Boston: Houghton Mifflin Company, 2007): 30 and 139, respectively. See also pp. 155–56.
22. Shreve, *Warm Springs*: 45–46. The italics are in the original text. See also Leonard Kriegel, *The Long Walk Home: An Adventure in Survival* (New York: Appleton-Century, 1964): 110–111.
23. Shreve, *Warm Springs*: 153–54. The italics are in the original.
24. Shell, *Polio and Its Aftermath*: 75.
25. Ellen Whelan Coughlin, "Parental Attitudes Toward Handicapped Children," *Child* 6 (1941): 41, 42, and 43, respectively. The cohort she studied consisted of 51 children with physical disabilities, ranging in age from five to twenty. Thirty-four of them were adolescents, 11 of whom were female and 2 African American. Nine had been disabled since birth, while the remaining 42 had become disabled because of an illness, usually because of polio. For child abandonment, also refer to Bruno, *The Polio Paradox*: 86. See Daniel J. Wilson, *Living with Polio: The Epidemic and Its Survivors* (Chicago: University of Chicago Press, 2005), Chapter 6, for a comprehensive treatment; his scope encompasses adults and children disabled by polio.
26. McDaniel to Flexner, March 7, 1912, Microfilm Roll Reel #92, Simon Flexner Papers, Rockefeller University Archives (RAC).
27. Barbara Welter, "The Cult of True Womanhood: 1820–1860," *American Quarterly* 18 (1966), 151–74, introduced me to the notion and experience of the women's sphere. Subsequent historiography has expanded women's roles as well as refined the domestic model of interpretation. According to Carol Ruth Berkin and Mary Beth Norton (*Women of America: A History* [Boston: Houghton Mifflin Company, 1979]), the "women's sphere" perspective represents a limited, one-dimensional analysis of women's roles (139–49). But Gerda Lerner, in her 1979 classic, *The Majority Finds Its Past: Placing Women in History* (New York: Oxford University Press, 1979), pp. 10–13, maps a complex historiographical agenda that takes into account the multiple roles of women. She recommends six fruitful areas of study for social historians, two of which clearly apply to this

context. First, women maintained hitherto hidden roles. During the past thirty years, many of these have been addressed, such as "teachers" and "civilizers," but others remain obfuscated, such as "the family's healer" or "nurse." Second, Lerner raises the issue of how to properly assess these achievements (pp. 10–13). Also see Lerner, p. 130. Finally, consult Sharla M. Fett, *Working Cures: Healing, Health, and Power on Southern Slave Plantations* (Chapel Hill: University of North Carolina Press, 2002): 118–20.

28. Samuel H. Preston and Michael R. Haines, *Fatal Years: Child Mortality in Late Nineteenth-Century America* (Princeton: University of Princeton Press, 1991): 12.
29. Nancy Tomes, *The Gospel of Germs: Men, Women, and the Microbe in American Life* (Cambridge: Harvard University Press, 1998): 146. These specific preventatives against polio can be found in a two-sided pamphlet published by the New York City Department of Health (hereafter cited as NYCDH), *Infantile Paralysis in Dangerous D* (New York: NYCDH, 1916 [NYCMA]). By all accounts, public health officials targeted maternal parents in matters of health. Since the home represented the woman's domain, prevention and care served as her responsibilities. See, among others, Barbara Bates, *Bargaining for Life: A Social History of Tuberculosis, 1876–1938* (Philadelphia: University of Pennsylvania Press, 1992): 234.
30. DiBona in Silver and Wilson, *Polio Voices*: 19.
31. NYCDH, *Circular of Information Regarding Acute Poliomyelitis (Infantile Paralysis): Information for the Public* (New York: NYCDH, 1913): 6–7; NYCDH issued an identical pamphlet the following year: *Circular of Information Regarding Acute Poliomyelitis (Infantile Paralysis): Information for the Public* (New York: NYCDH, 1914) (both NYCMA). See also J. N. Hays, *The Burdens of Disease: Epidemics and Human Response in Western History* (New Brunswick: Rutgers University Press, 1998): 165, 263; Preston and Haines, *Fatal Years*: 8; Naomi Rogers, *Dirt and Disease: Polio Before FDR* (New Brunswick, NJ: Rutgers University Press, 1996): 16.
32. National Foundation for Infantile Paralysis, *A Guide for Parents in the Nursing Care of Patients with Infantile Paralysis in the Home* (New York: NFIP, 1944): 5–9 (NYAM).
33. National Organization for Public Health Nursing (NOPHN) and National League of Nursing Education (NLNE), *Nursing for the Poliomyelitis Patient* (New York: NOPHN and NLNE, 1948): 76. See also pp. 32, 42, and 77. This booklet represented the authoritative guide to nursing care for "polios." Originally published in 1940, subsequent editions appeared in 1944 and 1948.
34. Seavey, Smith, and Wagner, *A Paralyzing Fear*: 262. Refer to p. 253 as well.
35. Jessie L. Stevenson, *The Nursing Care of Patients with Infantile Paralysis*, The National Organization for Public Health Nursing (New York: NFIP, 1940): 15–16, 28, and 33, respectively. Refer also to pp. 31–32, and 48–49 (NYAM). This 58-page guide, intended for public health nurses, maintained a comprehensive and detailed scope. See also Margarete Sandelowski, "Making the Best of Things: Technology in American Nursing, 1870–1940," *Nursing History Review* 5 (1997): 3–32.
36. Stone in Edmund J. Sass, George Gottfried, and Anthony Sorem, *Polio's Legacy: An Oral History* (Lanham, MD: University Press of America, 1996): 176–77.
37. Naomi Rogers, *Polio Wars: Sister Kenny and the Golden Age of American Medicine* (New York: Oxford University Press, 2014): 167 and 159, respectively.
38. Davis in Daniel and Robbins, *Polio*: 30–31.
39. Rogers, *Polio Wars*: 159. Emphasis is in the original.

40. Charles E. Rosenberg, *The Care of Strangers: The Rise of America's Hospital System* (Baltimore: Johns Hopkins University Press, 1987): 244 and 261, respectively. Also consult pp. 237 and 245–46.
41. Dominik in Sass, Gottfried, and Sorem, *Polio's Legacy*: 173. See also p. 71.
42. Grant, "Medical Social Work in an Epidemic of Poliomyelitis": 707.
43. Kehret, *Small Steps*: 35 and 37–38; Handel in Silver and Wilson, *Polio Voices*: 46–48; Joseph Greenblum, "The Control of Sick-Care Functions in the Hospitalization of a Child: Family versus Hospital," *Journal of Health and Human Behavior* 2 (Spring 1961): 32–38.
44. Schwartz in Sass, Gottfried, and Sorem, *Polio's Legacy*: 148. See Joel D. Howell, "Hospitals," in Roger Cooter and John Pickstone (eds.), *Medicine in the Twentieth Century* (Australia: Harwood Academic Publishers, 2000): 508.
45. Refer to the short oral testimony of Ernest Greenberg, an anesthesiologist employed in hospitals in Westchester County, New York, during the early 1950s, in Silver and Wilson, *Polio Voices*: 56. See also Shreve, *Warm Springs*: 155–56. Joe Jamelka's story can be found in Jason Chu Lee, "Poliomyelitis in the Lone Star State: A Brief Examination in Rural and Urban Communities" (MA thesis, Texas State University-San Marcos, 2005): 11, while Becker's recollection is in Gould, *A Summer Plague*: 290. See also Mee, *A Nearly Normal Life*: 33; Gullickson in Sass, Gottfried, and Sorem, *Polio's Legacy*: 40 and 42.
46. Phillips to Flexner, December 4, 1919, and a written response from Amoss to Phillips, December 11, 1919, Poliomyelitis Cases, Microfilm, Roll #90, Simon Flexner Papers, Rockefeller Institute for Medical Research (RAC).
47. *Report of the Department of Health of the City of Chicago for the Years of 1911 to 1918 Inclusive*: 179 and 211–13 (CPL).
48. Stevenson, *Nursing Care of Patients with Infantile Paralysis*: 47.
49. NFIP, *Guide for Parents in the Nursing Care of Patients with Infantile Paralysis in the Home*: 10–21.
50. Van Cleve in Sass, Gottfried, and Sorem, *Polio's Legacy*: 184; refer to page 71 as well. See also Mary Grimley Mason, *Life Prints: A Memoir of Healing and Discovery* (New York: Feminist Press, 2000): 16, 22; Shreve, *Warm Springs*: 37.
51. Vickery in Silver and Wilson, *Polio Voices*: 44.
52. Stevenson, *Nursing Care of Patients with Infantile Paralysis*: 44. See p. 9 as well.
53. Howard in Seavey, Smith, and Wagner, *A Paralyzing Fear*: 39–42. Refer also to Bruno, *The Polio Paradox*: 83; Williams, *Paralyzed with Fear*: 60–62.
54. Linda Eisenmann, "A Time of Quiet Activism: Research, Practice, and Policy in American Women's Higher Education, 1945–1965," *History of Education Quarterly* 45 (Spring 2005): 8–9; refer to p. 1 as well. Eisenmann's conclusions, although focused on educators, certainly encompass women involved in the Mothers' Marches: "In hindsight, the educators of the 1950s and the 1960s may seem gratuitously meek and self-effacing. In comparison to later efforts, their activism can appear unnecessarily limited and too adaptive. Yet, the nature of the advocacy practiced by the postwar educators suited itself to the opportunities and the thinking of an era filled with ambivalence about how women should balance home with career, community work with national service, and personal fulfillment with societal expectations" (17).
55. The loudspeaker slogan is quoted on p. 99 in Janice Flood Nichols, *Twin Voices: A Memoir of Polio, the Forgotten Killer* (Bloomington, IN: iUniverse, Inc., 2007). See also Lee, "Poliomyelitis in the Lone Star State": 49; David M. Oshinsky, *Polio: An American Story* (New York: Oxford University Press, 2005): 87–88; Daniel J. Wilson, *Polio* (Santa Barbara, CA: Greenwood Press, 2009): 47.

56. Oshinsky, *Polio*: 86–87; see also pp. 85 and 87–90. See also MOD, Medical Programs Records, Series 9: Human Resources, Biographical Data, Elaine Whitelaw, 1947–1992; Nichols, *Twin Voices*: 101; David W. Rose, *Images of America: March of Dimes* (Charleston, SC: Arcadia Publishing, 2003): 9, 16, 23, 43.
57. Charles Massey in Seavey, Smith, and Wagner, *A Paralyzing Fear*: 91. Also see p. 85. For another participant's view of these porch-light campaigns, refer to Ardean Marting, general chair of the mother's march on polio for San Diego County in 1951, in Seavey, Smith, and Wagner, *A Paralyzing Fear*: 81. See also Oshinsky, *Polio*: 87–90.
58. Stephen E. Mawdsley, "Polio and Prejudice: Charles Hudson Bynaum and the Racial Politics of the National Foundation for Infantile Paralysis, 1938–1954" (MA thesis, University of Alberta, 2008): 84–85. See also pp. 68–69.
59. Roy Porter, *The Greatest Benefit to Mankind: A Medical History of Humanity* (New York: Norton, 1997): 694–95; Nichols, *Twin Voices*: 103.
60. Mrs. Read is quoted on p. 100 in Nichols, *Twin Voices*. See also pp. 101 and 103.
61. Davis, *Passage through Crisis*: 126–128. See also Hugh Gregory Gallagher in Seavey, Smith, and Wagner, *A Paralyzing Fear*: 59.
62. Silver and Wilson, *Polio Voices*: 59.
63. Dixon is quoted in an editorial, "The Poliomyelitis Germ," *New York Times*, October 22, 1911, Section I: 14. A similar observation regarding siblings is asserted in "Infantile Paralysis Is a Dust Disease," *New York Times*, October 11, 1911: 3.
64. Durr in Silver and Wilson, *Polio Voices*: 65.
65. Seavey, Smith, and Wagner, *A Paralyzing Fear*: 30–31; Mason, *Life Prints*: 4–5.
66. The father is quoted on p. 125 in Davis, *Passage through Crisis*. Other quotes are, in order, on pp. 120–21 and 128. See also pp. 129–30.
67. Van Cleve in Sass, Gottfried, and Sorem, *Polio's Legacy*: 188–189.
68. Kellogg in Silver and Wilson, *Polio Voices*: 65. Consult also Shell, *Polio and Its Aftermath*: 80.
69. Diamond in Silver and Wilson, *Polio Voices*: 69. Also refer to p. 25.
70. Robert C. Huse, *Getting There: Growing Up with Polio in the 30's* (Bloomington, IN: 1stBooks, 2002): 8.
71. Rugh in Silver and Wilson, *Polio Voices*: 63.
72. Shreve, *Warm Springs*: 77; Diane Zemke, *Polio: A Special Ride?* (Minnetonka, MN: Diagnostic Center of Learning Patterns, Inc., 1997): 10–11.
73. Anne Finger, *Elegy for A Disease: A Personal and Cultural History of Polio* (New York: St. Martin's Press, 2006): 168; refer to p. 163 as well. Jacqueline Foertsch, in *Bracing Accounts: The Literature and Culture of Polio in Postwar America* (Teaneck, NJ: Farleigh Dickinson University Press, 2008), describes Finger's father as a "mentally unbalanced family tyrant" (62), surely the "most abusive father" portrayed in any memoir (62). Foertsch also shares some of the same quotes from Finger on p. 62.
74. Nichols, *Twin Voices*: 126 and 151, respectively. Italics are in the original. See pp. 30–31, 34–35, and 122 as well. The 1951 report is discussed in Bruno, *The Polio Paradox*: 50.
75. Both descriptions can be found in the oral history collection by Silver and Wilson, *Polio Voices*; Durr is on p. 82 and Esau on p. 42. See also Bruno, *The Polio Paradox*: 83.
76. Sass, Gottfried, and Sorem, *Polio's Legacy*: 58.
77. Kehret, *Small Steps*: 92 and 117–118. See also p. 116.
78. Mee, *A Nearly Normal Life*: 121; Kriegel, *Long Walk Home*: 129; Robert Lovering, *Out of the Darkness: Coping with Disability* (Phoenix, AZ: Associated Rehabilitation Counseling Specialists, 1993): 82; Nichols, *Twin Voices*: 83–84.

79. Davis in Daniel and Robbins, *Polio*: 36; Rogers in Seavey, Smith, and Wagner, *A Paralyzing Fear*: 30; Esau in Silver and Wilson, *Polio Voices*: 43; Kehret, *Small Steps*: 117; Huse, *Getting There*: 10; Nichols, *Twin Voices*: 72.
80. Richard Sennett, in *Families Against the City: Middle Class Homes of Industrial Chicago, 1872–1890* (New York: Vintage Books, 1974), pp. 62–68, provides an insightful theoretical framework that concisely addresses the nuclear family's intimate size, division of labor and spatial specialization, need to extend maturation, and significance of privacy (62–68). For Davis's experiences, refer to Daniel and Robbins, *Polio*: 31. *The New York Times* nonchalantly used its daily columns to advertise these names and addresses throughout July and August; for examples, see "Arrest in Hundreds to Check Infant Paralysis," *New York Times*, July 11, 1916: 1, and "Paralysis Increase Quickened by Heat," *New York Times*, August 7, 1916: 16. For Houston's practice, see Lee, "Poliomyelitis in the Lone Star State": 103.
81. Sass, Gottfried, and Sorem, *Polio's Legacy*: 59.
82. Regina Woods, *Tales from Inside the Iron Lung (and How I Got Out of It)*, with a forward by David E. Rogers, MD (Philadelphia: University of Pennsylvania Press, 1994): 2, 93.
83. Kangas's and Van Cleve's recollections are in Sass, Gottfried, and Sorem, *Polio's Legacy*, pp. 63 and 183, respectively. For these homebound instructional programs, refer to *Report to the Stockholders: Annual Statement of the General Superintendent Chicago Public Schools, 1951–52* (Chicago, 1952): 21 (CPL); Frischer in Daniel and Robbins, *Polio*: 71; *Annual Report of the Superintendent of the Pittsburgh Public Schools, 1949–50* (Pittsburgh: Board of Public Education 1950): 22 (CLP); Mee, *A Nearly Normal Life*: 153–54; Huse, *Getting There*: 15.
84. Paul K. Longmore and Lauri Umansky (eds.), *The New Disability History: American Perspectives* (New York: New York University Press, 2001): 7–8. Wilson, as previously noted in "A Crippling Fear," is more direct (467).
85. Alan Derickson, *Health Security for All: Dreams of Universal Health Care in America* (Baltimore: Johns Hopkins Press, 2005): 16–20. Dickerson quotes the commission on page 19.
86. Derickson, *Health Security for All*: 44; refer also to pp. 41–43 and 47. See also Nichols, *Twin Voices*: 66.
87. Derickson, *Health Security for All*: 52; Nancy Tomes, "Merchants of Health: Medicine and Consumer Culture in the United States, 1900–1940," *Journal of American History* 88 (September 2001): 529–30.
88. Wilson, *Living with Polio*: 483. However, Silver and Wilson, in *Polio Voices*, state that in 1940 "only 9.3 percent of the population had hospital insurance and only 4 percent had surgical insurance" (61). See also Grant, "Medical Social Work in an Epidemic of Poliomyelitis": 693, 701–02, and 705.
89. Derickson, *Health Security for All*: 113–14.
90. Silver and Wilson, *Polio Voices*: 61. Refer also to Wilson, *Living with Polio*: 466 and 483–484; Heather Green Wooten, *The Polio Years in Texas: Battling a Terrifying Unknown* (College Station: Texas A&M University Press, 2009): 85. For additional historical background on health insurance in the United States, refer to Jill Quadagno, *One Nation Uninsured: Why the U.S. Has No National Health Insurance* (New York: Oxford University Press, 2005), who corroborates Wilson's postwar figure, with only 22 percent of Americans covered by private medical insurers by 1946 (44); also refer to pp. 48–52. See also Nichols, *Twin Voices*: 103.

NOTES AND SOURCES   237

91. Rogers in Sass, Gottfried, and Sorem, *Polio's Legacy*: 57; Edward D. Berkowitz, "Rehabilitation: The Federal Government's Response to Disability, 1935–1954" (1976, reprinted New York: Arno Press, 1980: 7.
92. Davis, *Passage through Crisis*: 110–111; Shell, *Polio and Its Aftermath*: 68.
93. Kangas in Sass, Gottfried, and Sorem, *Polio's Legacy*: 65.
94. Amy L. Fairchild, Ronald Bayer, and James Colgrove, *Searching Eyes: The State, and Disease Surveillance in America* (Berkeley: University of California Press, 2007): 150; also see pp. 148–49 and 151. See also Porter, *Greatest Benefit to Mankind*: 646–47.
95. Lee, "Poliomyelitis in the Lone Star State": 79.
96. Daniel J. Wilson, "A Crippling Fear: Experiencing Polio in the Era of FDR," *Bulletin of History of Medicine* 72 (1998): 466, 483–84, 485; the last quote in this paragraph is on p. 484. For information about Warm Springs and the NFIP, see Gallagher, *FDR's Splendid Deception,* and Rose, *Images of America*. See also Fairchild, Bayer, and Colgrove, *Searching Eyes*: 151; Sass, Gottfried, and Sorem, *Polio's Legacy*: 73; Wooten, *Polio Years in Texas*: 85.
97. Davis, *Passage through Crisis*: 39 and 66, respectively; Schwartz in Seavey, Smith, and Wagner, *A Paralyzing Fear*:257; Kangas in Sass, Gottfried, and Sorem, *Polio's Legacy*: 64. Refer also to pp. 54 and 57.
98. Esau's recollection is on p. 42 while McKnight's is on p. 68 of Silver and Wilson, *Polio Voices*.
99. Edith Powell and John F. Hume, *A Black Oasis: Tuskegee Institute's Fight Against Infantile Paralysis, 1941–1975* (copyright, 2008): 58. Refer also to pp. 59–60 and 141.
100. Derickson, *Health Security for All*: 52. Also consult Jacqueline Foertsch, "'Heads, You Win': Newsletters and Magazine of the Polio Nation," *Disability Studies Quarterly* 27 (Summer 2007): 2, 4 (www.dsq-sds.org, accessed January 5, 2012).
101. "Day Shows 12 Dead by Infant Paralysis," *New York Times,* July 2, 1916: 6; "Warning Against Nostrums," *New York Times*, July 28, 1916: 5.
102. Dominik in Sass, Gottfried, and Sorem, *Polio's Legacy*: 172.
103. Lynette Iezzoni, *Influenza 1918: The Worst Epidemic in American History* (New York: TV Books, 1999): 17, 73–74, 119–20.
104. Porter, *Greatest Benefit to Mankind*: 389.
105. Anne Taylor Kirschmann, *A Vital Force: Women in American Homeopathy* (New Brunswick, NJ: Rutgers University Press, 2004).
106. Paul Starr, *The Social Transformation of American Medicine* (New York: Basic Books, 1982): 47–48.
107. Anne Hunsaker Hawkins, *Reconstructing Illness: Studies in Pathography* (West Lafayette, IN: Purdue University Press, 1993): 126–28.
108. Fett, *Working Cures*: 62.
109. Regina Morantz-Sanchez, *Sympathy and Science: Women Physicians in American Medicine* (Chapel Hill: North Carolina University Press, 2000): 11–12. Refer also to p. 17.
110. Kirschmann, *A Vital Force*: 7; also see pp. 119–20. See also Starr, *The Social Transformation of American Medicine*: 48–49 and 50–51.
111. Williams, *Paralyzed with Fear*: 255.
112. Kriegel, *Long Walk Home*: 144–47; Lee, "Poliomyelitis in the Lone Star State:" 70–71; Tomes, "Merchants of Health": 534–35; Williams, *Paralyzed with Fear*: 255.

113. Kangas in Sass, Gottfried, and Sorem, *Polio's Legacy*: 64. See also Oshinsky, *Polio*: 61–64; Shell, *Polio and Its Aftermath*: 63–64.
114. Davis, *Passage through Crisis*: 84–85, 94, and 95, respectively. Consult also pp. 83, 86–87, and 90–92. Davis provides wonderful insight into the struggle of one mother's gradual emotional adjustment (which I tap here), by providing oral testimony at periods of two and six weeks and four, eight, and fifteen months. Marvin's mother is quoted on pp. 96–97.
115. Mia Farrow, *What Falls Away: A Memoir* (New York: Nan A. Talese, 1997): 6. See also Huse, *Getting There*: 114–15; Rogers in Sass, Gottfried, and Sorem, *Polio's Legacy*, : 59; Mee, *A Nearly Normal Life*: 105–108; Sink, *The Grit Behind the Miracle*: 116; Louis Sternburg and Dorothy Sternburg, *View from the Seesaw* (New York: Dodd, Mead & Company, 1986): 90.
116. Kriegel, *Falling into Life*: 195.
117. Alice in Kehret, *Small Steps*: 75. For Kehret's description, see pp. 105–106. Refer also to pp. 60–98.
118. Woods, *Tales from Inside the Iron Lung*: 104.

Chapter 6

1. Peg Kehret, *Small Steps: The Year I Got Polio* (Morton Grove, IL: 1996): 67–68.
2. John R. Paul, *A History of Poliomyelitis* (New Haven: Yale University Press, 1971): 4.
3. Leonard Kriegel, "Uncle Tom and Tiny Tim: Some Reflections on the Cripple as Negro," *American Scholar* (Summer 1969): 417.
4. Tracie C. Harrison and Alexa Stuifbergen, "A Hermeneutic Phenomenological Analysis of Aging with a Childhood Onset Disability," *Health Care for Women International* 26 (September 2005): 737.
5. Daniel J. Wilson, in *Living with Polio: The Epidemic and Its Survivors* (Chicago: University of Chicago Press, 2005), offers a rare, but limited, glimpse into the world of students disabled by polio (179–89).
6. *John A. Watson City v. City of Cambridge*, 157 Mass. 561 (1893); *State ex. Rel. Beattie v. Board of Education of City of Antigo*, 176 Wisc. 231 (1919).
7. Robert C. Huse, *Getting There: Growing Up with Polio in the 30's* (Bloomington, IN: 1stBooks: 2002): 142; Davis in Thomas M. Daniel and Frederick C. Robbins (eds.), *Polio* (Rochester, NY: University of Rochester Press, 1997): 37; Susan Richards Shreve, *Warm Springs: Traces of a Childhood at FDR's Polio Haven* (Boston: Houghton Mifflin Company, 2007): 32; Mia Farrow, *What Falls Away: A Memoir* (New York: Nan A. Talese, 1997): 7; Yelder in Nina Gilden Seavey, Jane S. Smith, and Paul Wagner, *A Paralyzing Fear: The Triumph Over Polio in America* (New York: TV Books, 1998): 153–54, 156. For the widely used policy of relocating classes on the first floor, refer to Davis, *Passage through Crisis*: 87, as well as Robert Gurney in Edmund J. Sass, George Gottfried, and Anthony Sorem, *Polio's Legacy: An Oral History* (Lanham, MD: University Press of America, 1996): 27.
8. Alice Sink, *The Grit Behind the Miracle: A True Story of the Determination and Hard Work Behind an Emergency Infantile Paralysis Hospital, 1944–1945, Hickory, North Carolina* (Lanham, MD: University Press of America, 1998): 106.
9. Regina Woods, *Tales from Inside the Iron Lung (and How I Got Out of It)* (Philadelphia: University of Pennsylvania Press, 1994): 100. Refer also to pp. 1 and 10–11.

10. Owen in Seavey, Smith, and Wagner, *A Paralyzing Fear*: 236. Also see p. 241.
11. Brutger in Sass, Gottfried, and Sorem, *Polio's Legacy*, 73, 74, 75; Frischer in Daniel and Robbins, *Polio*: 72.
12. Huse, *Getting There*: 77–79 and 142, respectively. See also pp. 51–53, 140, and 143.
13. Kangas in Sass, Gottfried, and Sorem, *Polio's Legacy*: 65. Refer also to Reinette Lovewell Donnelly, "Watch Your Steps," *Polio Chronicle* Vol. 2, No. 7 (February 1933): 3–4 (RWSIR). In this Warm Springs newsletter, the author promotes the use of ramps in churches, colleges, government buildings, libraries, railway stations, and schools, recommending an 8 percent grade for a ten-foot ramp. Clearly individuals with disabilities knew of the need for such accommodations very early.
14. Owen in Sass, Gottfried, and Sorem, *Polio's Legacy*: 33; the second quote by him can be found in Seavey, Smith, and Wagner *A Paralyzing Fear*: 241. See Sharon Barnartt and Richard Scotch, *Disability Protests: Contentious Politics, 1970–1999* (Washington, DC: Gallaudet University Press, 2001), as well as Sass, Gottfried, and Sorem, *Polio's Legacy*: 53, for more information about school experiences.
15. Schwartz in Seavey, Smith, and Wagner, *A Paralyzing Fear*: 263.
16. This student is quoted in Richard L. Bruno, *The Polio Paradox: Understanding and Treating "Post-Polio Syndrome" and Chronic Fatigue* (New York: Warner Books, 2002): 84.
17. Davis, *Passage through Crisis*: 87; Kehret, *Small Steps*: 117.
18. Shreve, *Warm Springs*: 34–35; Harrison and Stuifbergen, "A Hermeneutic Phenomenological Analysis of Aging with a Childhood Onset Disability": 737.
19. Marc Shell, *Polio and Its Aftermath: The Paralysis of Culture* (Cambridge: Harvard University Press, 2005): 93.
20. Johnson in Sass, Smith, and Wagner, *Polio's Legacy*: 86.
21. Sharon L. Snyder and David T. Mitchell, *Cultural Locations of Disability* (Chicago: University of Chicago Press, 2006): 80. They add, on the same page, that the "physical body provided empirical evidence of an otherwise intangible disorder of the interior."
22. The information in these three paragraphs is summarized from David Manzo and Elizabeth C. Peters, *Cotting School* (Charleston, SC: Arcadia Publishing, 2008): 10, 8, and 10 again, respectively; consult also pp. 2, 7–8, 11, 13–14, 16–17, 24–28, 37–40, 48, and 78–79. See Barry M. Franklin's Chapter 4, "Private Philanthropy and the Education of Children," in *"Backwardness" to "At-Risk": Childhood Learning Difficulties and the Contradictions of School Reform* (Albany: State University of New York Press, 1994), for other examples.
23. Claire H. Liachowitz, *Disability as a Social Construct: Legislative Roots* (Philadelphia: University of Pennsylvania Press, 1988): 13, 14, 99–100. See also pp. 4 and 15. For additional context, refer to Franklin, *"Backwardness" to "At-Risk"*: 6–7; Robert L. Osgood, *For "Children Who Vary from the Normal Type": Special Education in Boston, 1838–1930* (Washington, DC: Gallaudet University Press, 2000); and Joseph L. Tropea, "Bureaucratic Order and Special Children: Urban Schools, 1890s–1940s," *History of Education Quarterly* 27 (Spring 1987): 29–53.
24. Margaret Winzer, *The History of Special Education: From Isolation to Integration* (Washington, DC: Gallaudet University Press, 1993): 331–32, 367.
25. Edith Reeves Solenberger, *Public School Classes for Crippled Children*, Department of the Interior, Bureau of Education, Bulletin No. 10 (Washington, DC: Government Printing Office, 1918): 27. See also pp. 13, 15, 16, 26, 30–33, and 39.

26. *Sixty-Fourth Annual Report of the Board of Education for the 1917–18 School Year* (Chicago, 1918): 269, 173, 271, 277, and 283, respectively. Refer also to pp. 269, 275–76, and 280–82 (CPL). Also see Shell, *Polio and Its Aftermath*: 99.
27. *Annual Report of the Superintendent of Schools for the 1938–39 School Year* (Chicago: 1939): 269, 173, 271, 277, and 283, respectively. Refer also to pp. 269, 275–76, and 280–82 (CPL).
28. *Sixty-Sixth Annual Report of the Board of Education of the City of Chicago for the 1930–31 School Year* (Chicago, 1931). No pagination appeared in this photocopy of the original report. See also *Annual Report of the Superintendent of Schools for the 1938–39 School Year* (Chicago, 1939): 275 (CPL). Also see Solenberger, *Public School Classes for Crippled Children*: 13 and 41.
29. Charles L. Mee, *A Nearly Normal Life* (Boston: Little, Brown & Co., 1999): 91.
30. Solenberger, *Public School Classes for Crippled Children*: 8, 11, 25, and 27, respectively. Also refer to pp. 10, 12, 22, 26, 30–33, and 39.
31. Liachowitz, *Disability as a Social Construct*: 103; Davis, *Passage through Crisis*: 93 and 149; Garland Thomson, *Extraordinary Bodies*: 23.
32. Paul K. Longmore and David Goldberger, "The League of the Physically Handicapped and the Great Depression: A Case Study in the New Disability History," *Journal of American History* 87 (December 2000): 893–894; Charlton Wallace, "Education of the Crippled Child." *Archives of Pediatrics* 27 (1910), in William R. F. Phillips and Janet Rosenberg (eds.), *The Origins of Modern Treatment and Education of Physically Handicapped Children* (New York: Arno Press, 1980): 345.
33. Winzer, *History of Special Education*: 370.
34. Diane Zemke, *Polio: A Special Ride?* (Minnetonka, MN: Diagnostic Center of Learning Patterns, Inc., 1997): 12.
35. Kehret, *Small Steps*: 166. Refer also to pp. 169–70. For Pugleasa's experience, refer to Seavey, Smith, and Wagner, *A Paralyzing Fear*: 128.
36. Rosemarie Garland Thomson, "Seeing the Disabled: Visual Rhetorics of Disability in Popular Photography," in Paul K. Longmore and Lauri Umansky (eds.), *The New Disability History: American Perspectives* (New York: New York University Press, 2001): 346–47. Also refer to Daniel J. Wilson, "A Crippling Fear: Experiencing Polio in the Era of FDR," *Bulletin of the History of Medicine* 72 (1998): 487.
37. Kriegel, *Long Walk Home*: 131–32 and 141, respectively. See also p. 137.
38. Bruno quotes James on p. 81 of *Polio Paradox*. Refer also to Davis, *Passage through Crisis*, 139, 140, 141, 143, 144, 145, 147, and 151. "Normals" is quoted on p. 140.
39. Mary Grimley Mason, *Life Prints: A Memoir of Healing and Discovery* (New York: Feminist Press, 2000): 3.
40. Huse, *Getting There*: 14.
41. Headley in Tony Gould, *A Summer Plague: Polio and Its Survivors* (New Haven: Yale University Press, 1995): 295. Also see Gail Bias in Sass, Gottfried, and Sorem, *Polio's Legacy*: 80.
42. Robert F. Murphy, *The Body Silent: The Different World of the Disabled* (New York: W. W. Norton, 1990): 86–87, 85, 110–11, and 108, respectively.
43. Joanna Bourke, *Dismembering the Male: Men's Bodies, Britain, and the Great War* (Chicago: University of Chicago Press, 1996): 13. For a fine analysis of how the schools explicitly socialized females and males, consult David Tyack and Elisabeth Hansot, *Learning Together: A History of Coeducation in American Public Schools* (New Haven: Yale University Press, 1990).

44. Thomas J. Gerschick and Adam S. Miller, "Coming to Terms: Masculinity and Physical Disability," in Donald F. Sabo and David F. Gordon (eds.), *Men's Health and Illnesses: Gender, Power, and the Body* (Thousand Oaks, CA: Sage, 1995): 185, 183, and 184, respectively. See also Bourke, *Dismembering the Male*: 11; Paul K. Longmore, *Why I Burned My Book and Other Essays on Disability*, edited by Robert Dawidoff (Philadelphia: Temple University Press, 2003): 11.

45. F. Scott Fitzgerald, *Flappers and Philosophers* (Champaign, IL: Book Jungle, undated): 7, 27, 29. Refer also to pp. 55 and 67.

46. James R. McGovern, "The American Woman's Pre-World War I Freedom in Manners and Morals," in Jean E. Friedman and William G. Shade (eds.), *Our American Sisters: Women in American Life and Thought* (Lexington, MA: D. C. Heath & Co., 1982): 480–82 and 484, respectively. See also pp. 487–88. The fashion commentator's observations are quoted on p. 486. McGovern engages this topic through a historiographic lens. Historians, to a certain extent, have debated the emergence of twentieth-century femininity. One school of thought has emphasized this as a postwar phenomenon (i.e., a sudden break with the past), while another has asserted that this transformation occurred more gradually, with early signs appearing with the Progressive Era, namely the very early 1900s (479–81).

47. Angela J. Latham, *Posing a Threat: Flappers, Chorus Girls, and Other Brazen Performers* (Hanover, NH: University Press of New England, 2000): 11 and 21, respectively. See also pp. 7, 20–21, 50, and 54–55.

48. Joshua Zeitz, in *Flapper: A Madcap Story of Sex, Style, Celebrity, and the Women Who Made America Modern* (New York: Three Rivers Press, 2006), seems to provide a more complex side of the flapper phenomenon, weaving it into that period's fashions, literature, music, and religious morality. Refer also to Paul K. Longmore and Paul Steven Miller, "'A Philosophy of Handicap': The Origins of Randolph Bourne's Radicalism," *Radical History Review* 94 (Winter 2006): 65.

49. Latham, *Posing a Threat*: 7, 96, 2, 88, and 90, respectively. Also see p. 3.

50. Mary Ryan, "The Projection of a New Womanhood: The Movie Moderns in the 1920s," in Friedman and Shade (eds.), *Our American Sisters*: 501, 508, 511, and 501, respectively. Refer also to pp. 500, 506, and 509–10. Also consult a fascinating film produced and directed by Laurie Block, *Fit: Episodes in the History of the Body* (Conway, MA: Straight Ahead Films, Inc., 1999).

51. Latham, *Posing a Threat*: 103 and 11, respectively. Also refer to p. 88. Joe Grixti, in "Desirability and Its Discontents: Young People's Responses to Media Images of Health, Beauty and Physical Perfection" (in Peter L. Twohig and Vera Kalitzkus [eds.], *Social Studies of Health, Illness and Disease: Perspectives from the Social Sciences and Humanities* [Amsterdam: Rodopi, 2008]), offers an in-depth analysis of this phenomenon; although he examines it in a more recent context, the social construction process and its outcomes remain the same (58–59).

52. Latham, *Posing a Threat*: 110, 126, and 127–28, respectively; also see pp. 101, 103, and 105. See also Zeitz, *Flapper*: 233, 261–62, and 265.

53. Rosemarie Garland Thomson, "Feminist Disability Studies," *Signs* 30 (Winter 2005): 1560.

54. Johnson in Gould, *A Summer Plague*: 278. The "neutered" quote can be found on p. 219, while Walker's recollections are on p. 284. Consult also Shell, *Polio and Its Aftermath*: 163–64.

55. Garland Thomson, *Extraordinary Bodies*: 25 and 27. See also Amy Rutstein-Riley, "Shifting Views of Self: Impact of Chronic Illness Diagnosis on Young

Emerging Adult Women," in Peter L. Twohig and Vera Kalitzkus (eds.), *Social Studies of Health, Illness and Disease: Perspectives from the Social Sciences and Humanities* (Amsterdam: Rodopi, 2008): 23. Jacqueline Foertsch, in *Bracing Accounts: The Literature and Culture of Polio in Postwar America* (Teaneck, NJ: Farleigh Dickinson University Press, 2008), provides a fine analysis of narratives by female authors (68–72).

56. Kehret, *Small Steps*: 57. She was not alone in feeling this way. Beatrice Yvonne Nau, who contracted polio at age 14 in Bremen, Kentucky, in 1943, maintained a hopeless outlook about marriage. Her experiences have been included in Julie Silver and Daniel Wilson, *Polio Voices: An Oral History from the American Polio Epidemics and Worldwide Eradication Efforts* (Westport, CT: Praeger, 2007): 46 and 67.
57. Frischer in Daniel and Robbins, *Polio*: 73.
58. Balbar in Silver and Wilson, *Polio Voices*: 66; Shell, *Polio and Its Aftermath*: 68 and 70. Mason, in *Life Prints*, notes that her father never fully accepted her disability, becoming "obsessive" about eliminating it (33). Refer also to pp. 31 and 38–39.
59. Donahue in Silver and Wilson, *Polio Voices*: 88.
60. Boarke, *Dismembering the Male*: 44 and 16, respectively. Refer to pp. 31 and 35 as well.
61. David A. Gerber, *Disabled Veterans in History* (Ann Arbor: University of Michigan Press, 2012): 5, 10, and 25, respectively; see also p. 6. Boarke, in *Dismembering the Male*, makes a similar point (74–75).
62. Boarke, *Dismembering the Male*: 44 and 43, respectively; see also p. 45. Also see Bentz Plagemann, *My Place to Stand* (New York: Farrar, Straus & Co., 1949): 168.
63. Peter L. Twohig and Vera Kalitzkus (eds.), *Social Studies of Health, Illness and Disease: Perspectives from the Social Sciences and Humanities* (Amsterdam: Rodopi, 2008): 1.
64. Gerschick and Miller, "Coming to Terms": 183, 184, and 185, respectively. See also Boarke, *Dismembering the Male*: 13; Susan L. Hutchinson and Douglas A. Kleiber, "Heroic Masculinity Following Spinal Cord Injury: Implications for Therapeutic Recreation Practice and Research," *Therapeutic Recreation Journal* 34 (2000): 43; Leonard Kriegel, *Falling into Life* (San Francisco: North Point Press, 1991): 55–56, 59; Murphy, *The Body Silent*: 95.
65. Boarke, *Dismembering the Male*: 11. Kriegel, in *Falling into Life*, writes that this fixed notion of manhood is deep-seated in American culture. "The image of manhood bequeathed to us by the major writers of the American Renaissance . . . was that of physical health and manly vigor. The writer's obligation was to affirm the virtue of man in the wilderness—and that virtue was predominantly physical" (26–27). Ahab, Melville's principal character in *Moby Dick*, serves as Kriegel's model of the disabled American male—"the essential cripple, a man whose sense of himself is dominated by physical insufficiency" (130–32).
66. Grixti, "Desirability and Its Discontents": 49.
67. Zanke in Silver and Wilson, *Polio Voices*: 83. Refer to pp. 21–22 as well.
68. Norkunas in Silver and Wilson, *Polio Voices*: 82–83.
69. Anne Finger, *Elegy for A Disease: A Personal and Cultural History of Polio* (New York: St. Martin's Press, 2006): 170.
70. Gerschick and Miller, "Coming to Terms": 191 and 199, respectively; refer also to pp. 193–94 and 201. See also Finger, *Elegy for A Disease*: 175; Hutchinson and Kleiber, "Heroic Masculinity Following Spinal Cord Injury": 43; Murphy,

The Body Silent: 95; Wilson, *Living with Polio*: 50. Curiously, in an analysis of narratives written by males, Foertsch, in *Bracing Accounts*, finds no pattern of how masculinity was expressed (63–68).

71. Davis, in *Passage through Crisis*, affords us a set of convenient categories to better understand the polio story, but it was not that simple. These did not function as discrete realities. His analysis merely represents a starting point for grasping this extremely complex and emotionally wrenching event in a person's life. As literary scholar Foertsch, in *Bracing Accounts*, reminds us, "elements of both denial and acceptance are widely locatable across the polio memoir canon and are most productively considered as the shifting, multivalent, pervasive phenomena that they are in the lived experience" (56). Consult also Arthur W. Frank, *The Wounded Storyteller: Body, Illness, and Ethics* (Chicago: University of Chicago Press, 1997): 33–35; Harrison and Stuifbergen, "A Hermeneutic Phenomenological Analysis of Aging with a Childhood Onset Disability": 738.
72. Charles L. Lowman and Morton A. Seidenfeld, "A Preliminary Report of the Psychosocial Effects of Poliomyelitis," *Journal of Consulting Psychology* 11 (1947): 30–32. Especially refer to Frank, *The Wounded Storyteller*: 33–35.
73. Mee, *A Nearly Normal Life*: 171 and 169, respectively. See also p. 167. Davis, *Passage through Crisis*: 139, 151.
74. Davis in Daniel and Robbins, *Polio*: 42.
75. Brenda Serotte, *The Fortune Teller's Kiss*, (Lincoln: University of Nebraska Press, 2006): 74.
76. Mee, *A Nearly Normal Life*: 168–69 and 171.
77. Mason, *Life Prints*: 12.
78. Garland Thomson, *Extraordinary Bodies*: 27. Consult Rita Charon, *Narrative Medicine: Honoring the Stories of Illness* (New York: Oxford University Press, 2006), Chapter 5, "The Patient, the Body, and the Self," for an analysis of this attempt at the separation of self from the body.
79. Davis, *Passage through Crisis*: 138, 139, 140, 141, 143, 144, 145, 147, 151, and 154. "Normals" is quoted on p. 140.
80. Lorenzo Wilson Milam, *The Cripple Liberation Front Marching Band Blues* (San Diego, CA: Mho & Mho Works, 1987): 95; Kriegel in Gould, *A Summer Plague*: 282.
81. Owen in Sass, Gottfried, and Sorem, *Polio's Legacy*: 33; Zemke, *Polio*: 26.
82. Bruno, in *Polio Paradox*, quotes this student on p. 81.
83. Bias in Sass, Gottfried, and Sorem, *Polio's Legacy*: 80, 80–81, and 82.
84. Wilson, "A Crippling Fear": 487.
85. Seavey, Smith, and Wagner, *A Paralyzing Fear*: 29; Gould, *A Summer Plague*: 77. See also Mee, *A Nearly Normal Life*: 44. Milam, in *The Cripple Liberation Front Marching Band Blues*, comments that thoughts of suicide proved to be prevalent among young people disabled by polio who sought an escape from anger, helplessness, shame, and pity (109).
86. New York Neurological Society, Collective Investigation Committee, *Epidemic Poliomyelitis: Report on the New York Epidemic of 1907* (New York: Journal of Nervous and Mental Diseases, 1910): 116.
87. Dominik and Jordan in Sass, Gottfried, and Sorem, *Polio's Legacy*: 173–74 and 131, respectively.
88. Seavey, Smith, and Wagner, *A Paralyzing Fear*: 59; Murphy, *The Body Silent*: 95.
89. Bruno, *Polio Paradox*: 99–100. Bruno quotes Margaret on p. 101. Consult also Shell, *Polio and Its Aftermath*: 219–21.

90. Heather Munro Prescott, *A Doctor of Their Own: The History of Adolescent Medicine* (Cambridge: Harvard University Press, 1998): 33. Also refer to George G. Deaver, "A Study of the Adjustment of 500 Persons Over Sixteen Years of Age With Disabilities Resulting from Poliomyelitis," *New York Medicine* 7 (April 1951): 16–18.
91. Schwartz in Seavey, Smith, and Wagner, *A Paralyzing Fear*: 264; Hoffman in Sass, Gottfried, and Sorem, *Polio's Legacy*: 140.
92. Kriegel, *Long Walk Home*: 56–57. Hugh Gregory Gallagher, *FDR's Splendid Deception: The Moving Story of Roosevelt's Massive Disability—and the Intense Efforts to Conceal It from the Public* (Arlington, VA: Vandamere Press, 1999): 16–18; Sink, *The Grit Behind the Miracle*: 15.
93. Gallagher, *FDR's Splendid Deception*: 11–12; Gould, *A Summer Plague*: 1–3 and 35; J. N. Hays, *The Burdens of Disease: Epidemics and Human Response in Western History* (New Brunswick: Rutgers University Press, 1998): 265; Lynette Iezzoni, *Influenza 1918: The Worst Epidemic in American History* (New York: TV Books, 1999): 75–76, 97; "F. D. Roosevelt Ill of Poliomyelitis," *New York Times*, September 16, 1921: 1; Naomi Rogers, "Race and the Politics of Polio: Warm Springs, Tuskegee, and the March of Dimes," *American Journal of Public Health* 97 (May 2007): 786; Seavey, Smith, and Wagner, *A Paralyzing Fear*: 47; James Tobin, *The Man He Became: How FDR Defied Polio to Win the Presidency* (New York: Simon & Schuster, 2013): 29, 38, 47–48, 50, 57–58, 66, 69, 73–76, 110; Daniel J. Wilson, *Polio* (Santa Barbara, CA: Greenwood Press, 2009): 24–26.
94. Gallagher, *FDR's Splendid Deception*: 24 and 27, respectively; see also pp. 20 and 22–23. Also see Tobin, *The Man He Became*: 145, 148, and 176.
95. Gallagher, *FDR's Splendid Deception*: 93–94 and 96, respectively. Also consult pp. 16–18, 59, and 104–05.
96. Longmore and Goldberger, "The League of the Physically Handicapped and the Great Depression": 897. Also consult Gould, *A Summer Plague*: 52–53 and 58; Ann Pointon and Chris Davies (eds.), *Framed: Interrogating Disability in the Media* (London: British Film Institute, 1997): 22.
97. Naomi Rogers, *Dirt and Disease: Polio Before FDR* (New Brunswick, NJ: Rutgers University Press, 1996): 166; Gould, *A Summer Plague*: 58 and 60.
98. Tobin, *The Man He Became*: 94–95; refer also to pp. 8, 84, 91, and 99–100. See also Doris Zames Fleischer and Frieda Zames, *The Disability Rights Movement: From Charity to Confrontation* (Philadelphia: Temple University Press, 2001): 1.
99. Tobin, *The Man He Became*: 195, 273, 295, and 306, respectively. Also consult pp. 191–92, 194, 298–99, and 302–03.
100. Tobin, *The Man He Became*: 287. See also pp. 192 and 285.
101. Gallagher, *FDR's Splendid Deception*: 101; refer also to pp. 59–60 and 161. See also Victor Cohn, *Four Billion Dimes* (Minneapolis, MN: Minneapolis Star and Tribune, 1955): 25; Turnley Walker, *Roosevelt and the Warm Springs Story* (New York: A. A. Wyn, Inc., 1953): 96, 100, 105, 114, 117, 159, 190; Department of Natural Resources, *Franklin D. Roosevelt's Little White House and Museum* (Atlanta, GA: Parks, Recreation and Historic Sites Division: undated): 40. See Wilson's superb analysis in "A Crippling Fear": 487–494.
102. Tobin, *The Man He Became*: 286.
103. "No Cure of Child Paralysis: Dr. Flexner Says the Only Control of Disease Lies in Prevention," *New York Times*, April 21, 1911: 3.
104. Barnartt and Scotch, *Disability Protests*: xxiii.
105. Frischer in Daniel and Robbins, *Polio*: 72.

106. Seavey, Smith, and Wagner, *A Paralyzing Fear*: 234; Fay S. Copellman, "Follow-Up of One Hundred Children with Poliomyelitis," *The Family* 25 (December 1944): 293–94; Deaver, "A Study of the Adjustment of 500 Persons Over Sixteen Years of Age With Disabilities Resulting from Poliomyelitis": 4–5; Foerstch, *Bracing Accounts*: 2; Milam, *Cripple Liberation Front Marching Band Blues*: 109.

Chapter 7

1. Edmund J. Sass, George Gottfired, and Anthony Sorem, *Polio's Legacy: An Oral History* (Lanham, MD: University Press of America, 1996). As I contemplated the title for this final chapter, I found myself repeatedly attracted by the title of this book. It seemed most appropriate, much better than anything I could imagine.
2. Kate Greenaway, *Mother Goose: Or, The Old Nursery Rhymes* (London: F. Warne, n.d.).
3. Roy Porter, *The Greatest Benefit to Mankind: A Medical History of Humanity* (New York: Norton, 1997): 238. Also refer to George Childs Kohn (ed.), *Encyclopedia of Plague and Pestilence: From Ancient Times to the Present* (New York: Checkmark Books, 2001): 196–202.
4. Iona Opie and Peter Opie (eds.), *Oxford Dictionary of Nursery Rhymes* (Oxford: Clarendon Press, 1951): 364–365.
5. The phrase "illusion of medical certainty" represents the basic argument in Gerald Markowitz and David Rosner's "The Illusion of Medical Certainty: Silicosis and the Politics of Industrial Disability, 1930–1960" (in Charles E. Rosenberg and Janet Golden [eds.], *Framing Disease: Studies in Cultural History* [New Brunswick: Rutgers University Press, 1992]): 185 and 202. These polio morbidity and mortality rates can be found in Naomi Rogers, *Dirt and Disease: Polio Before FDR* (New Brunswick, NJ: Rutgers University Press, 1996): 10, 11, and 13.
6. Sauer in Nina Gilden Seavey, Jane S. Smith, and Paul Wagner, *A Paralyzing Fear: The Triumph Over Polio in America* (New York: TV Books, 1998): 19 and 251, respectively. Also see pp. 245–46.
7. Edith Powell and John F. Hume, *A Black Oasis: Tuskegee Institute's Fight Against Infantile Paralysis, 1941–1975* (copyright 2008): 130.
8. Jacqueline Foertsch, "'Heads, You Win': Newsletters and Magazine of the Polio Nation," *Disability Studies Quarterly* 27 (Summer 2007): 2, 5 (www.dsq-sds.org, accessed January 5, 2012).
9. Hugh Gregory Gallagher, *Black Bird Fly Away: Disabled in an Able-Bodied World* (Arlington, VA: Vandamere Press, 1998): 9.
10. Foertsch, "Heads, You Win": 2.
11. Sharon Barnartt and Richard Scotch, *Disability Protests: Contentious Politics, 1970–1999* (Washington, DC: Gallaudet University Press, 2001): 14.
12. Joseph P. Shapiro, *No Pity: People with Disabilities Forging a New Civil Rights Movement* (New York: Three Rivers Press, 1994): 41, 48–49, 52, and 57–58, respectively; see also pp. 47, 50–51, and 53–56. Also see Ruth O'Brien, *Crippled Justice: The History of Modern Disability Policy in the Workplace* (Chicago: University of Chicago Press, 2001): 10.
13. Gallagher, *Black Bird Fly Away*: 107; refer also to pp. 105–06, 110, 112–17, and 120–22. See also Marc Shell, *Polio and Its Aftermath: The Paralysis of Culture* (Cambridge: Harvard University Press, 2005): 199–200.

Bibliography

Court Cases

State ex. Rel. Beattie v. Board of Education of City of Antigo, 176 Wisc. 231 (1919).
John A. Watson City v. City of Cambridge, 157 Mass. 561 (1893).

Government Documents

Board of Health of the State of New Jersey. *Thirty-Sixth Annual Report: 1912 Report of the Bureau of Vital Statistics.* Union Hill, NJ: Dispatch Printing Company, 1913. http://www.gfsmithlib1umdnj.edu/stockton/NJ1912A.pdf (accessed February 12, 2011).

Board of Health of the State of New Jersey. *Thirty-Seventh Annual Report: 1913 Report of the Bureau of Vital Statistics.* Patterson, NJ: News Printing Co., 1914. http://www.gfsmithlib1umdnj.edu/stockton/NJ1913A.pdf (accessed February 12, 2011).

Board of Health of the State of New Jersey. *Thirty-Eighth Annual Report: 1914 Report of the Bureau of Vital Statistics.* Patterson, NJ: News Printing Co., 1915. http://www.gfsmithlib1umdnj.edu/stockton/NJ1914A.pdf (accessed February 13, 2011).

Clark, Hannah B. "Sanitary Legislation Affecting Schools in the United States." In *Report of the Commissioner of Education for 1893 and 1894.* Vol. 2, pp. 1301–1349. Washington, DC: Government Printing Office, 1896.

Collective Investigation Committee. *Epidemic Poliomyelitis: Report on the New York Epidemic of 1907.* New York: Journal of Nervous and Mental Disease Publishing Co., 1910.

Department of Health of the City of New York. *Report of the Board of Health of the Department of Health of the City of New York for the Years 1910 and 1911.* New York: J. W. Pratt Co., 1912. http://www.tlcarchive.org/htm/home.htm (accessed August 28, 2007).

Department of Health of the City of New York. *Annual Report of the Board of Health of the Department of Health of the City of New York.* New York: 1912. http://www.tlcarchive.org/htm/home.htm (accessed August 28, 2007).

Department of Health of the City of New York. *Annual Report of the Board of Health of the Department of Health of the City of New York for the Calendar Year 1918.* New York: William Bratler, Inc., 1919. http://www.tlcarchive.org/htm/home.htm (accessed August 28, 2007).

Department of Health of the City of New York. *Annual Report of the Board of Health of the Department of Health of the City of New York for the Calendar Year 1919.* New York: 1920. http://www.tlcarchive.org/htm/home.htm (accessed August 28, 2007).

Department of Health of the City of New York. *Annual Report of the Board of Health of the Department of Health of the City of New York for the Calendar Year 1920.* New York: 1921. http://www.tlcarchive.org/htm/home.htm (accessed August 28, 2007).

Department of Health of the State of New Jersey. *Thirty-Ninth Annual Report: 1915 Report of the Bureau of Vital Statistics.* Patterson, NJ: News Printing Co., 1916. http://www.gfsmithlib1umdnj.edu/stockton/NJ1915A.pdf (accessed February 13, 2011).

Department of Health of the State of New Jersey. *Fortieth Annual Report: 1916 Report of the Bureau of Vital Statistics.* Trenton, NJ: State Gazette Publishing Co., 1917. http://www.gfsmithlib1umdnj.edu/stockton/NJ1916A.pdf (accessed February 13, 2011).

Department of Natural Resources. *Franklin D. Roosevelt's Little White House and Museum.* Atlanta, GA: Parks, Recreation & Historic Sites Division. Undated.

Emerson, Haven. *The Epidemic of Poliomyelitis (Infantile Paralysis) in New York City in 1916: Based on the Official Reports of the Bureau of the Department of Health.* 1917. Reprint, New York: Arno Press, 1977.

Frost, Wade H. *Epidemiologic Studies of Acute Anterior Poliomyelitis.* Treasury Department, U.S. Public Health Service, Hygienic Laboratory, Bulletin No. 90. Washington, DC: Government Printing Office, 1913.

Kendall, Henry O., and Florence P. Kendall. *Care during the Recovery Period in Paralytic Poliomyelitis.* U.S. Public Health Service Bulletin No. 242. Washington, DC: Government Printing Office, 1939.

Lavinder, C. H., Allen W. Freeman, and Wade H. Frost. *Epidemiologic Studies of Poliomyelitis in New York City and the Northeastern United States during the Year 1916.* U.S. Public Health Bulletin No. 91. Washington, DC: Government Printing Office, 1918.

Solenberger, Edith Reeves. *Public School Classes for Crippled Children.* Department of the Interior, Bureau of Education, Bulletin No. 10. Washington, DC: Government Printing Office, 1918.

U.S. Department of Education. *Digest of Education Statistics: Historical Summary of Public and Elementary and Secondary Statistics* http:/nces.ed.gov/programs/digest/d05/tables/dt05_032.asp (accessed April 23, 2007).

U.S. Department of Health and Human Services. *Morbidity and Mortality Weekly Report* 48 (April 2, 1999): 242–48. http://www.cdc.gov/mmwr/PDF/wk?mm 4812.pdf (accessed June 29, 2008).

White House Conference on Child Health and Protection. *Organization for the Care of Handicapped Children: Report of the Committee on National, State and Local Organization for the Handicapped.* New York: The Century Co., 1932.

Nonfiction Journal Articles

Abrams, Sarah E. "Brilliance and Bureaucracy: Nursing and Changes in the Rockefeller Foundation, 1915–1930." *Nursing History Review* 1 (1993): 119–37.

Affeldt, John E. "Recent Advances in the Treatment of Poliomyelitis." *Journal of the American Medical Association* 156 (September 1954): 12–15.

Altenbaugh, Richard J. "Polio, Disability, and American Public Schooling: An Historiographic Exploration." *Educational Research and Perspectives* 31 (December 2004): 137–55.

Altenbaugh, Richard J. "Where Are the Disabled in the History of Education?" *History of Education* 35 (November 2006): 705–30.

Anon. "Clinical Diagnosis of Poliomyelitis." *Therapeutic Notes* 92 (July–Aug. 1955): 181–85.
Anon. "Landmark Perspective: The Iron Lung." *Journal of the American Medical Association* 255 (March 1986): 1176–80.
Anon. "Medical News." *Journal of the American Medical Association* 113 (July 1939): 340.
Anon. "National Foundation for Infantile Paralysis." *American Journal of Public Health* 31 (1941): 1023.
Anon. "News on the Polio Front." *American Journal of Public Health* 36 (1946): 179.
Anon. "Poliomyelitis: A New Approach." *Lancet* (March 15, 1952): 552.
Anderson, Gaylord W. "Epidemiology of Poliomyelitis." *Journal of the Iowa State Medical Society* 37 (August 1947): 350–56.
Armstrong, David. "The Patient's View." *Social Science and Medicine* 18 (1984): 737–44.
Beck, Gustav J., George C. Graham, and Alvan L. Barach. "Effect of Physical Methods on the Mechanics of Breathing in Poliomyelitis." *Annals of Internal Medicine* 43 (September 1955): 540–66.
Benison, Saul. "Poliomyelitis and the Rockefeller Institute: Social Effects and Institutional Response." *Journal of the History of Medicine and Allied Sciences* 29 (January 1974): 74–92.
Blattner, Russell J. "Recent Advances in Clinical Aspects of Poliomyelitis." *Journal of the American Medical Association* 156 (September 4, 1954): 9–12.
Bredberg, Elizabeth. "Writing Disability History: Problems, Perspectives and Sources." *Disability and Society* 14 (March 1999): 189–201.
Calderwood, Carmelita. "Nursing Care in Poliomyelitis: Orthopedic Nursing Care of Patients in the Acute Stage of Poliomyelitis." *American Journal of Nursing* 40 (June 1940): 624–31.
Condran, Gretchen A., and Jennifer Murphy. "Defining and Managing Infant Mortality: A Case Study of Philadelphia, 1870–1920." *Social Science History* 32 (Winter 2008): 473–513.
Condrau, Flurin. "The Patient's View Meets the Clinical Gaze." *Social History of Medicine* 20 (December 2007): 525–40.
Copellman, Fay S. "Follow-Up of One Hundred Children with Poliomyelitis." *The Family* 25 (December 1944): 289–97.
Coughlin, Ellen Whelan. "Parental Attitudes Toward Handicapped Children." *Child* 6 (1941): 41–45.
Dauer, Carl C. "The Changing Age Distribution of Paralytic Poliomyelitis." *Annals of the New York Academy of Sciences* 61 (1955): 943–55.
Deaver, George G. "A Study of the Adjustment of 500 Persons Over Sixteen Years of Age With Disabilities Resulting from Poliomyelitis." *New York Medicine* 7 (April 1951): 16–18.
Dunphy, Lynne M. "'The Steel Cocoon': Tales of the Nurses and Patients of the Iron Lung, 1929–55." *Nursing History Review* 9 (2001): 3–33.
Eisenmann, Linda. "A Time of Quiet Activism: Research, Practice, and Policy in American Women's Higher Education, 1945–1965." *History of Education Quarterly* 45 (Spring 2005): 1–17.
Elkins, Earl C., and K. G. Wakim. "The Present Concept of Treatment of Poliomyelitis." *Journal of the Iowa State Medical Society* 37 (August 1947): 356–62.
Estabrooks, Carole A. "Lavinia Lloyd Dock: The Henry Street Years." *Nursing History Review* 3 (1995): 143–72.

Fairchild, L. McCarty. "Some Psychological Factors Observed in Poliomyelitis Patients." *American Journal of Physical Medicine* 31 (1952): 276–81.

Foertsch, Jacqueline. "'Heads, You Win': Newsletters and Magazine of the Polio Nation." *Disability Studies Quarterly* 27 (Summer 2007): 1–18. www.dsq-sds.org (accessed January 5, 2012).

Foreman, Phil. "Language and Disability." *Journal of Intellectual and Developmental Disability* (March 2005): 57–59.

Fox, Max J., and John Chamberlain. "Four Fatal Cases of Bulbar Poliomyelitis in One Family." *Journal of the American Medical Association* 151 (March 28, 1953): 1099–1101.

Frauenthal, H. W. "The Treatment of Infantile Paralysis Based on the Present Epidemic." *Journal of Electrotherapeutics and Radiology* 34 (October 1916): 506–29.

Garland Thomson, Rosemarie. "Feminist Disability Studies." *Signs* 30 (Winter 2005): 1557–87.

Ghormley, Ralph K. "History of Treatment of Poliomyelitis." *Journal of the Iowa State Medical Society* 37 (August 1947): 343–50.

Golden, Janet, and Naomi Rogers. "Nurse Irene Shea Studies the 'Kenny Method' of Treatment of Infantile Paralysis, 1942–1943." *Nursing History Review* 18 (2010): 189–203.

Grant, Alice A. "Medical Social Work in an Epidemic of Poliomyelitis." *Journal of Pediatrics* 24 (June 1944): 691–723.

Greenblum, Joseph. "The Control of Sick-Care Functions in the Hospitalization of a Child: Family versus Hospital." *Journal of Health and Human Behavior* 2 (Spring 1961): 32–38.

Harmon, Paul H. "The Racial Incidence of Poliomyelitis in the United States with Special Reference to the Negro." *Journal of Infectious Diseases* 58 (May–June 1936): 331–36.

Harrison, Tracie C., and Alexa Stuifbergen. "A Hermeneutic Phenomenological Analysis of Aging with a Childhood Onset Disability." *Health Care for Women International* 26 (September 2005): 731–47.

Heyd, Charles G. "Tribute to Haven Emerson, M. D.," *Bulletin of the New York Academy of Medicine* 31 (December 1955): 869–71.

Hirsch, Jerrold. "History and a Story of Polio: Using and Abusing Oral History Interviews." *Disability Studies Quarterly* 18 (1998): 264–66.

Hospital School Journal. "The Medical Department." 11 (March–April 1923): 1–6.

Hutchinson, Susan L., and Douglas A. Kleiber. "Heroic Masculinity Following Spinal Cord Injury: Implications for Therapeutic Recreation Practice and Research." *Therapeutic Recreation Journal* 34 (2000): 42–54.

Journal of the Indiana State Medical Association. "A Radical Improvement in Ether Anesthesia." 5 (October 15, 1912): 446–47.

Kelleher, W. Howlett, and R. K. Paraida. "Glossopharyngeal Breathing: Its Value in Respiratory Muscle Paralysis of Poliomyelitis." *British Medical Journal* 23 (September 1957): 740–43.

Kolmer, John A., and Anna M. Rule. "Concerning Vaccination of Monkeys Against Acute Anterior Poliomyelitis." *Journal of Immunology* 26 (June 1934): 505–15.

Kort, Michael. "The Delivery of Primary Health Care in American Public Schools, 1890–1980." *Journal of Social Health* 54 (December 1984): 453–57.

Kudlick, Catherine J. "Disability History: Why We Need Another 'Other.'" *American Historical Review* (June 2003), available at http://www.historycooperative.org?journals/ahr/108.3/kudlick.html (accessed April 29, 2004).

La Forge, Jan. "Preferred Language Practice in Professional Rehabilitation Journals." *Journal of Rehabilitation* 57 (Jan./Feb./Mar. 1991): 49–51.

Langford, William S. "Physical Illness and Convalescence: Their Meaning to the Child." *Journal of Pediatrics* 33 (1948): 242–50.

Longmore, Paul K., and David Goldberger. "The League of the Physically Handicapped and the Great Depression: A Case Study in the New Disability History." *Journal of American History* 87 (December 2000): 888–922.

Longmore, Paul K., and Paul Steven Miller. "'A Philosophy of Handicap': The Origins of Randolph Bourne's Radicalism." *Radical History Review* 94 (Winter 2006): 59–83.

Lowman, Charles L., and Morton A. Seidenfeld. "A Preliminary Report of the Psychosocial Effects of Poliomyelitis." *Journal of Consulting Psychology* 11 (1947): 30–37.

Maxwell, James H. "The Iron Lung: Halfway Technology or Necessary Step?" *Milbank Quarterly* 64 (1986): 3–29.

Merkel, Howard. "The Genesis of the Iron Lung: Philip Drinker, Charles F. McKhann, James L. Wilson, and Early Attempts at Administering Artificial Respiration to Patients with Poliomyelitis." *Archive of Pediatric and Adolescent Medicine* 148 (November 1994): 1174–80.

Moffat, Marilyn. "The History of Physical Therapy Practice in the United States." *Journal of Physical Therapy Education* 17 (Winter 2003): 15–25.

Montgomery, David. "History as Human Agency." *Monthly Review* 33 (October 1981): 42–48.

Porter, Roy. "The Patient's View." *Theory and Society* 14 (1985): 175–98.

Risse, Guenter B. "Revolt Against Quarantine: Community Responses to the 1916 Polio Epidemic, Oyster Bay, New York." *Transactions and Studies of the College of Physicians of Philadelphia* 14 (March 1992): 23–50.

Robinson, H. A., J. E. Finesinger, and J. S. Bierman. "Psychiatric Considerations in the Adjustment of Patients with Poliomyelitis." *New England Journal of Medicine* 254 (May 1956): 975–80.

Rogers, Naomi. "Race and the Politics of Polio: Warm Springs, Tuskegee, and the March of Dimes." *American Journal of Public Health* 97 (May 2007): 784–95.

Russell, Carol L. "How Are Your Person First Skills?" *Council for Exceptional Children* 40 (May/June 2008): 40–43.

Sandelowski, Margarete. "Making the Best of Things: Technology in American Nursing, 1870–1940." *Nursing History Review* 5 (1997): 3–32.

Scheer, Jessica, and Mark L. Luborsky. "The Cultural Context of Polio Biographies." *Orthopedics* 14 (November 1991): 1173–81.

Smith, Laura K., Dorothy M. Iddings, Eva-Marie Pfeiffer, and William A. Spencer. "Physical Therapy in the Poliomyelitis Respiratory Patient." *Physiotherapy* 41 (February 1955): 44–51.

Snow, Kathie. "To Ensure Inclusion, Freedom, and Respect for All, It's Time to Embrace People First Language." http://www.disabilityisnatural.com (accessed November 6, 2010).

Sullivan, Joe F. "Editorial." *Hospital School Journal* 8 (September–October 1919): 1.

Titchkosky, Tanya. "Disability: A Rose by Any Other Name? 'People-First' Language in Canadian Society." *Canadian Review of Sociology and Anthropology* 38 (May 2001): 125–37.

Welter, Barbara. "The Cult of True Womanhood: 1820–1860." *American Quarterly* 18 (1966): 151–74.

Wilson, Daniel J. "Covenants of Work and Grace: Themes of Recovery and Redemption in Polio Narratives." *Literature and Medicine* 13 (Spring 1994): 22–41.
Wilson, Daniel J. "A Crippling Fear: Experiencing Polio in the Era of FDR." *Bulletin of the History of Medicine* 72 (1998): 464–95.
Wilson, Daniel J. "Braces, Wheelchairs, and Iron Lungs: The Paralyzed Body and the Machinery of Rehabilitation in the Polio Epidemics." *Journal of Medical Humanities* 26 (Fall 2005): 173–90.

Booklets/Pamphlets/Reports

International Committee for the Study of Infantile Paralysis. *Poliomyelitis: A Survey.* Baltimore: Williams & Wilkins Co., 1932.
Knapp, A. C., E. S. Godfrey Jr., and W. L. Aycock. "An Outbreak of Poliomyelitis: Apparently Milk Borne." Chicago: American Medical Association, 1926.
National Foundation for Infantile Paralysis (NFIP). *The Tuskegee Institute Infantile Paralysis Center.* New York: NFIP, 1942.
National Foundation for Infantile Paralysis (NFIP). *A Guide for Parents in the Nursing Care of Patients with Infantile Paralysis in the Home.* New York: NFIP, 1944.
National Organization for Public Health Nursing (NOPHN) and National League of Nursing Education (NLNE). "Nursing for the Poliomyelitis Patient." New York: NOPHN and NLNE, 1948.
New York City Department of Health (NYCDH). *Circular of Information Regarding Acute Poliomyelitis (Infantile Paralysis): Information for the Public.* New York: NYCDH, 1913.
NYCDH. *Circular of Information Regarding Acute Poliomyelitis (Infantile Paralysis): Information for the Public.* New York: NYCDH, 1914.
Reconstruction Home for Infantile Paralysis. Ithaca, NY: Atkinson Press, 1937.

Nonfiction: Books, Chapters, Reports

100 Years of Free Public Schools in Pennsylvania: 1834–1934. Harrisburg: Department of Public Instruction, 1934.
Altenbaugh, Richard J. *The American People and Their Education: A Social History.* Upper Saddle River, NJ: Merrill/Prentice-Hall, 2003.
Alter, George. "Infant and Child Mortality in the United States and Canada." In Alain Bideau, Bertrand Desjardins, and Héctor Pérez Brignoli (eds.), *Infant and Child Mortality in the Past,* 91–108. Oxford: Clarendon Press, 1997.
Ariés, Philippe. *The Hour of Our Death: The Classic History of Western Attitudes Toward Death Over the Last One Thousand Years.* Translated by Helen Weaver. New York: Barnes & Noble Books, 1981.
Barnartt, Sharon, and Richard Scotch. *Disability Protests: Contentious Politics, 1970–1999.* Washington, DC: Gallaudet University Press, 2001.
Bartine, Oliver H. "History of the New York Society for the Relief of the Ruptured and Crippled Children." *American Journal of Care for Cripples* 3 (1916): 59–76. In William R. F. Phillips and Janet Rosenberg (eds.), *The Origins of Modern Treatment and Education of Physically Handicapped Children.* New York: Arno Press, 1980.
Bates, Barbara. *Bargaining for Life: A Social History of Tuberculosis, 1876–1938.* Philadelphia: University of Pennsylvania Press, 1992.
Berg, Roland H. *Polio and Its Problems.* Philadelphia: J. B. Lippincott, 1948.

Berkin, Carol Ruth, and Mary Beth Norton. *Women of America: A History*. Boston: Houghton Mifflin Company, 1979.

Bogdan, Robert. *Freak Show: Presenting Human Oddities for Amusement and Profit*. Chicago: University of Chicago Press, 1988.

Bourke, Joanna. *Dismembering the Male: Men's Bodies, Britain, and the Great War*. Chicago: University of Chicago Press, 1996.

Bruno, Richard L. *The Polio Paradox: Understanding and Treating "Post-Polio Syndrome" and Chronic Fatigue*. New York: Warner Books, 2002.

Byrom, Brad. "A Pupil and a Patient: Hospital Schools in Progressive America." In Paul K. Longmore and Lauri Umansky (eds.), *The New Disability History: American Perspectives*, 133–56. New York: New York University Press, 2001.

Carter, Richard. *The Gentle Legions: National Voluntary Health Organizations in America*. New Brunswick, NJ: Transaction Publishers, 1992.

Charon, Rita. *Narrative Medicine: Honoring the Stories of Illness*. New York: Oxford University Press, 2006.

Cohn, Victor. *Four Billion Dimes*. Minneapolis, MN: Minneapolis Star and Tribune, 1955.

Cohn, Victor. *Sister Kenny: The Woman Who Challenged the Doctors*. Minneapolis: University of Minnesota Press, 1976.

Cole, Wallace H., John F. Pohl, and Miland E. Knapp. *The Kenny Method of Treatment for Infantile Paralysis*. New York: NFIP, 1942.

Colgrove, James. *State of Immunity: The Politics of Vaccination in Twentieth-Century America*. Berkeley, CA: University of California Press, 2006.

Connolly, Cynthia A. *Saving Sickly Children: The Tuberculosis Preventorium in American Life, 1909–1970*. New Brunswick, NJ: Rutgers University Press, 2008.

Coontz, Stephanie. *The Way We Never Were: American Families and the Nostalgia Trap*. New York: Basic Books, 1992.

Cooter, Roger. "The Disabled Body." In Roger Cooter and John Pickstone (eds.), *Medicine in the Twentieth Century*, 367–83. Australia: Harwood Academic Publishers, 2000.

Cooter, Roger. "'Framing' the End of the Social History of Medicine." In John H. Warner and Frank Huisman (eds.), *Locating Medical History: The Stories and Their Meanings*, 309–37. Baltimore: Johns Hopkins University Press, 2004.

D'Antonio, Patricia. *American Nursing: A History of Knowledge, Authority, and the Meaning of Work*. Baltimore: Johns Hopkins University Press, 2010.

Daniel, Thomas M. *Captain of Death: The Story of Tuberculosis*. Rochester, NY: University of Rochester Press, 1997.

Davis, Fred. *Passage through Crisis: Polio Victims and Their Families*. Indianapolis, IN: Bobbs-Merrill, 1963.

Davis, Gwilym G. "Education of Crippled Children." *American Journal of Care for Cripples* 1 (1914): 5–13. In William R.F. Phillips and Janet Rosenberg (eds.), *The Origins of Modern Treatment and Education of Physically Handicapped Children*. New York: Arno Press, 1980.

Demos, John. *Past, Present, and Personal: The Family and the Life Course in American History*. New York: Oxford University Press, 1986.

Derickson, Alan. *Health Security for All: Dreams of Universal Health Care in America*. Baltimore: Johns Hopkins Press, 2005.

Draper, George. *Acute Poliomyelitis*. Philadelphia: P. Blakiston's Son & Co., 1927.

Fairchild, Amy L., Ronald Bayer, and James Colgrove. *Searching Eyes: The State, and Disease Surveillance in America*. Berkeley: University of California Press, 2007.

Fett, Sharla M. *Working Cures: Healing, Health, and Power on Southern Slave Plantations*. Chapel Hill: University of North Carolina Press, 2002.

Fleischer, Doris Zames, and Frieda Zames. *The Disability Rights Movement: From Charity to Confrontation*. Philadelphia: Temple University Press, 2001.

Foertsch, Jacqueline. *Bracing Accounts: The Literature and Culture of Polio in Postwar America*. Teaneck, NJ: Farleigh Dickinson University Press, 2008.

Frank, Arthur W. *The Wounded Storyteller: Body, Illness, and Ethics*. Chicago: University of Chicago Press, 1997.

Franklin, Barry M. *From "Backwardness" to "At-Risk:" Childhood Learning Difficulties and the Contradictions of School Reform*. Albany: State University of New York Press, 1994.

Freidel, Frank. *Franklin D. Roosevelt: The Ordeal*. Boston: Little, Brown and Company, 1954.

Gallagher, Hugh Gregory. *FDR's Splendid Deception: The Moving Story of Roosevelt's Massive Disability—and the Intense Efforts to Conceal It from the Public*. Arlington, VA: Vandamere Press, 1999.

Gamble, Vanessa Northington. *Making a Place for Ourselves: The Black Hospital Movement, 1920–1945*. New York: Oxford University Press, 1995.

Gardner, James B., and George Rollie Adams (eds.). *Ordinary People and Everyday Life: Perspectives on the New Social History*. Nashville, TN: American Association for State and Local History, 1983.

Garland Thomson, Rosemarie. *Extraordinary Bodies: Figuring Physical Disability in American Culture and Literature*. New York: Columbia University Press, 1997.

Garland Thomson, Rosemarie. "Seeing the Disabled: Visual Rhetorics of Disability in Popular Photography." In *The New Disability History: American Perspectives*, edited by Paul K. Longmore and Lauri Umansky. New York: New York University Press, 2001.

Gerber, David A. (ed.). *Disabled Veterans in History*. Ann Arbor: University of Michigan Press, 2012.

Gerschick, Thomas J., and Adam S. Miller. "Coming to Terms: Masculinity and Physical Disability." In Donald F. Sabo and David F. Gordon (eds.), *Men's Health and Illnesses: Gender, Power, and the Body*, 183–204. Thousand Oaks, CA: Sage, 1995.

Gordon, Linda. *Heroes of Their Own Lives: The Politics and History of Family Violence*. Urbana: University of Illinois Press, 2002.

Grixti, Joe. "Desirability and Its Discontents: Young People's Responses to Media Images of Health, Beauty and Physical Perfection." In Peter L. Twohig and Vera Kalitzkus (eds.), *Social Studies of Health, Illness and Disease: Perspectives from the Social Sciences and Humanities*, 49–74. Amsterdam, The Netherlands: Rodopi, 2008.

Guild for Crippled Children of the Poor of New York City, 1904. "Report of Work among the Tenements of New York City." *American Journal of Care for Cripples* 4 (1917): 37–54. In William R. F. Phillips and Janet Rosenberg (eds.), *The Origins of Modern Treatment and Education of Physically Handicapped Children*. New York: Arno Press, 1980.

Haggett, Peter. *The Geographical Structure of Epidemics*. New York: Oxford University Press, 2000.

Hammonds, Evelynn Maxine. *Childhood's Deadly Scourge: The Campaign to Control Diphtheria in New York City, 1880–1930*. Baltimore: Johns Hopkins University Press, 1999.

Harbison, Francis R. *D. T. Watson of Counsel*. Pittsburgh, PA: Davis & Warde, 1945.

Hawes, Joseph M. *The Children's Rights Movement: A History of Advocacy and Protection*. Boston: Twayne Publishers, 1991.

Hawkins, Anne Hunsaker. *Reconstructing Illness: Studies in Pathography*. West Lafayette, IN: Purdue University Press, 1993.

Hawkins, Joan. "'One of Us': Tod Browning's *Freaks*." In Rosemarie Garland Thomson (ed.), *Freakery: Cultural Spectacles of the Extraordinary Body*, 265–76. New York: New York University, 1996.

Hays, J. N. *The Burdens of Disease: Epidemics and Human Response in Western History*. New Brunswick: Rutgers University Press, 1998.

Hellman, Hal. *Great Feuds in Medicine: Ten of the Liveliest Disputes Ever*. New York: John Wiley & Sons, 2001.

Hofstadter, Richard. *Social Darwinism in American Thought*. Boston: Beacon Press, 1955.

Howell, Joel D. "Hospitals." In Roger Cooter and John Pickstone (eds.), *Medicine in the Twentieth Century*, 503–18. Australia: Harwood Academic Publishers, 2000.

Iezzoni, Lynette. *Influenza 1918: The Worst Epidemic in American History*. New York: TV Books, 1999.

Judd, Deborah, Kathleen Sitzman, and G. Megan Davis. *A History of American Nursing: Trends and Eras*. Sudbury, MA: Jones and Bartlett Publishers, 2010.

Karier, Clarence J., Paul Violas, and Joel Spring. *Roots of Crisis: American Education in the Twentieth Century*. Chicago: Rand McNally, 1973.

Karier, Clarence J. *Shaping the American Educational State, 1900 to the Present*. New York: Free Press, 1975.

Kenny, Elizabeth. *The Treatment of Infantile Paralysis in the Acute Stage*. Minneapolis: Bruce Publishing Co., 1941.

Kessler, Henry H. *The Crippled and the Disabled: Rehabilitation of the Physically Handicapped in the United States*. 1935, reprinted New York: Arno Press, 1980.

Kirschmann, Anne Taylor. *A Vital Force: Women in American Homeopathy*. New Brunswick, NJ: Rutgers University Press, 2004.

Klein, Aaron E. *Trial by Fury: The Polio Vaccine Controversy*. New York: Charles Scribner's Sons, 1972.

Kluger, Jeffrey. *Splendid Solution: Jonas Salk and the Conquest of Polio*. New York: G. P. Putnam's, 2004.

Koop, Steven E. *We Hold This Treasure: The Story of Gillette Children's Hospital*. Afton, MN: Afton Historical Society Press, 1998.

Kraut, Alan M. *Goldberger's War: The Life and Work of a Public Health Crusader*. New York: Hill and Wang, 2003.

Landon, John F., and Lawrence W. Smith. *Poliomyelitis: A Handbook for Physicians and Medical Students*. New York: Macmillan Company, 1934.

Latham, Angela J. *Posing a Threat: Flappers, Chorus Girls, and Other Brazen Performers*. Hanover, NH: University Press of New England, 2000.

Lerner, Gerda. *The Majority Finds Its Past: Placing Women in History*. New York: Oxford University Press, 1979.

Lewin, Philip. *Infantile Paralysis: Anterior Poliomyelitis*. Philadelphia: W. B. Saunders Co., 1941.

Liachowitz, Claire H. *Disability As a Social Construct: Legislative Roots*. Philadelphia: University of Pennsylvania Press, 1988.

Longmore, Paul K. *Why I Burned My Book and Other Essays on Disability*. Edited by Robert Dawidoff. Philadelphia: Temple University Press, 2003.

Longmore, Paul K., and Lauri Umansky (eds.). *The New Disability History: American Perspectives*. New York: New York University Press, 2001.
Lovett, Robert W. *The Treatment of Infantile Paralysis*. Philadelphia: P. Blakiston's Son & Co., 1917.
Lovett, Robert W. *Infantile Paralysis in Vermont, 1894–1922: A Memorial to Charles S. Caverly*. Burlington, VT: Vermont State Department of Health, 1924.
Macceca, Stephanie, E. *Wilma Rudolph: Against All Odds*. Huntington Beach, CA: Teacher Created Resources, 2011.
Manzo, David, and Elizabeth C. Peters. *Cotting School*. Charleston, SC: Arcadia Publishing, 2008.
Markel, Howard. *Quarantine! East European Jewish Immigrants and the New York City Epidemics of 1892*. Baltimore: Johns Hopkins University Press, 1997.
Markel, Howard. "For the Welfare of Children: The Origins of the Relationship between U.S. Public Health Workers and Pediatricians." In Alexandra Minna Stern and Howard Markel (eds.), *Formative Years: Children's Health in the United States, 1889–2000*, 47–65. Ann Arbor: University of Michigan Press, 2004.
McMurtrie, Douglas C. "A Study of the Character and Present Status of Provisions for Crippled Children in the United States." *American Journal of Care for Cripples* 2 (1916): 24–38. In William R. F. Phillips and Janet Rosenberg (eds.), *The Origins of Modern Treatment and Education of Physically Handicapped Children*. New York: Arno Press, 1980.
McNeil, William H. *Plagues and Peoples*. Garden City, NY: Anchor Books, 1976.
Morantz-Sanchez, Regina. *Sympathy and Science: Women Physicians in American Medicine*. Chapel Hill: North Carolina University Press, 2000.
Murphy, Robert F. *The Body Silent: The Different World of the Disabled*. New York: W. W. Norton, 1990.
Norden, Martin F. *The Cinema of Isolation: A History of Physical Disability in the Movies*. New Brunswick, NJ: Rutgers University Press, 1994.
O'Brien, Ruth. *Crippled Justice: The History of Modern Disability Policy in the Workplace*. Chicago: University of Chicago Press, 2001.
Offit, Paul A. *The Cutter Incident: How America's First Polio Vaccine Led to the Growing Vaccine Crisis*. New Haven: Yale University Press, 2005.
Osgood, Robert L. *For "Children Who Vary from the Normal Type": Special Education in Boston, 1838–1930*. Washington, DC: Gallaudet University Press, 2000.
Oshinsky, David M. *Polio: An American Story*. New York: Oxford University Press, 2005.
Paul, John R. *A History of Poliomyelitis*. New Haven: Yale University Press, 1971.
Persson, Sheryl. *Smallpox, Syphilis and Salvation: Medical Breakthroughs that Changed the World*. Wolloesbi, Australia: Exisle Publishing Limited, 2009.
Pointon, Ann, and Chris Davies (eds.). *Framed: Interrogating Disability in the Media*. London: British Film Institute, 1997.
Pohl, John F., in collaboration with Sister Elizabeth Kenny. *The Kenny Concept of Infantile Paralysis and Its Treatment*. Minneapolis: Bruce Publishing Co., 1943.
Porter, Roy. *The Greatest Benefit to Mankind: A Medical History of Humanity*. New York: Norton, 1997.
Powell, Edith, and John F. Hume. *A Black Oasis: Tuskegee Institute's Fight Against Infantile Paralysis, 1941–1975*. Copyright 2008.
Preston, Samuel H., and Michael R. Haines. *Fatal Years: Child Mortality in Late Nineteenth-Century America*. Princeton: University of Princeton Press, 1991.

Quadagno, Jill. *One Nation Uninsured: Why the U.S. Has No National Health Insurance*. New York: Oxford University Press, 2005.

Reagan, Leslie J., Nancy Tomes, and Paula A. Treichler. *Medicine's Moving Pictures: Medicine, Health, and Bodies in American Film and Television*. Rochester, NY: University of Rochester Press, 2007.

Rogers, Naomi. *Dirt and Disease: Polio Before FDR*. New Brunswick, NJ: Rutgers University Press, 1996.

Rogers, Naomi. "American Medicine and the Politics of Filmmaking: *Sister Kenny*." In Leslie J. Reagan, Nancy Tomes, and Paula A. Treichler (eds.), *Medicine's Moving Pictures: Medicine, Health, and Bodies in American Film and Television*, 199–238. Rochester, NY: University of Rochester Press, 2007.

Rogers, Naomi. *Polio Wars: Sister Kenny and the Golden Age of American Medicine*. New York: Oxford University Press, 2014.

Rollet, Catherine. "The Fight Against Mortality in the Past: An International Comparison." In Alain Bideau, Bertrand Desjardins, and Héctor Pérez Brignoli (eds.), *Infant and Child Mortality in the Past*, 38–60. Oxford: Clarendon Press, 1997.

Rose, David W. *Images of America: March of Dimes*. Charleston, SC: Arcadia Publishing, 2003.

Rosenberg, Charles E. *The Care of Strangers: The Rise of America's Hospital System*. Baltimore: Johns Hopkins University Press, 1987.

Rosenberg, Charles E. "Framing Disease: Illness, Society, and History." In Charles E. Rosenberg and Janet Golden (eds.), *Framing Disease: Studies in Cultural History*, xiii–xxvi. New Brunswick: Rutgers University Press, 1992.

Rothman, David J. *Beginnings Count: The technological Imperative in American Health Care*. New York: Oxford University Press, 1997.

Ruhräh, John, and Erwin E. Mayer. *Poliomyelitis in All Its Aspects*. Philadelphia: Lea & Febiger, 1917.

Rusk, Howard A. *Rehabilitation Medicine: A Textbook on Physical Medicine and Rehabilitation*. St. Louis, MO: C. V. Mosby Company, 1964.

Rusk, Howard A, and Eugene J. Taylor. *Living with A Disability: At Home—At Work—At Play*. Garden City, NY: Blakiston Company, 1953.

Rutstein-Riley, Amy. "Shifting Views of Self: Impact of Chronic Illness Diagnosis on Young Emerging Adult Women." In Peter L. Twohig and Vera Kalitzkus (eds.), *Social Studies of Health, Illness and Disease: Perspectives from the Social Sciences and Humanities*, 9–28. Amsterdam, The Netherlands: Rodopi, 2008.

Ryan, Mary P. "The Projection of a New Womanhood: The Movie Moderns in the 1920s." In Jean E. Friedman and William G. Shade (eds.), *Our American Sisters: Women in American Life and Thought*, 500–18. Lexington, MA: D. C. Heath & Co., 1982.

Sanderson, John P., Jr. "Crippled Children in Connecticut." *American Journal of Care for Cripples* 5 (1917): 303–05. In William R. F. Phillips and Janet Rosenberg (eds.), *The Origins of Modern Treatment and Education of Physically Handicapped Children*. New York: Arno Press, 1980.

Schweik, Susan M. *The Ugly Laws: Disability in Public*. New York: New York University Press, 2009.

Sennett, Richard. *Families Against the City: Middle Class Homes of Industrial Chicago, 1872–1890*. New York: Vintage Books, 1974.

Shapiro, Joseph P. *No Pity: People with Disabilities Forging a New Civil Rights Movement*. New York: Three Rivers Press, 1994.

Shell, Marc. *Polio and Its Aftermath: The Paralysis of Culture.* Cambridge: Harvard University Press, 2005.
Sills, David L. *The Volunteers: Means and Ends in a National Organization.* 1957, reprinted New York: Arno Press, 1980.
Sink, Alice. *The Grit Behind the Miracle: A True Story of the Determination and Hard Work Behind an Emergency Infantile Paralysis Hospital, 1944–1945, Hickory, North Carolina.* Lanham, MD: University Press of America, 1998.
Smith, Jane S. *Patenting the Sun: Polio and the Salk Vaccine.* New York: William Morrow and Co., 1990.
Snyder, Sharon L., and David T. Mitchell. *Cultural Locations of Disability.* Chicago: University of Chicago Press, 2006.
Solenberger, Edith Reeves. *Care and Education of Crippled Children in the United States.* 1914, reprinted New York: Survey Associates, 1974.
Sontag, Susan. *Illness As Metaphor and AIDS and Its Metaphors.* New York: Picador, 1989.
South Kingstown High School. *Hope, Fear and Rock 'n Roll: The Family in the Fifties* South Kingstown, RI: Rhode Island Historical Society, 1993.
Starr, Paul. *The Social Transformation of American Medicine.* New York: Basic Books, 1982.
Stedman, Ann B. L. "The History of a Hospital for Crippled Children in the Far West." *American Journal of Care for Cripples* 3 (1916): 3–9. In William R. F. Phillips and Janet Rosenberg (eds.), *The Origins of Modern Treatment and Education of Physically Handicapped Children.* New York: Arno Press, 1980.
Stevenson, Jessie L. *The Nursing Care of Patients with Infantile Paralysis.* The National Organization for Public Health Nursing. New York: NFIP, 1940.
Tobin, James. *The Man He Became: How FDR Defied Polio to Win the Presidency.* New York: Simon & Schuster, 2013.
Tomes, Nancy. *The Gospel of Germs: Men, Women, and the Microbe in American Life.* Cambridge: Harvard University Press, 1998.
Tomes, Nancy. "Celebrity Diseases." In Leslie J. Reagan, Nancy Tomes, and Paula A. Treichler (eds.), *Medicine's Moving Pictures: Medicine, Health, and Bodies in American Film and Television,* 36–67. Rochester, NY: University of Rochester Press, 2007.
Twohig, Peter L., and Vera Kalitzkus (eds.). *Social Studies of Health, Illness and Disease: Perspectives from the Social Sciences and Humanities.* Amsterdam, The Netherlands: Rodopi, 2008.
Tyack, David, and Elisabeth Hansot. *Learning Together: A History of Coeducation in American Public Schools.* New Haven: Yale University Press, 1990.
Valenza, Janet Mace. *Taking the Waters in Texas: Springs, Spas, and Fountains of Youth.* Austin: University of Texas Press, 2000.
Viner, Russell, and Janet Goldman. "Children's Experiences of Illness." In Roger Cooter and John Pickstone (eds.), *Medicine in the Twentieth Century,* 575–87. Australia: Harwood Academic Publishers, 2000.
Walker, Turnley. *Roosevelt and the Warm Springs Story.* New York: A. A. Wyn, Inc., 1953.
Wallace, Charlton. "Education of the Crippled Child." *Archives of Pediatrics* 27 (1910): 345–52. In William R.F. Phillips and Janet Rosenberg (eds.), *The Origins of Modern Treatment and Education of Physically Handicapped Children.* New York: Arno Press, 1980.
Wells, Robert. "Family History and Demographic Transition." In Michael Gordon (ed.), *The American Family in Social-Historical Perspective,* 516–32. New York: St. Martin's Press, 1978.

White, Elliot. "The Inception and Development of an Institute for Negro Crippled Children." *American Journal of Care for Cripples* 2 (1916): 171–74. In William R. F. Phillips and Janet Rosenberg (eds.), *The Origins of Modern Treatment and Education of Physically Handicapped Children.* New York: Arno Press, 1980.

Wickman, Ivan. *Acute Poliomyelitis.* 1913, reprinted New York: Johnson Reprint Corporation, 1970.

Williams, Gareth. *Paralyzed with Fear: The Story of Polio.* New York: Palgrave Macmillan, 2013.

Wilson, Daniel J. *Living with Polio: The Epidemic and Its Survivors.* Chicago: University of Chicago Press, 2005.

Wilson, Daniel J. *Polio.* Santa Barbara, CA: Greenwood Press, 2009.

Winzer, Margaret A. *The History of Special Education: From Isolation to Integration.* Washington, DC: Gallaudet University Press, 1993.

Wooten, Heather Green. *The Polio Years in Texas: Battling a Terrifying Unknown.* College Station: Texas A&M University Press, 2009.

Wright, Henry C. *Survey of Cripples in New York City.* New York: Committee on Survey of Cripples, 1920.

Zeitz, Joshua. *Flapper: A Madcap Story of Sex, Style, Celebrity, and the Women Who Made America Modern.* New York: Three Rivers Press, 2006.

Zelizer, Viviana A. *Pricing the Priceless Child: The Changing Social Value of Children.* New York: Basic Books, 1985.

Fiction

Barber, Elsie Oakes. *The Trembling Years.* New York: Macmillan Company, 1949.

Dickens, Charles. *A Christmas Carol and Other Christmas Stories.* New York: Signet Classic, 1984.

Fitzgerald, F. Scott. *Flappers and Philosophers.* Champaign, IL: Book Jungle, undated.

Kafka, Franz. Translated and edited by Stanley Corngold. *The Metamorphosis.* New York: Bantam Books, 1972.

Potok, Chaim. *In the Beginning.* Greenwich, CT: Fawcett Publications, Inc., 1975.

Roth, Philip. *Everyman.* Boston: Houghton Mifflin Company, 2006.

Roth, Philip. *Nemesis.* Boston: Houghton Mifflin Harcourt, 2010.

Theses/Dissertations

Berkowitz, Edward D. "Rehabilitation: The Federal Government's Response to Disability, 1935–1954." 1976, reprinted New York: Arno Press, 1980.

Lee, Jason Chu. "Poliomyelitis in the Lone Star State: A Brief Examination in Rural and Urban Communities." MA thesis, Texas State University-San Marcos, 2005.

Mawdsley, Stephen E. "Polio and Prejudice: Charles Hudson Bynaum and the Racial Politics of the National Foundation for Infantile Paralysis, 1938–1954." MA thesis, University of Alberta, 2008.

General Reference Works

Bowman, John S. (ed.). *The Cambridge Dictionary of American Biography.* Cambridge: Cambridge University Press, 1995.

Foner, Eric, and John A. Garraty (eds.). *The Reader's Companion to American History.* Boston: Houghton Mifflin Co., 1991.

Heilbron, J. L. (ed.). *The Oxford Companion to the History of Modern Science*. New York: Oxford University Press, 2003.
Kiple, Kenneth F. (ed.). *The Cambridge World History of Human Disease*. Cambridge: University of Cambridge Press, 1999.
Kohn, George Childs (ed.). *Encyclopedia of Plague and Pestilence: From Ancient Times to the Present*. New York: Checkmark Books, 2001.
Margotta, Roberto. *The History of Medicine*. New York: Smithmark Publishers, 1996.
Opie, Iona, and Peter Opie (eds.). *The Oxford Dictionary of Nursery Rhymes*. Oxford: Clarendon Press, 1951.
Porter, Roy (ed.). *The Cambridge Illustrated History of Medicine*. Cambridge: Cambridge University Press, 2001.

Newspapers

In addition to The New York Times
Baird, Woody. "Tennessee Woman Who Spent Life in Iron Lung Dies at Age 61." *Pittsburgh Post-Gazette*, Section A, May 29, 2008: 8.
Gregory, Cleburne. "Franklin Roosevelt Will Swim to Health." *Atlanta Journal*, October 26, 1924: 7.
Jacobs, Susan. "Watson Institute: Needs Have Changed, but Focus Is Still on Children with Disabilities." *Pittsburgh Post-Gazette*, January 16, 2002, Section N: 1–2.
"WHO Says Polio Virus Eliminated in Europe." *Pittsburgh Post-Gazette*, June 22, 2002, Section A: 2.

Autobiographies/Oral Histories/Memoirs

Alexander, Lawrence, as told to Adam Barnett. *The Iron Cradle: My Fight Against Polio*. New York: Thomas Y. Crowell Co., 1954.
Andrew, Charles H. *No Time for Tears: The Story of a Ten Year Old Boy's Desperate but Successful Battle to Survive Polio*. Garden City, NY: Doubleday & Company, 1951.
Bird, Patrick J. *A Rough Road*. Amazon.com: 2012.
Daggett, Richard L. *Not Just Polio: My Life Story*. Bloomington, IN: iUniverse, Inc., 2010.
Daniel, Thomas M., and Frederick C. Robbins (eds.). *Polio*. Rochester, NY: University of Rochester Press, 1997.
Dille, Jeane L. Curey. *Polio: A Dose of the Refiner's Fire*. Bloomington, IN: Author House Press, 2005.
Farrow, Mia. *What Falls Away: A Memoir*. New York: Nan A. Talese, 1997.
Finger, Anne. *Elegy for a Disease: A Personal and Cultural History of Polio*. New York: St. Martin's Press, 2006.
Gallagher, Hugh Gregory. *Black Bird Fly Away: Disabled in an Able-Bodied World*. Arlington, VA: Vandamere Press, 1998.
Gould, Tony. *A Summer Plague: Polio and Its Survivors*. New Haven: Yale University Press, 1995.
Hall, Robert F. *Through the Storm: A Polio Story*. St. Cloud, MN: North Star Press, 1990.
Hartnell, Carol A. *More Than a Pinch, Less Than a Bee Sting*. Garland, TX: Hannibal Books, 2008.

Huse, Robert C. *Getting There: Growing Up with Polio in the 30's*. Bloomington, IN: 1stBooks, 2002.
Kehret, Peg. *Small Steps: The Year I Got Polio*. Morton Grove, IL: Albert Whitman and Company, 1996.
Kenny, Elizabeth. *My Battle and Victory*. London: Robert Hale, Ltd., 1955.
Kriegel, Leonard. "Uncle Tom and Tiny Tim: Some Reflections on the Cripple as Negro." *American Scholar* (Summer 1969): 412–430.
Kriegel, Leonard. *The Long Walk Home: An Adventure in Survival*. New York: Appleton-Century, 1964.
Kriegel, Leonard. *Falling into Life*. San Francisco: North Point Press, 1991.
Kriegel, Leonard. *Flying Solo: Reimagining Manhood, Courage, and Loss*. Boston: Beacon Press, 1998.
Lake, Louise. *Each Day a Bonus: Twenty-Five Courageous Years in a Wheelchair*. Salt Lake City, UT: Deseret Book Company, 1971.
LeFan, Michael. *Patience, My Foot!* Joplin, MO: College Press, 1994.
Lovering, Robert. *Out of the Darkness: Coping with Disability*. Phoenix, AZ: Associated Rehabilitation Counseling Specialists, 1993.
Mason, Mary Grimley. *Life Prints: A Memoir of Healing and Discovery*. New York: Feminist Press, 2000.
McNellis, Helen, and Jerry McNellis. *"Don't Pick Him Up": Our Family's Experience with Polio*. Beaver Falls, PA: BrainTrain Press, 2011.
Mee, Charles L. *A Nearly Normal Life*. Boston: Little, Brown & Co., 1999.
Milam, Lorenzo Wilson. *The Cripple Liberation Front Marching Band Blues*. San Diego, CA: Mho & Mho Works, 1987.
Nichols, Janice Flood. *Twin Voices: A Memoir of Polio, the Forgotten Killer*. Bloomington, IN: iUniverse, Inc., 2007.
Plagemann, Bentz. *My Place to Stand*. New York: Farrar, Straus & Co., 1949.
Rivers, Thomas M. *Reflections on a Life in Medicine and Science: An Oral History Prepared by Saul Benison*. Cambridge: Massachusetts Institute of Technology, 1967.
Rusk, Howard A. *A World to Care for: The Autobiography of Howard A. Rusk, M.D.* New York: Random House, 1972.
Sass, Edmund J., with George Gottfried and Anthony Sorem. *Polio's Legacy: An Oral History*. Lanham, MD: University Press of America, 1996.
Seavey, Nina Gilden, Jane S. Smith, and Paul Wagner. *A Paralyzing Fear: The Triumph Over Polio in America*. New York: TV Books, 1998.
Serotte, Brenda. *The Fortune Teller's Kiss*. Lincoln: University of Nebraska Press, 2006.
Sheed, Wilfrid. *In Love with Daylight: A Memoir of Recovery*. New York: Simon & Schuster, 1995.
Shreve, Susan Richards. *Warm Springs: Traces of a Childhood at FDR's Polio Haven*. Boston: Houghton Mifflin Company, 2007.
Silver, Julie, and Daniel J. Wilson. *Polio Voices: An Oral History from the American Polio Epidemics and Worldwide Eradication Efforts*. Westport, CT: Praeger, 2007.
Sternburg, Louis, and Dorothy Sternburg. *View from the Seesaw*. New York: Dodd, Mead & Company, 1986.
Troan, John. *Passport to Adventure: Or, How a Typewriter from Santa Led to an Exciting Lifetime Journey*. Pittsburgh, PA: Geyer Printing, 2000.
Van Balen, Dee. *The Closing Door*. Pittsburgh, PA: CreateSpace, 2010.
Volk, Patricia. *Stuffed: Adventures of a Restaurant Family*. New York: Vintage Books, 2001.

Woods, Regina. *Tales from Inside the Iron Lung (and How I Got Out of It)*. With a forword by David E. Rogers, MD. Philadelphia: University of Pennsylvania Press, 1994.

Zemke, Diane. *Polio: A Special Ride?* Minnetonka, MN: Diagnostic Center of Learning Patterns, Inc., 1997.

Zola, Irving K. (ed.). *Ordinary Lives: Voices of Disability and Disease*. Cambridge, MA: Apple-wood Books, 1982.

Film

Tod Browning, producer and director. *Freaks*. Hollywood, CA: Metro-Goldwyn-Mayer, 1932.

Index

adolescence (and adolescents), xx, 74, 92, 96, 99, 162, 170–2, 175–80
Abramovitz, Hyman, *see* League of the Physically Handicapped
Afghanistan, *see* World Health Organization
Africa, *see* World Health Organization
African Americans, 2, 3, 13, 15, 30–1, 62, 87–8, 105, 164, 190
   and Elizabeth Kenny, 48–9
   medical care of, 30–1, 53, 68, 85–6, 118
   and National Foundation for Infantile Paralysis, 31, 67–8, 142
   see also Bynum, Charles H., poster child, Tuskegee Institute, Warm Springs
Afro-American Medical Association, 118
aftercare, *see* Committee on Aftercare, convalescence, physical therapy, rehabilitation, surgery, Vermont Plan
Ager, Louis C., 56
AIDS, 141
Alabama Department of Pensions and Security, 151
Alabama State Crippled Children's Service, 120
Alaska, 6
Alger, Horatio, *see* Rusk, Howard A.
Allen, James Clark, 70
alternative medicine, 152–4, 156
   see also folk remedies
Alter, George, 4
ambulances, 24, 31, 53
American Congress of Physical Therapy, 47
American Journal of Nursing, The, 48

American Legion, 24, 150
   see also philanthropies
American Lung Association, *see* National Tuberculosis Association
American Medical Association, 4, 6, 47, 48, 81
   and Howard Carter, 44
American Orthopedic Association, 63
American Public Health Association, 49
American Red Cross, 24, 39
American Society of Physical Medicine, 81–2
Americans with Disabilities Act of 1990, *see* disability rights movement, Gallagher, Hugh Gregory
Amoss, H. L., 138
anesthesia, 97
   general, 33, 40, 100
   local, 28
antibiotics 28, 37, 191
Architectural Barriers Act of 1968, *see* disability rights movement, Gallagher, Hugh Gregory.
Arizona, 141
Arkansas, 14, 39, 68, 142
arthrodesis, *see* surgery
artificial respirator, *see* chesperator, iron lung(s), rocking bed
Asia, *see* World Health Organization
asylums, 77, 78, 85–7, 153
Australia, *see* Kenny, Elizabeth
Axtell, James, xx

baby boomers, 142
Bailyn, Bernard, xxi
Balbar, Ellen, 174–5
Baltimore, 2, 6, 13, 141
Banks, Charles E., 18

Baron, Charlotte, 39
Barton, Clara, *see* Kenny, Elizabeth
Baxter, Donald A., 56
Bayer, Ronald, 56
Baylor University, 39, 78
Beattie, Merritt, 160
Becker, Lawrence, 92–3, 138
Benny, Jack, 65
Berle, Milton, 65
Bias, Gail, 100–01, 103, 179
Bird, Paddy, 84
Bissell, Emily, *see* Christmas Seal.
Blue, Rupert, as Surgeon General 5–6
Boche, Karen (Bruber), 91
Bodian, David, xviii
Boston 2, 6, 41, 63, 164, 165, 166, 182
   Children's Hospital, 27, 35, 89
Bourke, Joanna, 176
Bousfield, Midian O., 119, 120
Boy Scouts, 179, 181
Boyer, Carol, 26, 40, 70
braces, 27, 56, 57, 59, 66, 67, 70, 71, 78, 79, 80, 84, 87, 90, 93–7, 102, 106, 113, 115, 119, 120, 124, 128, 146, 151, 154, 161, 162, 163, 165, 168, 169, 170, 178, 179, 182, 184
Bradford frame, 42, 135
Bredberg, Elizabeth, xxiv
Bridgeman, Laura, *see* Freeberg, Ernest
Brooklyn 5, 12–13, 18, 56, 59, 137
   Seaside Hospital, 113
Bronx 20, 70, 73, 87, 115, 127, 129, 143
Brown, Jerry, *see* Roberts, Edward.
Bruno, Richard L., xviii, 94, 99, 129, 181
Brutger, Kay, 101–02, 162
bubonic plague, 1–2, 12, 15, 189
Buffalo, 6
Burns, George and Gracie, 65
Bynum, Charles H., 68, 70
   and *Mother's March on Polio,* 142
   see also March of Dimes, National Foundation for Infantile Paralysis, poster child, Tuskegee Institute.

Cagney, James, 65
California, 6, 39, 93, 149
   Department of Rehabilitation, 142
   see also to Hollywood, Los Angeles, San Francisco.

Calderwood, Carmelita, 32
Cameroon, *see* World Health Organization.
Carnegie, Andrew, 81
Carver, George Washington, 120
Caverly, Charles S., 6, 90
Center for Independent Living, *see* Roberts, Edward.
charities, *see* philanthropies.
Charon, Rita, xxvi-xxvii, 26
Chenault, John, W. 68, 120
chesperator, 39
Chicago, 10–11, 13, 44, 73, 76, 79, 114, 119, 138, 141, 147, 165
   and Association for the Prevention of Infantile Paralysis, 11
   Department of Health, 13, 15, 18–19, 20, 41
   public library, 167
   public schools, 85, 167
   see also Fallon School, Spalding School for Crippled Children
children, xx, xxii, 180
   abandonment of, 125, 151, 156
   abuse of, 84–5, 125, 129
   and childhood, xx, xxi, 24, 30, 53, 162
   diseases of, xx-xxi, xxiii, 2, 189
   morbidity rates of, 2 124, 189
   mortality rates of, 2, 35, 124, 189
   and peers, 26, 53, 162, 163, 169–77, 180, 186
   as refugees, 16–20
   and ward culture, xxiii 31, 80, 82, 83–4, 95–6, 102–09, 155, 190
   see also braces, iron lung(s), wheelchair(s)
Children's Brace Fund for Victims of Infantile Paralysis, 57
   see also philanthropies
Children's Community Center, 110
Children's House of the Home for Incurables (Philadelphia), 78
chiropractor(s), *see* alternative medicine
Christian Scientists, 153
Christmas Carol, see Tiny Tim
Christmas Seals, 60
Christy, Howard Chandler, 65
cinema, 64, 66, 68, 77, 107–09, 141, 142, 143–4, 173, 175, 190, 191

Index

City Committee of the Unemployed Council, *see* League of the Physically Handicapped
Cleveland, Grover, 65
Clinic of Orthopedic Hospital (Los Angeles), 177–8
Cole, Wallace H., 44, 45, 46, 51, 82
Coler, Bird S., 105
Colgrove, James, 56
Committee on the Cost of Medical Care, *see* family
Committee on Crippled Children of the Brooklyn Bureau of Charities, 56
 see also philanthropies
Connecticut, 93, 151
 Asylum for the Education and Instruction of Deaf and Dumb Persons, 85
 Bethel, 18
 Hartford, 85
 Newington, xvii
 Stephney, 58
 also see New Haven
convalescence, 55, 56, 57, 68, 89
 institutions for, 77, 79–85, 119, 121, 156, 167, 178, 181
 see also physical therapy, rehabilitation, Rusk, Howard A., surgery, Vermont Plan
Convalescent Home for Crippled Children, 79
Cooter, Roger, and John Pickstone, xxi
Cote, Alice, 129
Cotting School, 164–5
Coughlin, Ellen Whelen, 131–2
 see also family
Crawford, Joan, 65
Cremin, Lawrence A., xxi-xxii
cripple, xix, 55, 56, 84, 87, 97, 102, 107, 108, 113, 114, 128, 135, 144, 156, 163, 167, 178, 179, 183, 184
 see also disability
Crippled Children's East Side Free School (New York City), 168
Crosby, Bing, 48, 151
Crutch, The, *see* Warm Springs
Curie, Madame, *see* Kenny, Elizabeth
cyanosis, *see* iron lung(s)

Dallas, 30, 141
Daniel, Thomas M., 36, 41
Davis, Bette, 65
Davis, Fred, 76, 103, 109, 143–4, 150–1, 154–5, 175
Davis, Michael W. R., 24, 26, 40, 49, 84, 108, 130, 136, 146, 147, 160–1, 178
Dawidoff, Robert, xx
Day Home and School for Crippled Children, 57
DDT (dichloro-diphenyl-trichloroethane), 128
death, xviii, 27, 29–30, 31, 40, 53, 124–5, 133, 138, 142, 143, 145, 151, 155, 159
 also see suicide
defeminization, xxii, 107, 114
 see also disability, femininity
deformity, 42, 43, 46, 73, 76, 77, 98, 99, 113, 175
 see also cripple, disability
de Kruif, Paul, 64, 119
Delaware, 60
 Wilmington, 61
Democratic Party, *see* Roosevelt, Franklin D.
Denmark, 51, 60, 164
Dentist(s), 80, 168
Denver, 44
 Children's Hospital, 32
Derickson, Alan, 148–9
Detroit, 14, 73, 190
 Orthopedic Clinic, 131
Diamond, Steven, 144
DiBona, Anthony, 133
Dickens, Charles, *see* Tiny Tim
Diehl, Howard, 45, 51
Dior, Christian, 141
diphtheria, xx, 2, 4, 61–2
Disabled in Action, *see* Heumann, Judy.
disability, xxi, xxiii, 15, 49, 55, 57, 58, 59, 62, 79, 84, 90, 93, 103, 106–12, 129, 140, 142, 143, 144, 154–5, 159, 175
 adaptations for, 73, 116, 117–18, 135, 186, 192
 and architectural/physical impediments, 75, 87, 117, 146–7, 155

disability (*continued*)
  and community formation, 106
  defined, 91
  and desexing, 107, 114, 173–5, 186
  discrimination, 53, 75, 87–8, 91, 169–77, 180, 183 184, 192
  as an economic problem, 56, 107, 109, 112, 114, 115, 132, 151
  as "human wreckage," 66
  language, 194–5n.
  laws, 75–6
  portrayals of, 71, 72, 73
  as a social construct, 73–77, 88, 96, 107, 160, 165, 178, 179, 185, 186
  and socializing, 53, 169
  statistics, 41
  stereotypes, 106–07, 111, 148, 181–5
  see also defeminization, disability rights movement, education, public school(s), schooling, teaching, Tiny Tim, Warm Springs
disability rights movement, xxiii, 73, 185, 191–2
  see also Gallagher, Hugh Gregory, Heumann, Judy, Roberts, Edward
Dixon, Samuel C., 143
doctors, 24, 35, 38, 41, 42, 44, 46, 47, 49, 50, 68, 70, 79, 119, 120, 142, 150
  and parents, 25, 31, 56, 89, 124, 128, 131, 136, 138, 139, 151, 155
  and patients, 27, 28, 29, 32, 34, 39, 40, 53, 55, 74, 78, 85, 86, 90, 92, 94, 145, 167, 168, 179, 182, 190
  see also hospital(s), surgery
domesticity, 133, 142, 153
  see also mothers, Welter, Barbara
Dominik, Jack, 136, 152, 180
Donahue, Emily, 175
Donoho, Randy, 70
Doty, Alvah H., 9, 59
Draper, George, 47, 182, 184
Drinker, Philip, *see* iron lung(s)
Durr, George, 121, 143, 145

East Side Settlement House, 57
Easter Seal Society, 73
education, 60, 66, 90, 147–8, 156
  defined, xxi

  see also health education, public school(s), schooling, Tomes, Nancy
Eiben, Robert M., 36, 37, 39, 40
Eisenmann, Linda, 141
Elkins, Earl C., 34
Elks, 150
  see also philanthropies
Ellison, Ralph, and *Invisible Man*, 87
Emerson, Haven, 6, 9, 56, 57, 58, 59, 148, 152
  and *The Epidemic of Poliomyelitis (Infantile Paralysis) in New York City in 1916*, 11–12, 13
  and Hospital for Deformities and Joint Disease, 56
  and Hospital of the New York Society for the Relief of Ruptured and Crippled, 56
  and New York Orthopedic Hospital, 56
emotional maladjustment, 109–112, 115, 177–85
  see also psychological treatments
emotional trauma, 25, 26, 27, 33, 36, 37, 38, 40, 53, 102–03, 106, 125, 144, 145, 170, 171, 179, 186
Episcopalians, 85
Equatorial Guinea, *see* World Health Organization
Esau, Ruth, 145, 146, 151
ether, *see* anesthesia
Ethopia, *see* World Health Organization.
Europe (and European), xviii, 1, 3, 5, 6, 12, 62, 67, 164

Fallon School (Chicago), 166
family, xx-xxi, xxiii, 25, 27, 32, 33, 37, 38, 39, 49, 50, 56, 61, 79, 83, 84, 85, 89, 90, 93, 94, 103, 117, 121, 126, 148, 153, 156, 161, 162
  and disability, 71, 109, 125, 128–31, 143, 145–7, 154–5, 166, 174–5, 190
  and *A Guide for Parents in the Nursing Care of Patients with Infantile Paralysis in the Home*, 134
  income, 125, 129, 149, 150
  and medical bills, 101, 129, 132, 148–50, 156, 190
  quarantine, 26, 53, 83, 127–8

Index

violence, 125, 129
  see also death, father(s), mother(s)
Fairchild, Amy L., 56
Fairchild, L. McCarty, 53
Farrow, Mia, 24, 25, 29, 55, 161
fasiotomy, *see* surgery.
father(s), 101, 125, 128, 129–30, 132, 133, 138, 143–44, 149, 150, 151, 174–5
  see also family, mother(s)
Federation of Women's Clubs, *see* Bynum, Charles H.
femininity, xxii, xxv, 114, 159, 171–5, 181, 190
  see also defemininization, disability, flapper
Finger, Anne, xviii, 50, 71, 89, 99–100, 144
Fitzergald, F. Scott, *see* flapper.
flapper, 171–2
  see also femininity
Flexner, Simon, 9, 10, 29, 57, 58, 59, 73, 132, 185
Flick, Margaret Ann, 115
flies, 10, 11, 16
Foertsch, Jacqueline, xxv
folk remedies, 133, 152
Fontaine, Joan, 141
Ford, Edsel, 63
Ford, Elise, *see* Christy, Howard Chandler
France, 6, 45
Frankenstein, images of 17, 97, 100
Freaks, 108
freak show(s), 74, 77, 108, 109
  see also disability, *Freaks*
Frick, Henry, C. 81
Freeberg, Ernest, xx
Frischer, Ruth E., 162, 174, 186
frog breathing, *see* glossopharyngeal breathing.

Gallagher, Hugh Gregory, 27, 28, 29, 33, 37, 76–7, 78, 87, 92, 124, 126, 183, 191, 192
Gamble, Vanessa Northington, 119–20
Garland Thomson, Rosemarie, 72–3, 74–5, 107, 169, 173
gender, 53
  see also defeminization, disability, femininity, masculinity.
General Education Board, 120
Genoa, *see* quarantine
Georgia, 30, 62, 68, 82, 118, 119, 142
  see also Warm Springs
Georgia Warm Springs Foundation, 48, 59, 64
  see also March of Dimes, National Foundation for Infantile Paralysis, President's Birthday Ball Commission, Warm Springs
Gerber, David A., 175–6
germ theory, *see* Koch, Robert
Germany, 6, 60, 62, 112, 153, 164
Gerschick, Thomas J., and Adam S. Miller, 176–7
Gillespie, Dizzy, 49
Gillette, Arthur J., *see* Gillette State Hospital for Crippled Children
Gillette State Hospital for Crippled Children, 25, 31, 45, 79–80, 86, 91, 95
Girl Scouts, 179
glossopharyngeal breathing, 92
Goldberger, Joseph, 10, 59
Golden, Janet, xx, xxii, xxiv-xxv
Goldthwait Unit, *see* Wallace H. Cole
Gonzales Warm Springs Rehabilitation Hospital for Crippled Children, 62, 121
Grant, Cary, 48
Great Britain, 45, 112
Great Depression, 4, 63, 111, 125, 149, 150
Greenberg, Ernest, 36, 40
Grixti, Joe, 175
Gross, Samuel D., 41
Guckin, Justine, xvii
Gudakunst, Donald W., 46, 50, 126
Guggenheim family, *see* philanthropies
Gullickson, Ray K., 47, 138
gulping, *see* glossopharyngeal breathing.
Gurney, Robert, 24, 46, 89

Halloween, 145, 186
Handel, Ken, 137
Hamlin, Marian, 17
handicapped, *see* disability

Harlow, Jean, 66
Harriman, Mrs. Averill, *see* philanthropies
Harvard University, 27, 33, 81, 89, 90, 184
  Infantile Paralysis Committee, 52
Haverstock, Henry, Sr., 51
Haverstock, Henry, Jr., 51
Hawkins, Ann Hunsaker, xxiii, xxiv, xxvi, 153
Hayes, Helen, 141
Haynes Memorial Infectious Disease Hospital, 41
Headley, Joan, 170
health education, 60
  see also education, public school(s), schooling, Tomes, Nancy
health insurance, 148–50, 190
health mobiles, 61
Heine-Medin's disease, *see* poliomyelitis.
Henderson, Melvin, *see* Kenny, Elizabeth
Henie, Sonja, 65
Henry Street Settlement (New York City), 57, 58
Herzog, Maximillan, 11
Heumann, Judy 192, *see* disability rights movement, Roberts, Edward.
Hirsch, Jerrold, xxv
historiography, xix-xx, 7–9
Hoffman, Mary Ann, 23, 181
Holt, Luther Emmett, 133
Hollywood, 48, 64, 65
Home for Destitute Crippled Children (Chicago), 85
Homeopathy, 152–3
Hopkins, Harry, *see* League of the Physically Handicapped
Hoppin, W. W., *see* Opposite House
hospital(s), xxiii, 24, 32, 35, 55, 56, 61, 67, 68, 74, 77–9, 82, 129, 132, 133, 135, 138, 148, 152–3, 155, 156, 161, 182, 191
  and outpatient care, 58, 78, 90, 93, 119, 161, 162
  rules, 25, 53, 136–7, 143
  smell, of xix, 25, 39, 49
  see also doctor(s), nurse(s), surgery
Hospital for Crippled and Deformed Children (Boston), 58

Hospital School Journal, The, 112
hot packs, *see* Kenny, Elizabeth, mother(s)
House of the Annunciation for Crippled and Incurable Children (New York City), 85
House of St. Giles the Cripple (Brooklyn), 78
House of Saint Michael and All Angels, 85
Houston, 30, 39, 78, 105, 118, 138, 156
Houston Chronicle, The, 147
Howard, Josephine, 140
Howard University, 120
Howell, Juanita, 37
Hudson River, *see* New York City
human capital, *see* vocational education.
Huse, Robert, 94, 104, 144, 155, 160, 162, 170
hydrotherapy, 52, 62, 93, 120, 121
  see also physical therapy, rehabilitation
hygiene, 61
  in the family, 133
  see also public health, sanitation

Illinois, 48, 70, 120
  Barington, 74, 148, 178
  see also Chicago
immigrants, 61
  Italian, 3, 19
immobilization, *see* Kenny, Elizabeth, plaster casts, rehabilitation, splints.
India, *see* World Health Organization
Indiana, 5, 148
  University Hospital, 49
industrial education, *see* manual training, vocational education
Industrial School for Crippled and Deformed Children (Boston), 168
infantile paralysis, *see* poliomyelitis
influenza, 2
  pandemic of 1918, 15, 98, 152, 181
Institute of Physical Medicine and Rehabilitation, 52
  See also Rusk, Howard A., New York University
International Health Board, 58
Iowa, 5, 6, 124

iron lung(s), 29, 33–41, 66, 67, 70, 78, 87, 104–05, 125, 126, 128, 145, 146, 151, 155
  and Collins respirator, 35
  and Emerson respirator, 35
  weaning from, 38, 91–3
  see also March of Dimes, National Foundation for Infantile Paralysis, respiratory failure
Israel, *see* World Health Organization

Jacobi, Mary Putnam, 41
Jamelka, Joe, 138
Jefferson Davis Hospital, 30–1, 39, 78
Jefferson Medical College (Philadelphia), 41
Jersey City Medical Center, 48, 49, 137, 139
  see also Kenny Elizabeth
Jim Crow, 119–20
Johns Hopkins University, xviii
Johnson, Barb, 164
Johnson, Bobby, 31
Johnson, Jean, 104, 173
Joint Disease Hospital, 78
Jolson, Al, 65
Jones, Cyndi, 71–2
Jones, Robert, and *Modern Methods in the Surgery of Paralysis, with Special Reference to Muscle-Grafting, Tendon-Transplantation and Arthrodesis*, 98
Jordan, Len 104, 180
Journal of the Indiana State Medical Association, The, 100

Kafka, Franz, *The Metamorphosis*, 123–4, 155, 179
Kangas, David, 147, 150, 151, 154, 162–3
Kansas State Meeting of Colored Women, *see* Charles H. Bynum
Kehret, Peg, 27–8, 32, 37, 47, 83, 95, 96–7, 104, 106, 130, 136–7, 145–6, 156, 159, 169, 174
Keller, Helen, xxiv
Kellogg, Ted, 144
Kelly, Grace, 141
Kennedy Center, *see* Gallagher, Hugh Gregory

Kenny, Elizabeth, 8, 43–53, 82, 102, 135–6, 139
  Foundation, 49, 51
  Institute, xxvi, 50, 51, 52, 82–3, 105, 135
  Kenny Concept of Infantile Paralysis and Its Treatment, 48
  Kenny Method of Treatment for Infantile Paralysis, 46
Kentucky, 24, 49, 68, 136, 142, 161, 178
  see also Louisville
Kessler, Henry H., 113
Kingston Avenue Hospital, 56
Kirkpatrick, Bill, 26–7
Kitt, Ertha, 41
Kiwanis, 150
  see also philanthropies
Kline, Marvin L., 51
Knapp, Miland E., 45, 46, 51, 82
Koch, Robert, 60
Kosair Crippled Children's Hospital (Louisville), 24, 26, 49
Kriegel, Leonard, 29, 71, 74, 87, 91, 95–6, 102, 121, 146, 153, 155, 169–70, 179, 181

Landon, John F., and Lawrence W. Smith, and *Poliomyelitis: A Handbook for Physicians and Medical Students*, 114
Latham, Angela J., 172–3
Latinos/as, 121
League of the Physically Handicapped, 111–12, 192
Lederer, Susan E., xx
Lee, Gypse Rose, 141
Lewin, Philip, 89–90, 98–9
  and *Infantile Paralysis: Anterior Poliomyelitis*, 24, 35, 52, 73, 91
Lewis, Jerry, 77
Liachowitz, Claire H., 76
Library of Congress, *see* Gallagher, Hugh Gregory
Life magazine, *see* Kenny, Elizabeth
Lions Clubs, *see* philanthropies
Lister, Joseph, 3
London (UK), 1, 189
Longmore, Paul K., xx
Longmore, Paul K., and David Goldberger, 111–12, 183

Los Angeles, 24, 31, 35, 42, 44, 82, 183
  General Hospital, 25
Louisiana, 5, 39
  New Orleans, 135
Louisville, 24, 26, 38, 147, 160
Lovering, Robert, 146
Lovett, Robert W., 58, 98, 112, 139, 183
  and Harvard Infantile Paralysis Commission, 182
  and Roosevelt, Franklin D., 182
  and *The Treatment of Infantile Paralysis*, 27, 41, 42, 138
  and Vermont Plan, 89–90

Madison Avenue, 142
manual training, 81, 83, 85, 86, 112–16, 165, 166, *see also* industrial education, vocational education.
March of Dimes, xix, 7, 8, 59, 61, 64–8, 78, 149, 191
  and Eddie Cantor, 64
  and *The Crippler*, 64
  see also Kenny, Elizabeth, National Foundation for Infantile Paralysis
Marshall, Margaret, 71
Martin, Ernest G., 90
Marx Brothers, 65
masculinity, xxv, 114, 133, 175–7, 180, 181
mass media, *see* cinema, radios, television
Massachusetts, xix, 6, 32, 62, 85, 93, 148
  Asylum for the Blind (later the Perkins Institution), 85
  Attleboro, 129
  Cambridge, 160
  Lowell 94, 104, 162
  School for Idiotic and Feeble-Minded Youth, 85
  Shrewsbury, 71
  State Board of Health, 98
  Worcester, 177
  see also Boston
massage, *see* physical therapy
Mason, Mary Grimley, 111, 117, 143
Massey, Charles, 142

Maternity and Infancy Act, *see* Sheppard-Towner Act
Mathewson, Christy, 65
Mawdsley, Stephen E., 31, 66–8
Mayo Clinic, xxvi, 44, 48, 81
McCarroll, Henry R., 49
McDaniel, Carolyn, 132
McKnight, Samuel, 151
McNellis, Jerry, 31, 80, 95
Mee, Charles L., 28, 74, 87, 103–4, 125, 146, 147–8, 178
Meehan, Norma, 129–30
Meharry Medical College, 31, 119, 120
mental hygiene, 110, 180
  see also emotional maladjustment
Merman, Ethel, 65
Metro-Golden-Mayer, *see Freaks*
Mexico, 12
miasma theory, 3
Michigan, 39, 70, 93
  Battle Creek, 95
  Cass City, 145
  Flint, 14
  State Board of Health, 14
  see also Detroit
Milam, Lorenzo W., 71, 117, 179
Albert G. Milbank, and Milbank Memorial Fund, 61
milk, 10–11
Minneapolis, xviii, xxvi, 44, 46, 47, 50, 82, 135, 156
  General Hospital, 45, 138
Minnesota, 44, 45, 50, 87, 95, 105, 135, 150–1, 159
  Austin, 27, 145
  Bethesda, 79
  State Hospital for Crippled and Deformed Children, *see* Gillette State Hospital for Crippled Children
  State Hospital for Indigent Crippled and Deformed Children, *see* Gillette State Hospital for Crippled Children
  Virginia, 169
  see also Minneapolis, St. Paul
Miss America, 173
Mississippi, 30
Mitchel, John, Mayor, 141
Monroe, Marilyn, 141
Moore, H. Frank, *see* Bethel, CT

mother(s), xxii, 132, 145, 146, 151, 156, 162, 174, 175
  and acute care, xxii, 132–8, 150
  education of, 4
  and emotional stress, 37, 84, 89, 127, 129–30, 132, 135, 138, 139, 154, 190
  and hospital personnel, 26
  and rehabilitation, 57, 58, 78, 94, 101, 129, 132, 135, 138–40, 142, 150
  see also family, father(s), hygiene
Mothers Marches, 140–2
movies, see cinema
Murphy, Robert F., 171
myotomy, see surgery

narrative medicine, see Charon, Rita
National Association for Colored Women, 118
National Association for the Study and Prevention of Tuberculosis, see National Tuberculosis Association
National Association of Colored Graduate Nurses, see Bynum, Charles H.
National Association of Negro Business and Professional Women's Clubs, see Bynum, Charles H.
National Council of Negro Women, see Bynum, Charles H.
National Foundation for Infantile Paralysis, xxiii, 8, 12, 24, 38–9, 58, 59, 82, 140–2
  and Walt Disney, 66
  and education, 65–6, 142
  and fundraising, 142, 190
  and *A Guide for Parents in the Nursing Care of Patients with Infantile Paralysis in the Home*, 134, 139
  income of, 141–2
  and medical bills, 51, 66, 126, 150–1
  and National Research Council, 51
  organization of 64, 90
  and Polio Emergency Volunteers, 141
  and research, 110–1
  and Self-Help Device Research Project, 116
  and "Story of the Kenny Method," 50
  and Warner Brothers, 66
  see also African Americans, Bynum, Charles H., Georgia Warm Springs Foundation, Kenny, Elizabeth, poster child, March of Dimes, Mothers Marches, O'Connor, Basil, Tuskegee Institute
National Gallery of Art, see Gallagher, Hugh Gregory.
National League of Nursing Education, and *Nursing for the Poliomyelitis Patient*, 134–5
National Medical Association, 119
National Organization for Public Health Nursing, and *Nursing for the Poliomyelitis Patient*, 134–5
National Tuberculosis Association, 60–1, 65–6, 70
  see also Society for the Prevention of Tuberculosis, Pennsylvania Society for the Prevention of Tuberculosis.
Nebraska, 6, 92, 138
Nelson, Alice, 83
New England
  Hospital for Women and Children (Boston) 90
  and Puritans, xx, 5
New Haven 17, 126, 136
  Hospital 110, 160
Newington Home for Crippled Children, 110
New Jersey, 5, 13, 15, 17, 18, 48, 77, 137, 182
  Atlantic City, 48, 173
  health department, 19
  Orange, 127
New Mexico, 39
New York, 12, 18, 39, 41, 61, 120, 126, 148, 183, 184
  DeWitt, 142
  Ithaca, 175
  Long Island, 17, 127
  Peekskill, 121
  Poughkeepsie, 5
  Syracuse, 145
  Utica, xviii, 99
  West Haverstraw, 84, 96
  Westchester County, 17, 36
  White Plains, 79

New York City, 2, 5, 6–7, 44, 48, 51, 56, 57, 61, 62, 63, 77, 78, 79, 84, 111–12, 114, 146, 147, 162, 166, 171, 182, 183, 190, 192
   1916 outbreak, xix, 7, 9–14, 16–17, 20, 55, 59, 89, 90, 93, 96, 124, 127, 133, 147
   Babies Hospital of, 133
   Carnegie Hall in, 33
   Commissioner of Public Welfare, 105–6
   Committee on Aftercare of Infantile Paralysis Cases, 58, 59
   Hospital for Deformities and Joint Disease, 93
   Waldorf-Astoria Hotel in, 63, 64
   See also Bronx, Brooklyn
New York City Department of Health, 6, 10, 57, 59, 61, 148, 152
   and 1916 polio outbreak, 7, 55, 56, 124, 133
   and *Circular of Information Regarding Acute Poliomyelitis (Infantile Paralysis): Information for the Public*, 16–17, 133–4
   see also Emerson, Haven
New York City Emergency Relief Board, *see* League of the Physically Handicapped
New York Globe, The, 56
New York Hospital for the Ruptured and Crippled, 78
   and James Knight, 79
New York Neurological Society, 190
New York Orthopedic Dispensary and Hospital, 5, 6, 7, 8, 79
New York State Reconstruction Home, 84, 91, 96
New York State School for the Blind, 85
New York Times, The, 5–6, 7, 9, 10, 17, 18, 47, 55, 56, 57, 105, 124, 127, 147
New York Tribune, The, 57
New York University, 48, 52, 73, 115
Nichols, Janice Flood, 144–5, 146
Nigeria, *see* World Health Organization
Nightingale, Florence, *see* Kenny, Elizabeth
Norkunas, Bill, 177
North Carolina, 82, 144
   Charlotte, 24

Hickory, 24, 67, 126, 161
North Dakota, 23
Northwestern University, 48, 81, 91, 119
Norway, 164
nurses, 32–3, 44, 66, 70, 79, 90, 95, 96, 104–5, 136, 290
   and hospital care, 24, 28, 29, 53, 78, 80, 85, 86, 91, 98, 99, 100, 119, 126
   in intensive care, 31, 33, 131
   and parents, 25, 52, 57, 58, 137, 175
   public health, 9, 134, 135, 138, 139, 140
   school, 160, 165, 166, 167, 168
   training of, 32, 43, 46, 48, 49, 102–3, 110, 120
   see also doctor(s), iron lung(s)s, Visiting Nurse Association
Nursing Care of Patients with Infantile Paralysis, 139

occupational therapy, 79, 80, 83, 91, 92, 115, 116, 140
O'Connor, Basil, 44, 45, 48, 50, 51, 63
   see also Georgia Warm Springs Foundation, Kenny, Elizabeth, March of Dimes, National Foundation for Infantile Paralysis, Roosevelt, Franklin D., Tuskegee Institute
O'Connor, Edward, 129
Odell, Diane, 33
Ohio, 82, 93, 120, 148
   Cincinnati, 6
   Elyria, 95
   Toledo, 139
   see also Cleveland
Oklahoma, 39, 82, 152
open-air classroom, 164
Opposite House, 57
orthopedics, 27, 41, 45, 49, 52, 56, 57, 58, 62, 66, 77, 79, 81, 82, 83, 91, 94, 114, 120, 135, 138, 139
   see also doctor(s), plaster casts, splints, surgery.
Owen, Richard, xxvi, 49, 161, 163, 179

Pakistan, *see* World Health Organization
parents, *see* family, father(s), mother(s), sibling(s)

Pasteur, Louis, 3
Pasteur Institute, 61
pathography, *see* Hawkins, Ann Hunsaker
Paul, John R., 4, 43
Peabody Home for Crippled Children (Massachusetts) 85
Pennsylvania, 5, 6, 15, 17, 19, 81, 143, 148, 165
  Belle Vernon, 144
  Chambersburg, 128
  Department of Public Welfare, 86
  Harrisburg, 86
  Ridgway, 5
  Society for the Prevention of Tuberculosis, 60, 62
  Washington, 81
  see also Philadelphia, Pittsburgh
Philadelphia, 2, 13, 41, 60, 62, 67, 77, 85
  Almshouse, 30
  health department, 15
Philadelphia Inquirer, The, 117
philanthropies, xix, 7, 55, 56, 57, 59–64, 70, 77, 78, 106, 108, 112, 113, 119, 131, 142, 146, 148, 150–1, 176
  see also March of Dimes, National Foundation for Infantile Paralysis, Rockefeller Foundation, Rosenwald Fund
physical therapy, 27, 41, 50, 52, 53, 55, 66, 78, 80, 81–2, 86, 93–7, 110, 119–20, 131, 161, 166, 167, 182, 183
  see also Kenny, Elizabeth, rehabilitation, Rusk, Howard A., Wright, Jessie
Pinza, Enzio, 141
Pitcairn, John, 81
Pittsburgh, 39, 48, 67, 86, 104, 147
  Municipal Hospital, 24, 26, 39
plaster casts, 27, 41, 42, 44, 45, 53, 89, 94, 98–9, 113, 162, 168
  see also Kenny, Elizabeth, rehabilitation, splints, surgery
Pohl, John F., 45, 46, 48, 51
police, 17, 128, 142
Polio Chronicle, The, *see* Warm Springs

poliomyelitis, xxii, 5, 59, 62, 73, 77, 78, 80
  and boys, 13, 14
  defined, xvii-xviii
  and girls, 13, 14
  and pain, 24, 25, 26, 27, 28, 32, 49, 50, 103, 159
  and paralysis, xvii-xviii, 23, 27–8, 29, 42–3, 53, 57, 73, 85, 121, 145, 174
  and Post-Polio Syndrome, xxv-xxvi
  rural outbreaks of, 6, 10, 14, 148
  statistics, xxv, xviii, xix, 6, 7, 12–15, 18–19, 33, 34, 35, 39, 41, 42, 52, 66–8, 73–4, 80, 81, 114, 124, 129, 138, 139, 144, 159, 166, 167, 168, 182, 184, 190, 191
  symptoms, xvii, 23, 124, 147
  types, xvii-xviii, 28, 33, 34, 52, 125, 138
  urban outbreaks of, 5, 6, 14, 20, 148, 165–6
  see also New York City
Polk State School for the Feeble-Minded, 86–7
Porter, Roy, xx, 8–9
poster child, xxiii, 58, 59, 68–73, 108, 191
  and Charles Massey, 68–9
  and Richard M. Nixon, 70
Potok, Chaim, 19–20
President's Birthday Ball Committee, 12, 50, 63–4, 118
  and *President's Birthday Magazine*, 64
  see also March of Dimes, National Foundation for Infantile Paralysis
Preston, Samuel H., and Michael R. Haines, 2
private school(s), 162, 164, 166
  see also Quaker school
Progressive education, 165
  and mandatory attendance, xxiii, 3, 112, 159–60
  see also education, manual training, public school(s), schooling
psychological treatment(s), 53, 91, 114, 115
  see also emotional trauma, emotional maladjustment, National Foundation for Infantile Paralysis

public health, 66, 127, 134, 140, 143, 190
  see also Chicago, flies, Mexico, New York City, New Jersey, Pennsylvania, quarantine, sanitation
public library, see education
public school(s), xxi, xxii, 3, 63, 80, 83, 87, 91, 103, 105–6, 112, 126, 147, 168, 186, 191
  administrators, xxii, 160–1, 163, 166, 169
  and health, 18, 20, 26, 60, 61
  see also education, schooling, special education, teachers
Pugleasa, Charlene, 169
Putnam, Nina Wilcox, 65

Quaker school, 161
quarantine, 1, 10, 15, 16, 53, 55, 126, 127, 140, 143, 147
  and automobiles, 9, 15, 20
  as defensive isolation, 15
  and railroads, 9, 15, 19, 20
  as spatial barrier, 15
  and surveillance, 10
  and wharves, 18, 19
  see also public health

radio(s), 84, 104, 120, 141
Rathbone, Basil, 48
Reader's Digest, see Elizabeth Kenny
rehabilitation, 30, 53, 66, 77, 79, 85, 90–102, 113–14, 121, 125, 128, 138–40, 143, 146, 147, 150, 169, 180, 190, 191
  See also National Foundation for Infantile Paralysis, physical therapy, Rusk, Howard A., Warm Springs
religious miracles, 154
  see also alternative medicine
respiratory failure, xvii, 29, 91–2
  Also see to glossopharyngeal breathing, iron lung(s), rocking bed, tracheotomy
Riley, Thomas J., 58
Rivers, Thomas M., 12
Roberts, Edward, 191–2
Robertson, John D., 10–11, 18
Robinson, Jackie, 49

Rockefeller Foundation, 59, 113
  and Jerome D. Greene, 57, 59
Rockefeller Institute for Medical Research, 9, 12, 57, 132, 138, 185
  see also Flexner, Simon
Rockefeller, John D., Sr., 81
Rockefeller, John D., Jr., 59, 63
Rockefeller, John D., Jr., Mrs., 64
rocking bed, 39–40, 78, 92
  see also iron lung(s)
Rockwell, Norman, 145
Rogers, Ginger, 66
Rogers, Marilynne, 38, 50, 75, 87, 93, 105, 143, 146, 179
Rollet, Catherine, 3–4
Roman Catholic(s), 51
Roosevelt, Eleanor, 48, 63, 117, 119, 182, 183
Roosevelt, Franklin D., 7, 8, 45, 48, 50, 62–4, 73, 141
  at Campobello, 182
  and disability, 76, 107, 112, 181–5
  and George Draper, 47
  and Louis Howe, 182, 183–4
  as President, xix, 112, 117, 119, 181, 183
  see also Gallagher, Hugh Gregory, Longmore, Paul K., and David Goldberger, March of Dimes, National Foundation for Infantile Paralysis, Presidents Birthday Ball, Tobin, James, Warm Springs
Roosevelt, Theodore, 65
Roosevelt, Sara, 182, 183–4
Rose, Wickliffe, 57
Rosenberg, Charles E., xxii
Rosenwald Fund, 119–20
Rotarians, see philanthropies
Rothman, David J., 34
Rudolph, Wilma, 8, 197
Rugh, George, 144
Rusk, Howard A., 115–16
  see also rehabilitation, physical therapy
Russell, Rosalind, 65
  in *Sister Kenny*, 48

Sabin, Albert, xvii, 8, 190
St. Louis, 49, 115, 124

St. Paul, 6, 25, 44, 45, 47, 79, 91
  See also Minneapolis, Minnesota
Salk, Jonas E., xvii, xviii, xix, xxv, 7, 8, 52, 82, 86, 190
Salomon, George S., 95
San Francisco, 43
sanitation, 4, 6, 10, 11, 19, 61
  see also flies, public health
Sass, Edmund J., 108
Sauer, Mark, 190
Second International Poliomyelitis Conference, 52
schooling, 12, 61, 72, 86, 143, 157, 159–60, 190
  home, 140, 147–8, 161, 162, 186
  hospital, 77, 78, 105, 116, 147, 167, 186
  during rehabilitation, 58, 84, 85, 113, 186
  see also education, public school(s), special education
Schwartz, Arvid, 103, 105, 135, 137, 150, 163, 181
Schweik, Susan M., 75–6
scoliosis, 42, 80, 89, 94, 135
Scotland, 1
Scrooge, *see* Tiny Tim
segregation, *see* African Americans, disability, special education
Seidenfeld, Morton A., *see* psychological treatment(s)
Serotte, Brenda, 70–1, 115–16, 127, 178
Shannon Hospital, 31, 36, 49
Shell, Marc, 126, 131, 159, 163–4
Shelley, Mary, *see* Frankenstein.
Sheltering Arms, 82–4, 95, 156
Sheppard-Towner Act, 4
Shreve, Susan Richards, 43, 87, 99, 104, 116–17, 130–1, 138, 139, 161, 163
Shriners, 150
  Hospital for Crippled Children, 45, 104
  See also philanthropies
Siblings, 124, 130, 132, 143–5, 155, 156, 161, 175, 190
Sigmon, Shelby, 161
Silver, Julie, and Daniel J. Wilson, 151

smallpox, xx, 2, 61
Smith, Alfred E., *see* Roosevelt, Franklin D.
Smith, Kate, 48, 65
Smith, Lawrence W., *see Poliomyelitis: A Handbook for Physicians and Medical Students*
Smith-Hughes Act of 1917, *see* manual training, vocational education
Snyder, Sharon L., and David T. Mitchell, 164
Social Darwinism, 74
Social Security, 149, 150, 151
Solenberger, Edith Reeves, 77–8, 79
Somalia, *see* World Health Organization
South Carolina, 30
South Dakota, 82
Southwestern Poliomyelitis Respiratory Center, 39, 78, 93, 105
Spalding School for Crippled Children (Chicago), 166–8
special education, xxi, xxiii, 77, 85, 109, 114, 120, 148, 164–9
splints, 27, 41, 42, 44, 45, 53, 90, 93, 94, 135
  see also Kenny, Elizabeth, rehabilitation
Stanford University, 48
Steiff, Margarete, 131
Stone, Charles A., 135
suicide, 24, 179–80, 186
  see also death
Suite, Fred, Jr., 154
surgery, 33, 66, 78, 84, 89, 90, 97–102, 194, 125, 132, 138, 144, 149, 152, 154, 162, 175
Sweden, 6, 13, 164
Syria, *see* World Health Organization.

tachycardia, 93
Taylor, Robert, 66
teacher(s), 72, 80, 86, 91, 120, 147, 160, 161, 163–4, 167, 168, 186
teddy bears, 31, 131
  see also Steiff, Margarete, toys
telethons, 72, 106–07
television, 77, 84, 106–07, 147
Tennessee, 31, 33
tentomy, *see* surgery

Texas, 12, 30, 39, 106, 120, 121, 138
  San Angelo epidemic in, 31, 36, 49
  Scottish Rite Hospital for Crippled
    Children
  see also Dallas, Houston
Thrall, Alice R., 96
Time magazine, xix
Tiny Tim, 58–9, 106, 108, 159, 190
Tisdale, William, 32
Tobin, James, 183–5
Tomes, Nancy
  and "celebrity diseases," 65–6
  and "popular health education," 60
toys, 30, 31, 49, 49, 131, 134,
    155, 170
  see also teddy bears
tracheotomy, 29, 33, 40, 145
  see also surgery
Tubbey, Alfred H., and *Modern
    Methods in the Surgery of Paralysis,
    with Special Reference to Muscle-
    Grafting, Tendon-Transplantation
    and Arthrodesis*, 2, 55, 60–1, 79,
    80, 81, 166, 167
tuberculosis, 2, 4, 55, 60–1, 62, 77 79,
    80, 81, 166, 167
  see also National Tuberculosis
    Association
Tunney, Gene, 65
Tuskegee Institute. *Also see* Chenault,
    John W., National Foundation for
    Infantile Paralysis.
  and John A. Andrew Memorial
    Hospital, 119, 120
  and Infantile Paralysis Center, 31, 68,
    119–21, 160

United States, 43, 44, 60, 62, 63,
    159, 189
  Army Air Corps, 45, 81, 115, 126
  Army Medical Corps, 45
  Bureau of Education, 77, 165, 166
  Children's Bureau, 3, 41, 118
  Congress, 191
  Department of Agriculture, 152
  Navy, 82
  Public Health Service, 17, 18, 19, 61
University of Berlin, 61
University of California-Berkeley, *see*
    Roberts, Edward

University of Chicago, 120
University of Iowa, 120
University of Maryland, 97
University of Minnesota, xviii, 32, 45,
    48, 52, 79, 120
University of Pittsburgh, 52, 81
University of Rochester, 48
University of Texas, 30

vaccination(s) (and vaccines), xix, 61,
    72, 141, 170
Van Cleve, Bill, 139, 144, 147
Vanderbilt, William H., 81
Vaughn, Sarah, 49
Venice, *see* quarantine
Vermont, 6, 90, 112–13
veterans, *see* disability
Veteran's Administration, *see* Rusk,
    Howard A., Wright, Jessie
Vermont Plan. *Refer* to Lovett,
    Robert W.
Vickery, Margo, 139–40
Viner, Russell, xx, xxiv-xxv xx, xxii,
    xxiv-xxv
Visiting Nurse Association, 138–9
vocational education, 79, 91, 112–16,
    164, 166, 167
  see also industrial training, manual
    training
Vocational Rehabilitation Act of
    1920, 76

Wakim, K. C., 34
Wald, Lillian D., 57, 59
Walker, Josephine, 174
ward culture, *see* children
Waring, Mary F., *see* National
    Association for Colored
    Women
Warm Springs, 45, 62, 63, 73,
    77, 95, 96, 116–18, 119
    161, 183
  Also Roosevelt, Eleanor, Roosevelt,
    Franklin D., O'Connor, Basil,
    Tuskegee Institute
Washington, 6
Washington, DC, 6, 70, 111–12, 161,
    192
Washington Doctors Hospital, 49
Washington University, 49

D. T. Watson Home for Crippled Children, 27, 39, 48, 81–2, 104–5
Watson, John A., 160
Weaver, Harry, 51
Welter, Barbara, 133
wheelchair(s), 32, 71, 73, 75, 80, 83, 87, 92, 94–6, 97, 103, 104, 105, 106, 115, 118, 131, 141, 146, 147, 162–3, 168, 170, 174, 183, 185, 186, 192
Wheelchair Review, The, *see* Warm Springs
Whitelaw, Elaine, 141–2
  See also Bynum, Charles, H., Mothers Marches, National Federation for Infantile Paralysis
Wickman, Ivan, 13
Williams, Gareth, 102
Williams, Linsley, 58
Wilson, Daniel J., 8, 14, 38, 97, 149
  see also Silver, Julie

Wilson, Robert Edward, 123, 124
Wilson School (Cleveland), 166, 168
Wisconsin, 125, 138, 160
Woltje, Hilda, 127
Woman's American Supply League, 57
Women's Medical College, 41
Woods, Regina, 35, 38, 147, 156, 161
Wooten, Heather Green, 106
World Health Organization, xviii-xvix
World War I, 44, 45, 56, 65, 90, 136, 167, 175
World War II, xxv, 32, 39, 44, 67, 114, 125, 141, 175, 181, 191
Wright, Jessie, 39–40, 81–2

Yelder, Clara, 120, 160

Zanke, William, 176
Zemke, Ron, 169, 179
Ziegfeld *Follies*, 173
zymotic theory, 30, 31

Printed and bound in Great Britain by
CPI Group (UK) Ltd, Croydon, CR0 4YY